Neurology Image-Based
Clinical Review

Neurology Image-Based Clinical Review

Jonathan Howard, MD
Assistant Professor of Neurology and Clerkship Director
Clinical Neurological Sciences
NYU Langone Medical Center
New York, New York

Anuradha Singh, MD
Clinical Associate Professor
Chief of Neurology
Director of Clinical Neurophysiology/EEG Laboratory
Bellevue Epilepsy Center
Bellevue Hospital Center
New York, New York

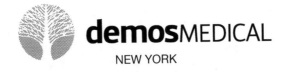

demosMEDICAL

NEW YORK

Visit our website at www.demosmedical.com

ISBN: 9781620701034
e-book ISBN: 9781617052804

Acquisitions Editor: Beth Barry
Compositor: Exeter Premedia Services Private Ltd.

Library of Congress Cataloging-in-Publication Data

Names: Howard, Jonathan, 1975- , author. | Singh, Anuradha, author.
Title: Neurology image-based clinical review / Jonathan Howard, Anuradha
  Singh.
Description: New York, NY : Demos Medical Publishing, [2016] | Includes
  bibliographical references and index.
Identifiers: LCCN 2016013927| ISBN 9781620701034 | ISBN 9781617052804 (e-book
  ISBN)
Subjects: | MESH: Diagnostic Techniques, Neurological | Nervous System
  Diseases—therapy | Neuroimaging | Clinical Medicine—methods | Neurologic
  Examination | Diagnosis, Differential | Case Reports
Classification: LCC RC346 | NLM WL 141 | DDC 616.8/0475—dc23
LC record available at https://lccn.loc.gov/2016013927

Special discounts on bulk quantities of Demos Medical Publishing books are available to corporations, professional associations, pharmaceutical companies, health care organizations, and other qualifying groups. For details, please contact:

Special Sales Department
Demos Medical Publishing
11 West 42nd Street, 15th Floor, New York, NY 10036
Phone: 800-532-8663 or 212-683-0072; Fax: 212-941-7842
E-mail: specialsales@demosmedical.com

Printed in the United States of America by Edwards Brothers Malloy.
16 17 18 19 20 / 5 4 3 2 1

We dedicate this book to our patients who have taught us so much through the years and our colleagues who have always been a great support to us. We would like to express our eternal gratitude to our parents and other loved ones for their everlasting love and support.

Contents

AA	Anaplastic astrocytoma
ABRA	Amyloid beta-related angiitis
ACA	Acute cerebellar ataxia
ACA	Anterior cerebral artery
AC	Arachnoid cyst
ACE	Angiotensin converting enzyme
ACTH	Adrenocorticotropic hormone
AD	Alzheimer's disease
ADC	Apparent diffusion coefficient
ADEM	Acute disseminated encephalomyelitis
ADP	Adenosine diphosphate
AEDs	Antiepileptic drugs
AIDP	Acute inflammatory demyelinating polyneuropathy
ALS	Amyotrophic lateral sclerosis
AML	Angiomyolipoma
AMN	Adrenomyeloneuropathy
Anti-TPO	Anti-thyroid peroxidase
AOP	Artery of Percheron infarction
AP	Anteroposterior
APBD	Adult polyglucosan body disease
ApoE e4	Apolipoprotein E epsilon 4
ASA	Anterior spinal artery
AS	Ankylosing spondylitis
AS	Aqueductal stenosis
AVM	Arteriovenous malformation
B-HCG	B-human chorionic gonadotropin
BOEC	Benign occipital epilepsy of childhood
BOLD	Blood oxygen level dependent
BP	Blood pressure
BRAO	Branch retinal artery occlusion
CAA	Cerebral amyloid angiopathy
CADASIL	Cerebral autosomal dominant arteriopathy with sub-cortical infarcts and leukoencephalopathy
CAR	Carcinoma-induced retinopathy
CBC	Complete blood count
CBD	Corticobasal degeneration
CBF	Cerebral blood flow
CBGD	Cortical basal ganglionic degeneration
CBV	Cerebral blood volume
CC	Corpus callosum
CCM	Cerebral cavernous malformation
CDC	Centers for Disease Control and Prevention
CDM	Copper deficiency myelopathy
CDMS	Clinically definite MS
CEA	Carcinoembryonic antigen
Chemo	Chemotherapy
CIDP	Chronic inflammatory demyelinating polyneuropathy
CIS	Clinically isolated syndrome
CJD	Creutzfeldt–Jakob disease
CM	Cavernous malformation
CMI	Chiari malformation type I
CMII	Chiari malformation type II
CNS	Central nervous system
CO	Carbon monoxide
COMT	Catechol-O-methyltransferase
CPA	Cerebellopontine angle
CPM	Central pontine myelinolysis
CPR	Cardiopulmonary resuscitation
CPS	Complex partial seizures
CSF	Cerebrospinal fluid
CSM	Cervical spondylotic myelopathy
CTA	Computed tomography angiography
CVA	Cerebrovascular accident
DAI	Diffuse axonal injury
DBS	Deep brain stimulation
DI	Diabetes Insipidus
DIS	Dissemination in space
DM	Dermatomyositis
DM	Diabetes mellitus
DNET	Dysembryoplastic neuroepithelial tumor
DVA	Developmental venous anomaly
DWI	Diffusion-weighted image
DWS	Dandy–Walker Syndrome
ED	Emergency department
EEC	El Escorial Criteria
EEG	Electroencephalogram
EEG–fMRI	Electroencephalography–functional magnetic resonance imaging
EGFR	Endothelial growth factor receptor
EMA	Epithelial membrane antigen
EMG	Electromyography
ER	Emergency room
ERM	Ezrin, radixin, moesin
ESR	Erythrocyte sedimentation rate
ETLE	Extratemporal lobe epilepsy
FALS	Familial ALS
FCDs	Focal cortical dysplasias
FDA	Food and Drug Administration
FDG-PET	Fludeoxyglucose-PET
FFI	Familial fatal insomnia
FLAIR	Fluid-attenuated inversion recovery
fMRI	Functional magnetic resonance imaging

FMSE	Focal motor SE	LFFEBRT	Limited field fractionated external beam radiotherapy
FS	Febrile seizures	LGIT	Low glycemic index treatment
FSRT	Fractionated stereotactic radiosurgery	LGS	Lennox–Gastaut syndrome
FTD	Frontotemporal dementia	LH	Lymphocytic hypophysitis
GBM	Glioblastoma multiforme	LINAC	Linear accelerator
GBS	Guillain–Barré syndrome	LOLA	L-ornithine and L-aspartate
GCI	Glial cytoplasmic inclusion	LPA	Lopogenic progressive aphasia
GCSE	Generalized convulsive SE	MAD	Modified Atkins diet
GCW	Glasgow Coma Scale	MAP	Mean arterial pressure
Gd	Gadolinium	MAR	Melanoma-associated retinopathy
GFAP	Glial fibrillary acidic protein	MBP	Myelin basic protein
GH	Growth hormone	MCA	Middle cerebral artery
GI	Gastrointestinal	MCT	Medium chain triglyceride
GPFA	Generalized paroxysmal fast activity	MEB	Muscle–eye–brain
GTC	Generalized tonic–clonic seizure	MEG	Magnetoencephalogram
GTR	Gross total resection	MELAS	Mitochondrial encephalomyopathy, lactic acidosis, and stroke-like episodes
H&E	Hematoxylin and eosin		
HAART	Highly active antiretroviral therapy	MERCI	Mechanical Embolus Removal in Cerebral Ischemia
HCG	Human chorionic gonadotropin		
HD	Huntington's disease	MERRF	Myoclonus epilepsy and ragged red fibers
HDL	High-density lipoprotein		
HH	Hypothalamic hamartoma	MGMT	O6-methylguanine-DNA methyltransferase
HIE	Hypoxic-ischemic encephalopathy		
HIVD	HIV dementia complex	MLD	Metachromatic leukodystrophy
HS	Hippocampal sclerosis	MMN	Multifocal motor neuropathy
HSV	Herpes simplex virus	MMPH	Multifocal micronodular pneumocyte hyperplasia
HTN	Hypertension		
HU	Hounsfield units	MP-RAGE	Magnetization prepared rapid acquisition gradient echo
Hz	Hertz		
IBM	Inclusion body myositis	MProsV	Prosencephalic vein of Markowski
ICA	Internal carotid artery	MRA	Magnetic resonance angiography
ICP	Intracranial pressure	MRI	Magnetic resonance imaging
ICU	Intensive care unit	MRS	Magnetic resonance spectroscopy
IDH1	Isocitrate dehydrogenase	MRV	Magnetic resonance venography
IGF	Insulin growth factor	MSA	Multiple system atrophy
IHC	Immunohistochemistry	MS	Multiple sclerosis
IHC	Initial immunohistochemistry	MTS	Mesial temporal sclerosis
IIH	Idiopathic intracranial hypertension	MTT	Mean transit time
ILAE	International League Against Epilepsy	NCSE	Nonconvulsive SE
IMRT	Intensity modulated RT	NF I	Neurofibromatosis I
INR	International normalized ratio	NF II	Neurofibromatosis II
IPH	Intraparenchymal hemorrhage	NIDDK	National Institute of Diabetes and Digestive and Kidney Diseases
IRIS	Immune reconstitution inflammatory syndrome		
		NIV	Noninvasive ventilation
IS	Infantile spasms	NMD	Neuronal migrational disorder
ITP	Immune thrombocytopenic purpura	NMO	Neuromyelitis optica
IVH	Intraventricular hemorrhage	NPH	Normal pressure hydrocephalus
IVIG	Intravenous immunoglobulin	NSE	Neuron specific enolase
IV	Intravenous	NSR	Normal sinus rhythm
JC	John Cunningham virus	NYULMC	New York University Langone Medical Center
JME	Juvenile myoclonic epilepsy		
JPA	Juvenile pilocytic astrocytoma		
KD	Ketogenic diet	ON	Optic neuritis
LAM	Lymphangioleiomyomatosis	PCA	Posterior cerebral artery
LDL	Low-density lipoprotein	PCD	Paraneoplastic cerebellar degeneration
LE	Limbic encephalitis		

PCNSL	Primary CNS lymphoma
PCR	Polymerase chain reaction
PD	Parkinson's disease
PEA	Pulseless electrical activity
PEG	Percutaneous endoscopic gastrostomy
PEIR	Pathology Education Instructional Resource
PET	Positron emission tomography
PFC	Prolonged febrile convulsion
PGE	Primary generalized epilepsy
PICA	Posterior inferior cerebellar artery
PLED	Periodic lateralized epileptiform discharge
PMEs	Progressive myoclonic epilepsies
PMG	Polymicrogyria
PML	Progressive multifocal leukoencephalopathy
PM	Polymyositis
PNFA	Progressive nonfluent aphasia
PNS	Peripheral nervous system
PPA	Primary progressive aphasia
PPMS	Primary progressive MS
PRES	Posterior reversible encephalopathy syndrome
PSA	Posterior spinal artery
PSP	Progressive supranuclear palsy
RBC	Red blood cell
RE	Rasmussen's encephalitis
RIS	Radiographically isolated syndrome
RRMS	Relapsing–remitting MS
RT	Radiation therapy
SAH	Subarachnoid hemorrhage
SBH	Subcortical band heterotopia
SCA	Superior cerebellar artery
SCD	Sickle cell disease
SDH	Subdural hematoma
SEA	Spinal epidural abscess
SEDH	Spinal epidural hematoma
SEGA	Subependymal giant cell astrocytoma
SE	Status epilepticus
SI	Sacroiliac

SISCOM	Subtraction ictal SPECT co-registered to MRI
SOD	Septo-optic dysplasia
SPECT	Single photon emission computed tomography
SPMS	Secondary progressive MS
SPS	Simple partial seizure
SRS	Stereotactic radiosurgery
SSEP	Somatosensory evoked potential
STIR	Short tau inversion recovery
SV	Semantic variant
SVT	Sinus venous thrombosis
SWS	Sturge–Weber syndrome
t-PA	Tissue Plasminogen Activator
T1WI	T1-weighted image
T2WI	T2-weighted image
TBI	Traumatic brain injury
TB	Tuberculosis
TIA	Transient ischemic attack
TLE	Temporal lobe epilepsy
TMP–SMX	Trimethoprim–sulfamethoxazole
TNF	Tumor necrosis factor
TSC	Tuberous sclerosis complex
TSI	Thyroid stimulating immunoglobulin
TS	Tuberous sclerosis
TTF-1	Thyroid transcription factor-1
UBO	Unidentified bright object
VA	Vertebral artery
VD	Vascular dementia
VEEG	Video EEG
VEGF	Vascular endothelial growth factor
VEP	Visual evoked potential
VGM	Vein of Galen malformation
VHL	Von Hippel–Lindau
VLCFA	Very long chain fatty acid
VM	Vacuolar myelopathy
VNS	Vagal nerve stimulator
VZV	Varicella zoster virus
WBRT	Whole brain radiation therapy
WD	Wilson's disease
WK	Wernicke–Korsakoff

The ability to properly interpret and develop independence and proficiency in neuroradiological studies is crucial for all neurologists. Various lesions often produce peculiar visual patterns on MRI and CT scans; these narrow the broad list of potential differential diagnoses, thus obviating the need for more invasive tests such as brain biopsies or angiograms. At the same time, neurologists need to understand the strengths and limitations of these studies and to appreciate the relevance of neuroradiological findings in the larger clinical context.

If a picture is worth a thousand words, a visual memory of a clinical case is retained and absorbed in a way traditional text readings are not. We introduce each topic in this book with a brief clinical scenario to reinforce this connection, and populate the text with a broad array of neuroimages, including CT, MRI, MRA, and angiography, to familiarize readers with the interpretation of various modalities, and to demonstrate how these findings influence treatment.

For the sake of readability, each condition is presented in a uniform and straightforward manner. Every topic begins with a brief case scenario and image-based diagnosis, and is followed by a short introduction to the disorder, clinical presentation, radiographic appearance, diagnostic hallmarks, differential diagnosis, and treatment. Each section also includes selected references for further study. The bulleted template presents readers with the most relevant and necessary clinical information and deliberately avoids long exposition. We hope that this approach will facilitate the use of this book as a handy reference at the point of care, or as a visual study guide for self-assessment and test review.

This abundantly illustrated volume covers all the major areas of neurology including epilepsy; vascular neurology; infectious, autoimmune, and demyelinating diseases; traumatic brain injuries; neurodegenerative diseases; neuro-oncology, and more. The format enables readers to explore more than 1,500 images depicting the full spectrum of neurological disorders, complete with accompanying tables, gross and microscopic neuropathology images, and EEG illustrations. As readers move through the topics, we hope they will use the key takeaway points summarized in every section to hone their clinical skills.

As clinicians, we build on our experiences with previous patients to formulate our approaches to the diagnosis and treatment of future patients. We designed this book to support that process. We believe that students and neurologists across all levels of training will find this guide of value as they apply neuroradiological findings to clinical care decisions for their patients.

Acknowledgments

Our deepest thanks go out to Dr. Robin Mitnick who, with painstaking attention to detail, created legends for the neuroradiology images. Without her contributions, portions of this book would not have been possible.

We are grateful to Drs. Dimitri Agamanolis, Roberta Seidman, and Seema Shroff, who graciously agreed to share their collection of neuropathology images to make this book more colorful.

We would also like to thank Drs. Dhanashri Miskin and Shavonne Massey for providing the text for numerous spine and pediatric topics. Our heartfelt thanks go out to Drs. Ritvij Bowry and Keith DeSousa for polishing the entries related to vascular neurology. Thanks to Dr. Aaron Nelson for his contributions to the management of infantile spasms. We owe Dr. Dana Price our thanks for providing an extensive review of the medical and surgical management of Lennox–Gastaut syndrome. Our thanks and appreciation go to Drs. Stephen Trevick, Alexandra Lloyd-Smith, Jessica Lin, Danielle Stember, and Deepti Anbarasan for proofreading several chapters and offering valuable suggestions.

Last but not least, we would like to express our sincere gratitude to the medical students, neurology residents, fellows, attending physicians, and Demos Medical Publishing, who made this work possible.

CHAPTER 1

ISCHEMIA

1.1   Ischemic Stroke

Case History

A 77-year-old woman presented with the sudden onset of left-sided weakness and numbness. On examination, in addition to the weakness and sensory loss, she had a left homonymous hemianopsia and was unaware of her deficits, denying that there was anything wrong with her. Her eyes were deviated to the right.

Diagnosis: Ischemic Stroke

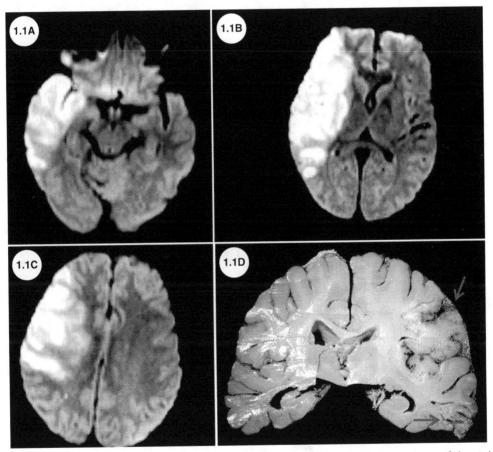

Images 1.1A–1.1C: Diffusion-weighted axial images demonstrate infarction in the territory of the right middle cerebral artery (MCA). **Image 1.1D:** Gross picture of a subacute right MCA infarction.

Introduction

■   The brain receives its blood supply from two paired arteries, the internal carotid arteries (ICAs) and vertebral arteries (VAs). The right common carotid artery arises from the brachio-cephalic artery, while the left common carotid artery arises directly from the aortic arch. The common carotid artery divides into the external carotid artery and the ICA.

■ Intracranially, the ICA gives rise to the ophthalmic artery, the anterior choroidal artery, and the posterior communicating artery. It then divides into the anterior cerebral artery (ACA) and middle cerebral artery (MCA). The VAs arise from the subclavian artery and run through the transverse foramen of the cervical vertebrae.

The posterior inferior cerebellar arteries (PICA) arise from the VAs, which then fuse at the pontomedullary junction to form the basilar artery. The anterior inferior cerebellar arteries (AICAs) and the superior cerebellar arteries (SCAs) arise from the basilar artery, which then divides into the paired posterior cerebral arteries (PCAs).

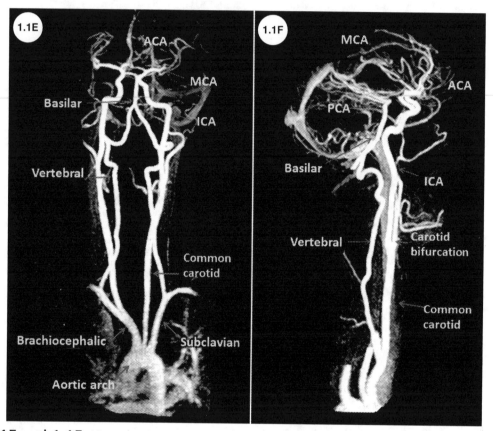

Images 1.1E and 1.1F: Normal magnetic resonance (MR) angiogram of the neck and head demonstrates the intracranial and extracranial vasculature.

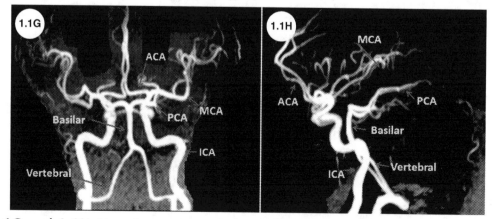

Images 1.1G and 1.1H: Normal magnetic resonance angiographies of the head demonstrate the intracranial vasculature.

The anterior and posterior circulations are connected via the circle of Willis, which is composed of the ACAs, a single anterior communicating artery, the ICAs, the PCAs, and the posterior communicating arteries. A complete circle of Willis is present in less than half of the population, however.

The anterior circulation refers to those brain areas supplied by the ICAs, MCAs, and ACAs. This includes the frontal lobes, lateral temporal lobes, parietal lobes, caudate and lentiform nuclei, and internal capsule. The posterior circulation refers to those brain areas supplied by the vertebral, basilar, and PCAs. This includes the brainstem, cerebellum, occipital lobes, medial temporal lobes, and thalami.

An ischemic stroke occurs when there is a focal neurological deficit, usually of very sudden onset, lasting at least 24 hours, due to an occlusion of a blood vessel supplying the central nervous system (CNS). By definition, any deficit

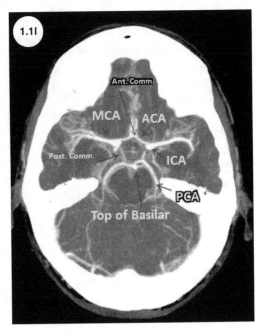

Image 1.1I: Normal CT angiogram of the head demonstrates the circle of Willis.

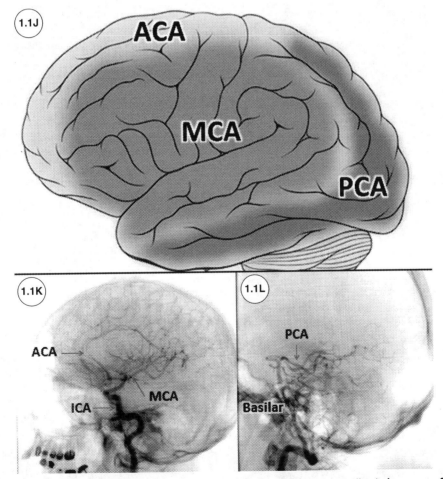

Image 1.1J: Illustration of the cortical vascular territories (image credit Dr. Frank Gaillard). **Images 1.1K and 1.1L:** Catheter angiography of the internal carotid artery (ICA) and vertebral artery demonstrates normal intracranial vasculature.

that lasts less than 24 hours is termed a transient ischemic attack (TIA), though most TIAs are much shorter than this. Stroke is the third leading cause of death in the United States, and is the leading cause of disability in adults. There are nearly 750,000 strokes in the United States annually causing 200,000 deaths. Eighty percent of strokes are ischemic and 20% are hemorrhagic.

Clinical Presentation

■ The clinical presentation depends on which vessel is occluded.

Anterior Cerebral Artery

■ The ACA supplies the medial portion of the frontal lobe, anterior parietal lobe, as well as the corpus callosum and cingulate gyrus. Occlusions of the ACA stem may be well tolerated as long as there is sufficient collateral flow through the anterior communicating artery.

■ Infarctions of the ACA produce contralateral weakness and sensory loss primarily of the leg as this part of the motor homunculus is located within the interhemispheric fissure. Urinary incontinence, to which patients are often indifferent, can be seen due to disruption of the micturition inhibition center. Patients can become disinhibited or abulic. Left-sided lesions may result in a transcortical motor aphasia, while right-sided lesions may produce hemineglect.

Middle Cerebral Artery

■ Infarctions of the entire MCA produce contralateral weakness, sensory loss, and a homonymous hemianopsia. Left-sided lesions result in global aphasia, while right-sided lesions cause

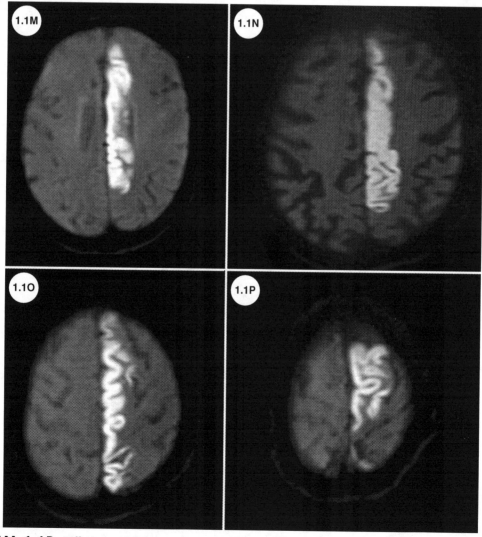

Images 1.1M–1.1P: Diffusion-weighted axial images demonstrate an acute infarction in the territory of the left ACA.

hemineglect and lack of prosody. The eyes will be deviated to the side of the lesion due to injury to the frontal eye fields. Examples are shown in **Images 1.1A–1.1C**.

■ The MCA has three divisions: the superior division, the inferior division, and the deep branches. The superior division supplies the lateral frontal lobe above the Sylvian fissure. Infarctions of the superior division produce contralateral weakness. Infarctions on the left produce a Broca's aphasia, while infarctions on the right produce neglect.

■ The inferior division supplies the posterior frontal lobe, anterior parietal lobe, and lateral temporal lobe. Infarctions on the left cause a Wernicke's aphasia, while on the right cause left hemineglect. With either side, there will be contralateral

visual field deficits due to disruption of the optic radiations, though this may be difficult to detect in patients with significant neglect or aphasia. With parietal lobe lesions, there will be cortical sensory loss. There are usually minimal to no motor findings.

■ The deep territory consists of the subcortical white matter and basal ganglia. Infarctions in this territory produce contralateral weakness and sensory loss. Large lesions may be associated with aphasia or neglect.

Posterior Cerebral Artery

■ The PCA supplies the inferior medial temporal lobe and the occipital lobe. Small penetrating branches supply parts of the midbrain and thalamus. PCA infarctions produce a contralateral

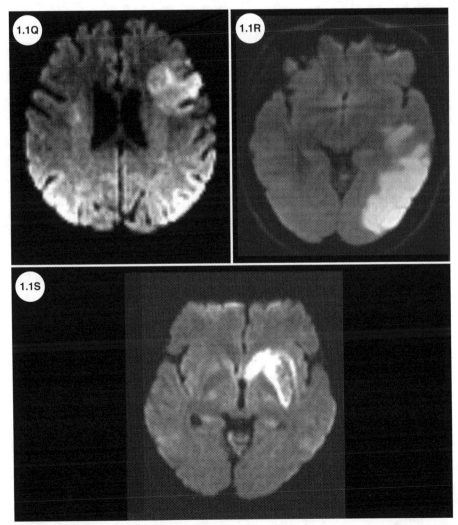

Image 1.1Q: Diffusion-weighted axial image demonstrates an acute infarction in the superior division of the MCA.
Image 1.1R: Diffusion-weighted axial image demonstrates an acute infarction in the inferior division of the MCA.
Image 1.1S: Diffusion-weighted axial image demonstrates an acute infarction of the deep branches of the MCA.

homonymous hemianopsia. There may be sparing of the central vision (macular sparing) due to collateral supply to the occipital pole from the MCA. There will be sensory deficits if the thalamus is affected. Involvement of the midbrain can lead to motor deficits, upper cranial nerve palsies, vertical gaze impairment, or coma. Infarctions on the left cause alexia without agraphia if there is involvement of the splenium of the corpus callosum.

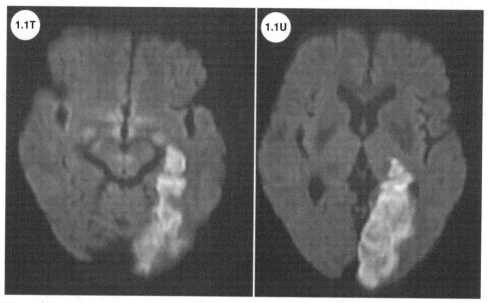

Images 1.1T and 1.1U: Diffusion-weighted axial images demonstrate an acute infarction of the left posterior cerebral artery (PCA).

■ A fetal origin of the PCA occurs when the posterior communicating artery is larger than PCA. It is a common variant, occurring in 20% to 30% individuals. With pathology of the anterior circulation, there may be infarction in territories normally supplied by the posterior circulation.

Radiographic Appearance and Diagnosis

■ A CT scan without contrast is required for any patient who presents with the sudden onset of a neurological deficit to rule out intracranial bleeds or mass lesions that might mimic ischemic strokes. The brain parenchyma will be normal in cases of hyperacute ischemic stroke, though a clot within the lumen of the large arteries may appear hyperdense, a finding known as the "dense MCA sign." Within the brain parenchyma itself, blurring of the distinction between the gray and white matter becomes visible after 6 to 12 hours.

■ After several days, the infarcted tissue becomes markedly hypodense. Swelling and edema are evident as well.

■ Within the core of the infarction, there is neuronal death within minutes. The ischemic penumbra refers to tissue that is at risk of infarction but can be preserved if blood flow is promptly restored. CT perfusion scans can be used acutely to determine the mean transit time (MTT), the cerebral blood flow (CBF), and the cerebral blood volume (CBV) to help determine if there is an ischemic penumbra.

■ **Within the infarct core there will be:**

  ▪ Prolonged MTT or Tmax

  ▪ Markedly decreased CBF

  ▪ Markedly decreased CBV

■ **Within the ischemic penumbra there will be:**

  ▪ Prolonged MTT or Tmax

  ▪ Moderately decreased CBF

  ▪ Near normal or even increased CBV

■ MRIs are more sensitive than CTs for acute stroke, especially smaller infarctions.

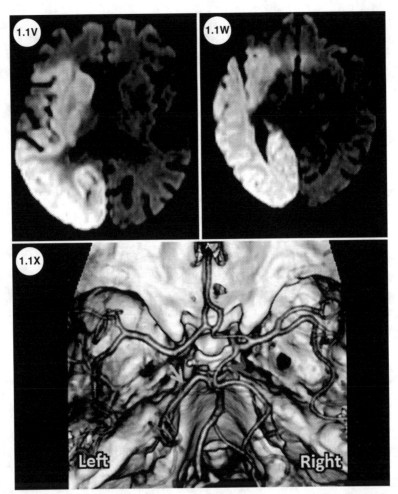

Images 1.1V and 1.1W: Diffusion-weighted axial images demonstrate an acute infarction of the right MCA and PCA. **Image 1.1X:** CT angiogram demonstrates a fetal PCA (red arrow) on the right. A normal PCA is seen on the left (blue arrow).

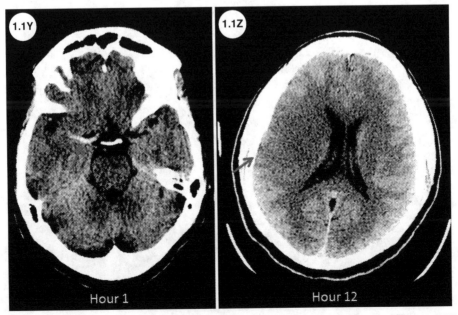

Image 1.1Y: Axial CT image demonstrates a dense right MCA (red arrow). **Image 1.1Z:** Axial CT image demonstrates blurring of the gray–white junction on the right (red arrow).

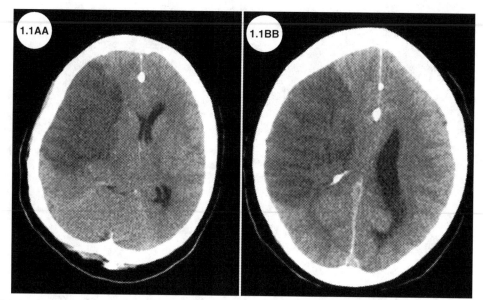

Images 1.1AA and 1.1BB: Axial CT images demonstrate hypodensity in the MCA territory on the right with midline shift and compression of the lateral ventricle.

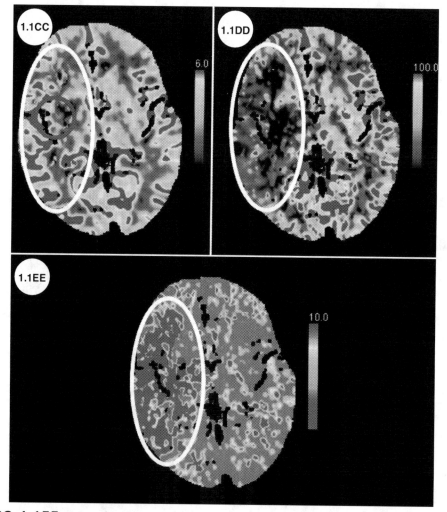

Images 1.1CC–1.1EE: CT perfusion images demonstrate an acute right MCA infarction. In this case, the ischemic core is delineated by the red circle while the penumbra is delineated by the white oval.

Diffusion-weighted sequences, which reveal abnormal movements of water, are the most sensitive sequence for detecting acute ischemic events. If there is corresponding hypointensity (referred to as "drop-out") on the apparent diffusion coefficient (ADC) map, then the diagnosis is confirmed in the appropriate clinical setting. Importantly, other diseases, such as active multiple sclerosis (MS) lesions, abscesses, or tumors such as primary CNS lymphoma can also demonstrate restricted diffusion. In the acute setting, the advantage of using an MRI to confirm a stroke diagnosis has to be weighed against delaying thrombolytic therapy. On magnetic resonance angiographies (MRAs), the occluded vessel can be seen.

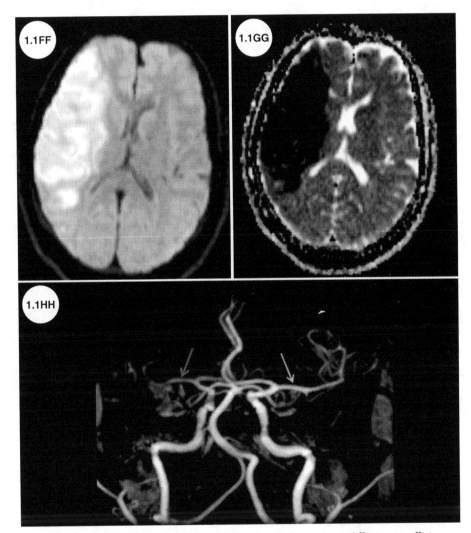

Images 1.1FF and 1.1GG: Diffusion-weighted axial image and apparent diffusion coefficient map demonstrate restricted diffusion in the territory of the right MCA infarct. **Image 1.1HH:** Magnetic resonance angiogram demonstrates occlusion of the right MCA (red arrow). The normal MCA is seen (blue arrow).

■ A stroke should be the presumed diagnosis in any patient who presents with the sudden onset of focal neurological deficits. However, it is important to keep in mind potential stroke mimics. Possible stroke mimics include:

   ■ **Seizures:** Patients in status epilepticus or those suffering from postictal paralysis, termed Todd's paralysis, may present with focal neurological findings. Though motor deficits are the most common postictal deficit, patients also may present with aphasias.

   ■ **Migraines:** Patients may present with focal neurological deficits, in which case the migraine is referred to as a complicated migraine.

- **Tumors**: Neoplasms may present with the sudden onset of focal symptoms, especially if there is hemorrhage into the tumor.

- **Multiple sclerosis:** Patients with MS might develop acute neurological symptoms or wake up with new symptoms. Active areas of demyelination in MS may also show diffusion restriction making the radiographic appearance similar to infarction as well.

- **Psychiatric disturbances:** Patients with a wide variety of psychiatric disturbances may present with neurological deficits that resemble strokes. Patients may consciously feign symptoms, termed factitious disorder (or malingering if for secondary gain), or may do so unconsciously in cases of conversion disorder.

- **Toxic/metabolic abnormalities:** Patients with toxic or metabolic abnormalities may present with focal neurological findings. This is most classically present in patients who have had a prior stroke whose symptoms reappear or worsen in the setting of systemic illness, which can be easily confused with new symptoms.

Treatment

Acute Stroke Treatment

- An acute ischemic stroke is a neurological emergency. The goal of acute treatment is to preserve the ischemic penumbra. Tissue Plasminogen Activator (t-PA), a thrombolytic agent, should be given to all patients who can be treated within 3 hours, assuming there are no contraindications. Newer data indicates the time window in which treatment is effective can be extended to 4.5 hours. Without blood supply, brain tissue dies rapidly, and the earlier it is given, the greater the potential benefit. With t-PA, there is a 30% risk reduction for disability at 3 months compared to placebo. The major risk is intracranial hemorrhage, which occurs in 6% of patients. The risk for bleeding increases with larger infarctions, longer times from stroke onset, and deviation from the t-PA protocol. Aspirin is the treatment of choice for stroke patients not eligible for t-PA, and it has been shown to reduce mortality if given within the first 48 hours.

- Interventional procedures can be used to mechanically remove the clot or deliver thrombolytics directly to the clot. The Mechanical Embolus Removal in Cerebral Ischemia (MERCI) trial investigated the use of a corkscrew device to mechanically remove clots within intracranial arteries within 8 hours of stroke onset. The Penumbra System is another interventional device used to aspirate and extract a clot from within the lumen of an artery.

- The MR CLEAN trial demonstrated effectiveness of these interventions if done within a 6-hour window. Multiple other recent trials (SWIFT PRIME, EXTEND-IA, ESCAPE, REVASCAT) with variable inclusion criteria demonstrated unequivocal positive benefit of acute endovascular treatment of ischemic stroke in select patients with significant increase in bleeding risk. Some studies also demonstrated a trend in reduction of mortality. The likelihood of good outcome increases with higher degree of recanalization, and patients who receive earlier treatment fare better. Outcomes are best in strokes of anterior circulation.

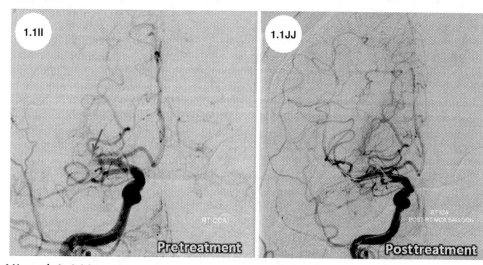

Images 1.1II and 1.1JJ: Catheter angiogram of a patient with a large MCA infarction shows loss of flow in the MCA (red arrow). Some flow is restored in the occluded artery after removal of the thrombus.

▓ Large infarctions of the MCA, sometimes called malignant MCA infarctions, may cause swelling, herniation, and death. The swelling peaks on days 3 to 5, and younger patients with less brain atrophy are most vulnerable. Osmotic agents such as mannitol and hyperventilation are used

to lower intracranial pressure (ICP). In certain cases, removal of the skull (hemicraniectomy) may be a lifesaving procedure.

▓ Protection against deep vein thrombosis, dysphagia screening to prevent aspiration, nursing care

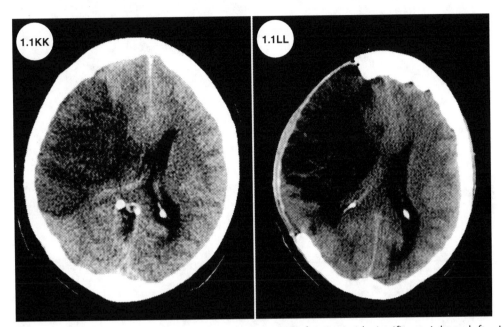

Image 1.1KK: Axial CT image demonstrates a large right MCA infarction with significant right to left midline shift.
Image 1.1LL: Axial CT image from the same patient after a right hemicraniectomy demonstrates partial resolution of the mass effect.

to prevent skin breakdown, the prevention of contractures, and the early institution of physical, occupational, and speech therapy are all crucial.

Secondary Stroke Prevention

▓ Once patients have been stabilized, treatment involves determining the stroke mechanism, preventing a second stroke, and rehabilitation. All patients should have the following risk factors addressed:

▓ **Hypertension:** Hypertension is the most important risk factor for both ischemic and hemorrhagic strokes. The risk of stroke correlates directly with blood pressure elevation, even in patients who do not meet criteria for hypertension. The goal blood pressure in stroke patients is 120/80.

▓ **Lipids:** An elevated cholesterol and low-density lipoprotein (LDL) are risk factors for ischemic stroke. An elevated high-density lipoprotein (HDL) is protective. Stroke patients should be started on an HMG-CoA reductase inhibitor, even in the absence of elevated LDL.

▓ **Diabetes:** Diabetes is a strong risk factor for all subtypes of stroke. Despite this, strict glycemic control has not been shown to prevent stroke.

▓ **Lifestyle:** Cigarette smoking, obesity, heavy alcohol consumption, and a sedentary lifestyle should all be addressed.

▓ **Carotid stenosis:** About 30% of ischemic strokes are due to artery-to-artery thromboembolism. Any vessel that precedes the intracranial vasculature may be a source of emboli, including the aortic arch, the common carotid artery, the ICAs, or the VAs. Of these, carotid bifurcation is the most common source of emboli. Patients with carotid stenosis greater than 70% benefit from intervention either by a carotid endarterectomy or stenting of the stenotic artery. This is best done as soon as patients are medically stable, as the highest risk for a second stroke is within the first 72 hours after the initial event.

▓ **Atrial Fibrillation:** About 20% of ischemic strokes are cardioembolic. The most common cause is atrial fibrillation, which has a 5% risk of annual stroke. Stasis within the left atrium

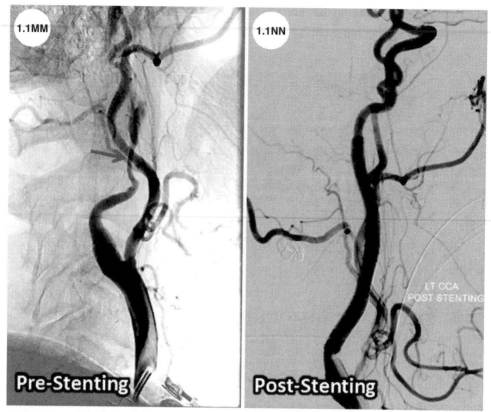

Images 1.1MM and 1.1NN: Catheter angiogram demonstrates significant stenosis of the ICA (red arrow). The ICA is shown after the placement of a stent (blue arrow).

allows for clot formation. The clot can then dislodge to occlude an intracranial vessel.

- Congestive heart failure, endocarditis, coronary artery disease, intracardiac tumors, and cardiac wall motion abnormalities, especially after a myocardial infarction, are also risk factors for cardioembolism.

- Patients with a possible cardioembolic event should have a transesophageal echocardiogram to screen for an intracardiac thrombus

and an electrocardiogram (EKG) to screen for atrial fibrillation. In patients with a normal EKG, prolonged cardiac monitoring should be used, as patients may have paroxysmal atrial fibrillation that is not detected on a single EKG.

- In patients with an intracardiac thrombus or atrial fibrillation, anticoagulation is indicated. Using warfarin to maintain an international normalized ratio (INR) from 2 to 3 for a patient with atrial fibrillation leads to

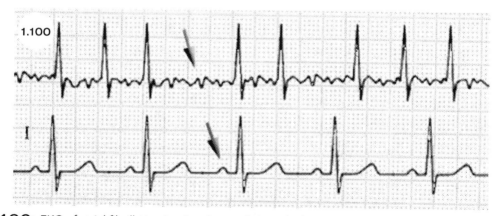

Image 1.1OO: EKG of atrial fibrillation (top) and normal sinus rhythm (bottom). The purple arrow indicates a P wave, which is lost in atrial fibrillation (image credit J. Heuser).

a 66% reduction in stroke, which outweighs the 1% annual bleeding rate from anticoagulation. Alternatives to warfarin are available. Dabigatran is a direct thrombin inhibitor, which has been shown to be superior to warfarin in patients with atrial fibrillation with equal rates of bleeding. Unlike warfarin, there is no way to reverse the medication in patients who experience bleeding events. Apixaban is a direct factor Xa inhibitor. In comparison with warfarin, it prevented 21% more strokes, and resulted in 31% fewer incidents of major bleeding over an average of

1.8 years. Rivaroxaban is also a direct factor Xa inhibitor. It has shown efficacy in preventing strokes in patients with atrial fibrillation. Anticoagulation is also indicated for patients with a number of different types of mechanical heart valves.

- **Antiplatelet agents:** In patients with atherosclerotic disease, antiplatelet agents are indicated (**Table 1.1.1**).

- About 20% of strokes are either cryptogenic or due to other mechanisms. These other mechanisms include:

Table 1.1.1 Antiplatelet Agents

Antiplatelet Agent	Dose	Mechanism	Side Effects	Notes
Aspirin	50–325 mg daily	Acetylates platelet cyclooxygenase, which inhibits platelet aggregation via inhibition of thromboxane A2	Is inexpensive and widely available, but can cause gastric discomfort, ulceration, and hemorrhage, which can be fatal	IST and CAST trials found that aspirin given in the first 48 hours of stroke reduced recurrent stroke risk and had a minimal impact on mortality as well.
Clopidogrel	75 mg daily	Blocks adenosine diphosphate (ADP) receptor on platelets, preventing fibrinogen binding to platelets and platelet aggregation	Minimal	CAPRIE study found clopidogrel was only slightly superior to aspirin in stroke prevention. MATCH study found no benefit to combination of clopidogrel and aspirin, with a higher bleeding rate.
Aspirin/ Dipyridamole	50–200 mg twice daily	Inhibits uptake of adenosine and increases cyclic AMP levels, which both inhibit platelet aggregation	Main side effect is headaches, GI upset, and bleeding from aspirin	PRoFESS study found it was equal to clopidogrel in stroke prevention, ESPS-2, and showed combination of aspirin and dipyridamole was superior to aspirin alone.

- **Hypercoagulable states:** Inherited coagulation cascade disorders usually present with strokes before the age of 30, most commonly of the venous system. Such disorders include antithrombin III deficiency, protein C and S deficiency, activated protein C resistance/ factor V Leiden mutation, and prothrombin gene mutation. The antiphospholipid syndrome is a hypercoagulable state that is more common in women and may present with recurrent, spontaneous abortions. It can be screened for by testing lupus anticoagulant and anticardiolipin antibodies. Inherited coagulation cascade disorders should be treated with warfarin. Systemic malignancies can also lead to hypercoagulable states as can the use of oral contraceptive medications, particularly in women who smoke.

- **Paradoxical embolus:** A paradoxical embolus occurs when there is atrial septal

defect or patent foramen ovale allowing a venous clot to bypass the lungs and enter the left side of the heart and arterial system, eventually reaching the intracranial arteries. There is debate about the role these play in strokes, as they are not uncommon incidental findings. Surgical repair of the defect is indicated if it is felt to be the stroke mechanism.

- **Remote infarctions** appear as encephalomalacia of affected brain areas. Compensatory enlargement of the ventricles due to destruction of the adjacent brain tissue is termed hydrocephalus ex vacuo.

- With damage to the motor tracts in the cerebral cortex, there will be degeneration of the corticospinal tract throughout its course in the CNS, a finding termed Wallerian degeneration.

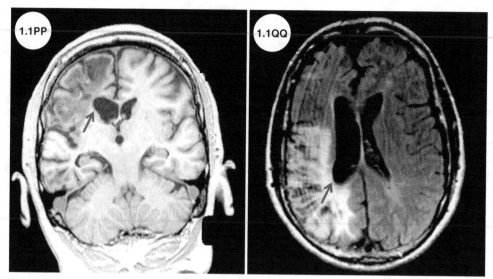

Images 1.1PP and 1.1QQ: Coronal T1-weighed and axial fluid-attenuated inversion recovery (FLAIR) images demonstrate an old infarct in the right MCA territory. There is corresponding dilation of the lateral ventricle adjacent to the infarct (red arrow).

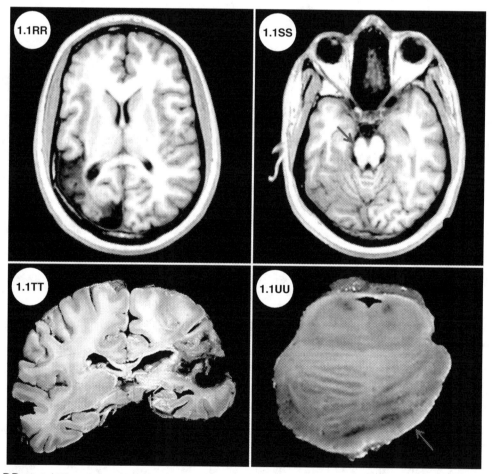

Image 1.1RR: Axial T1-weighted image demonstrates an old infarction in the right posterior MCA and PCA territories. **Image 1.1SS:** Axial T1-weighted image from the same patient demonstrates atrophy of the right cerebral peduncle (red arrow) due to Wallerian degeneration. **Images 1.1TT and 1.1UU:** Gross pathology demonstrates an old right MCA infarction and resultant atrophy of the pons.

References

1. Berkhemer OA, Fransen PS, Beumer D, et al. A randomized trial of intraarterial treatment for acute ischemic stroke. *N Engl J Med*. January 2015;372(1):11–20.
2. Powers WJ, Derdeyn CP, Biller J, et al. 2015 American Heart Association/American Stroke Association focused update of the 2013 guidelines for the early management of patients with acute ischemic stroke regarding endovascular treatment: A guideline for healthcare professionals from the American Heart Association/American Stroke Association. *Stroke*. October 2015;46(10):3020–3035.
3. Jauch EC, Saver JL, Adams HP Jr, et al. Guidelines for the early management of patients with acute ischemic stroke: a guideline for healthcare professionals from the American Heart Association/American Stroke Association. *Stroke*. March 2013;44(3):870–947.

1.2 Brainstem Stroke Syndromes

Case History

A 66-year-old man presented with the acute onset of double vision imbalance. On examination, he had a left abducens nerve palsy and ataxia of his left arm. He had some mild weakness of his right side.

Diagnosis: Brainstem Stroke

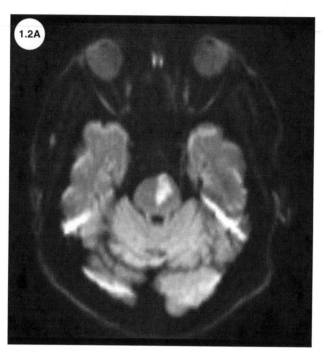

Image 1.2A: Diffusion-weighted axial image demonstrates an infarction of the medial pons.

Introduction

■ The brainstem consists of the midbrain, pons, and medulla. It contains cranial nerves 3 to 12 and the motor, sensory, and cerebellar pathways, and it is the site of production for many neurotransmitters. It also contains the reticular activating system, which is responsible for the maintenance of consciousness. Blood supply to the brainstem comes from the VAs and basilar artery.

Clinical Presentation

■ Infarctions of the brainstem produce numerous different clinical syndromes depending on the size and location of the infarction. They can be devastating events resulting in coma and death or produce only minimal symptoms and findings. Typical signs and symptoms include dizziness, vertigo, ataxia, nausea, imbalance, diplopia, nystagmus, dysarthria, and dysphagia. Brainstem pathology often produces a pattern of findings known as "crossed deficits." This means cranial nerve findings on the same side of the lesion with motor and/or sensory findings on the opposite side of the lesion, as these pathways run contralateral in the brainstem while cranial nerves exit ipsilaterally. The reticular activating system, which is responsible for the maintenance of consciousness, is located in the brainstem, and patients can be made comatose from lesions there.

■ **Midbrain:** Infarctions of the medial midbrain result from occlusions of small penetrating

1.2.1

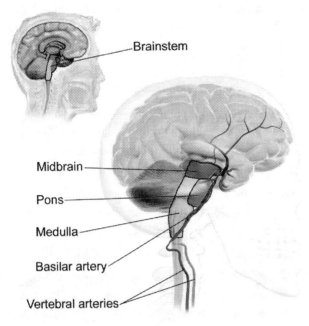

Brainstem

Midbrain

Pons

Medulla

Basilar artery

Vertebral arteries

Illustration 1.2.1: Vascular supply to the brainstem (Blausen.com staff. "Blausen gallery 2014." *Wikiversity Journal of Medicine*).

arteries that arise from upper basilar artery, while infarctions of the lateral midbrain result from occlusions of the proximal PCA. The symptoms include various combinations of an ipsilateral oculomotor nerve palsy, contralateral hemiataxia and tremor (due to involvement of the red nucleus and cerebellar pathways), and contralateral weakness (due to involvement of the corticospinal tract within the cerebral peduncle).

■ **Pons:** Infarctions of the pons result from occlusions on the paramedian branches of the basilar artery. The symptoms depend on whether stroke occurs in the upper or lower pons and whether it is medial or lateral. Medial infarctions of the upper pons result in ipsilateral ataxia, internuclear ophthalmoplegia, and contralateral motor deficits. Lateral infarctions of the upper pons produce ipsilateral ataxia, dizziness, nausea, vomiting, nystagmus dysconjugate gaze, Horner's syndrome, and contralateral sensory deficits if there is involvement of the spinothalamic tract or medial lemniscus. Medial infarctions of the lower pons result in ipsilateral ataxia, nystagmus, conjugate gaze to the side of the lesion, a sixth nerve palsy, and contralateral motor deficits. Lateral infarctions of the lower pons produce ipsilateral ataxia, dizziness, nausea, vomiting, nystagmus, dysconjugate gaze, sensory deficits of the face, facial paralysis, auditory dysfunction if there is involvement of the cochlear nucleus, and contralateral sensory deficits if there is involvement of the spinothalamic tract or medial lemniscus.

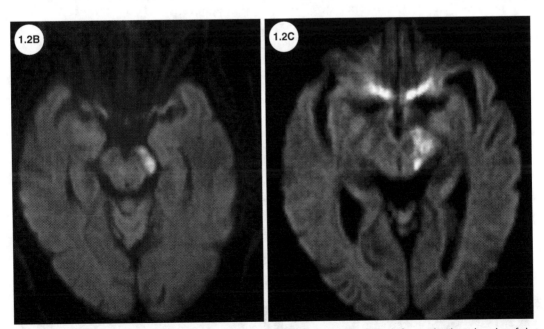

Image 1.2B: Diffusion-weighted axial image demonstrates an infarction of the left cerebral peduncle of the midbrain in a patient who presented with an ipsilateral oculomotor palsy and contralateral weakness (Weber's syndrome). **Image 1.2C:** Diffusion-weighted axial image demonstrates an infarction of the left midbrain affecting both the red nucleus and the cerebral peduncle in a patient who presented with a left oculomotor nerve palsy as well as contralateral weakness and ataxia (Claude's syndrome). (*continued*)

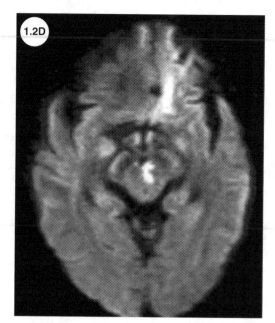

Image 1.2D: (*continued*) Diffusion-weighted axial image demonstrates an infarction of the left paramedian midbrain in a patient who presented with a left oculomotor palsy, contralateral ataxia, and mild contralateral weakness (Benedikt's syndrome).

■ **Medulla:** Occlusion of the vertebral artery or the PICA results in the lateral medullary (Wallenberg) syndrome. Its features are dysphagia, hoarseness, dizziness, nausea and vomiting, nystagmus, problems with balance, gait coordination, and loss of pain and temperature sensation on the *contralateral* side of the body and *ipsilateral* side of the face. Horner's syndrome due to disruption of the sympathetic pathways in the brainstem is often seen. Infarctions of the medial medulla are less common. These result in

ipsilateral paralysis of the tongue due to damage to the hypoglossal nerve and nucleus and contralateral weakness of the arm and leg due to damage to the corticospinal tract. Involvement of the medial lemniscus results in contralateral impairment of proprioception and light touch of the contralateral body.

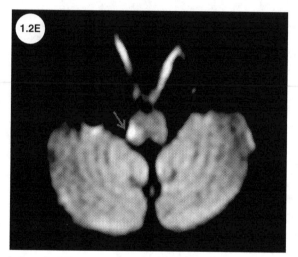

Image 1.2E: Diffusion-weighted axial image demonstrates an infarction of the right lateral medulla (red arrow).

■ **Basilar occlusion:** An embolism that occludes the basilar artery can produce an infarction of the entire pons. This can cause what is known as "locked-in syndrome," a condition where patients have preserved consciousness with no voluntary movements other than vertical eye movements, which are controlled by vertical gaze centers in the midbrain.

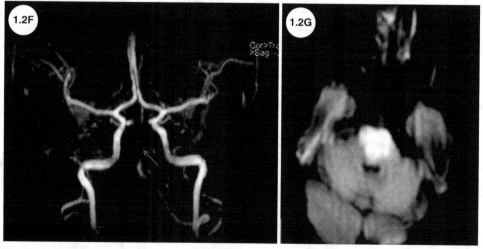

Image 1.2F: MR angiogram demonstrates absence of flow in the basilar artery (red arrow). **Image 1.2G:** Diffusion-weighted axial image demonstrates restricted diffusion of the entire pons.

■ **Artery of Percheron infarction:** The artery of Percheron (AOP) is a variant of thalamic and midbrain vasculature characterized by a solitary arterial trunk that arises from the proximal segment of either PCA to supply the bilateral thalami and midbrain. Its occlusion may result in bilateral, symmetric paramedian thalamic infarctions. Symptoms include disorientation, confusion, hypersomnolence, deep coma, akinetic mutism, amnesia, dysarthria, aphasia, hypophonia, or dysprosody. It also supplies the rostral midbrain where infarction produces bilateral oculomotor nerve palsies.

Radiographic Appearance and Diagnosis

■ As with any suspected stroke, CT scans are required to rule out hemorrhage, and diffusion-weighted imaging is the most sensitive modality to detect ischemia.

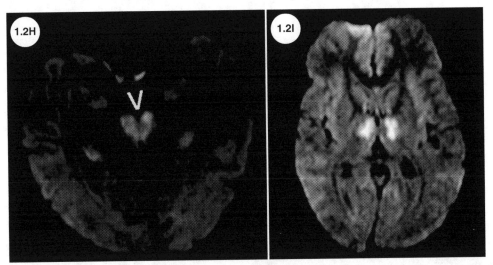

Image 1.2H: Diffusion-weighted axial image demonstrates restricted diffusion of the bilateral rostral midbrain, the "V sign." **Image 1.2I:** Diffusion-weighted axial image demonstrates bilateral paramedian thalamic infarctions.

Treatment

■ Treatment is as per ischemic stroke. As with large-vessel infarctions, thrombolysis is effective as an acute treatment in lacunar strokes. Treating hypertension, along with antiplatelet agents and other medical comorbidities, is the mainstay of treatment.

Case History

A 30-year-old male presented with an acute onset of nausea, vertigo, and ataxia. On examination, he had Horner's syndrome on the left and was unable to walk due to his imbalance.

Diagnosis: Cerebellar Infarction

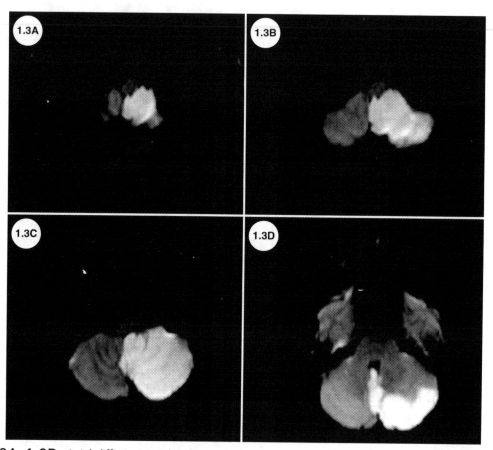

Images 1.3A–1.3D: Axial-diffusion-weighted images demonstrate an acute infarct of the left posterior inferior cerebellar artery.

Introduction

■ Blood supply to the cerebellum comes from three major arteries.

■ The PICAs arise from each vertebral artery just before they fuse together to form the basilar artery. They supply the lateral medulla and most of the inferior part of the cerebellar hemispheres and vermis.

■ The AICAs arise from the basilar artery. They supply the inferolateral pons, the middle cerebellar peduncle, and a small part of the anterior cerebellum. They also give off the labyrinthine arteries, which supply the structures of the inner ear.

■ The SCAs arise from the top of the basilar artery just before it splits to form the PCAs. They supply the upper lateral pons, the superior cerebellar peduncle, and the superior part of the vermis and cerebellar hemispheres.

Clinical Presentation

■ PICA infarctions present with a combination of vertigo, gait ataxia, and nausea and vomiting.

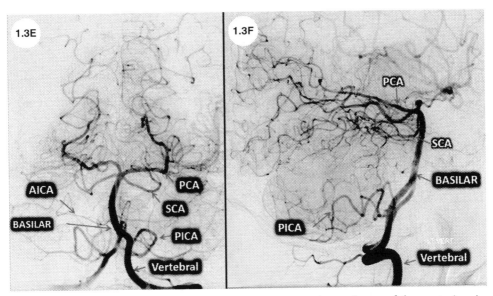

Images 1.3E and 1.3F: Catheter angiogram demonstrating normal vasculature of the posterior circulation.

The *lateral medullary* (Wallenberg) *syndrome* is common as well, especially when the underlying cause is a vertebral dissection. Large PICA infarctions may cause enough swelling of the cerebellum to obstruct the fourth ventricle and cause fatal obstructive hydrocephalus. Swelling tends to peak several days after the initial stroke.

■ AICA infarctions present with a combination of vertigo, nausea and vomiting, nystagmus, falling to the side of the lesion due to injury to vestibular nuclei, ipsilateral hearing loss or tinnitus, and ipsilateral facial weakness and sensory loss.

■ SCA infarctions, though rare, present with a combination of vertigo, nausea and vomiting, headache, gait ataxia, and diplopia.

Radiographic Appearance and Diagnosis

■ Although CT scans are needed to rule out hemorrhages, diffusion weighted images (DWI) is the preferred imaging modality to evaluate suspected ischemic stroke. This reveals restricted diffusion in the ischemic area.

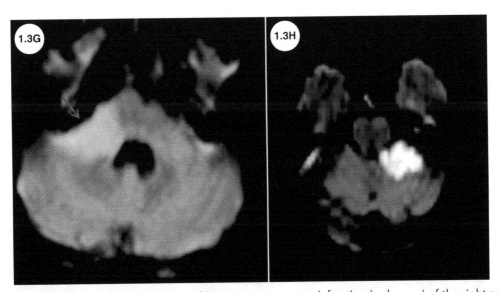

Image 1.3G: Axial diffusion-weighted image demonstrates an acute infarction (red arrow) of the right anterior inferior cerebellar artery. **Image 1.3H:** Axial diffusion-weighted image demonstrates an acute infarction of the left superior cerebellar artery.

Treatment

■ A ventricular drain may be lifesaving in PICA infarctions and obstruction of the fourth ventricle.

References

1. Erdemoglu AK, Duman T. Superior cerebellar artery territory stroke. *Acta Neurol Scand*. October 1998;98(4):283–287.
2. Montgomery AK, Maixner WJ, Wallace D, Wray A, Mackay MT. Decompressive craniectomy in childhood posterior circulation stroke: a case series and review of the literature. *Pediatr Neurol*. September 2012;47(3):193–197.
3. Tsitsopoulos PP, Tobieson L, Enblad P, Marklund N. Surgical treatment of patients with unilateral cerebellar infarcts: clinical outcome and prognostic factors. *Acta Neurochir (Wien)*. October 2011;153(10):2075–2083.
4. Nouh A, Remke J, Ruland S. Ischemic posterior circulation stroke: a review of anatomy, clinical presentations, diagnosis, and current management. *Front Neurol*. April 2014;5:30.

1.4 Lacunar Strokes

Case History

A 60-year-old smoker with uncontrolled hypertension presented with the acute onset of numbness of his left arm and leg. On exam, he had decreased sensation to all sensory modalities on the entire left side, including his face.

Diagnosis: Lacunar Stroke

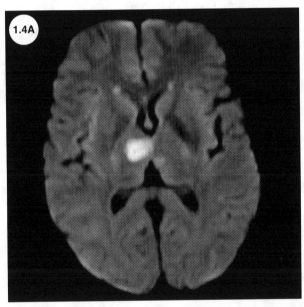

Image 1.4A: Diffusion-weighted axial image reveals an area of restricted diffusion in the right thalamus.

Introduction

- Lacunar infarctions are due to occlusions in small, single arteries that penetrate to supply the deep structure of the brain. The pathological term used to describe the changes in these small arteries is lipohyalinosis, and prolonged, uncontrolled hypertension is the main risk factor.

- Overall, these comprise about 20% of all ischemic strokes.

Clinical Presentation

- There are several presentations:
    - **Pure motor hemiparesis**: This localizes to the posterior limb of the internal capsule, subcortical white matter, or the pons.
    - **Pure sensory symptoms**: This localizes primarily to the thalamus.
    - **Ataxic hemiparesis**: This localizes primarily to the base of the pons.
    - **Clumsy hand/dysarthria**: This localizes primarily to the base of the pons or genu of the posterior limb of the internal capsule.

- They are generally not associated with the higher cortical function abnormalities, such as aphasia and neglect syndrome. Strokes in the thalamus are an exception to this, however, and can be associated with behavioral and cognitive abnormalities.

- Many are clinically silent or present with cognitive decline or parkinsonism when they accumulate in large numbers.

Radiographic Appearance and Diagnosis

- As with any suspected stroke, CT is the imaging modality of choice to rule out hemorrhage.

Restricted diffusion on DWIs is the most sensitive MRI sequence for revealing ischemia.

▪ Lacunar strokes occur due to occlusions of the lenticulostriate arteries of the MCA that supply the basal ganglia, internal capsule, and white matter in the corona radiata, the thalamoperforating branches of the PCA supplying the thalamus, or the penetrating branches of the basilar artery supplying the pons. The cerebellum is also vulnerable to such strokes.

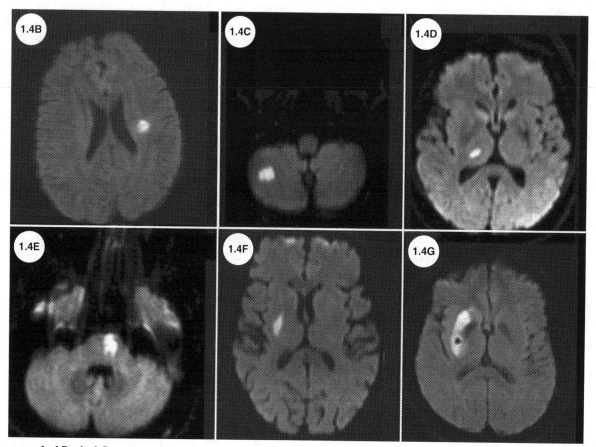

Images 1.4B–1.4G: Lacunar strokes in common locations are seen on the axial-diffusion-weighted images. These are: the subcortical white matter (1.4B), cerebellum (1.4C), the thalamus (1.4D), the pons (1.4E), the internal capsule (1.4F), and the basal ganglia (1.4G).

Treatment

▪ Acute treatment is as per ischemic stroke. As with large-vessel infarctions, thrombolysis is effective as an acute treatment in lacunar strokes.

▪ As uncontrolled hypertension is the leading risk factor for lacunar strokes, managing hypertension, along with antiplatelet agents and other medical comorbidities, is the mainstay of treatment.

References

1. Caplan LR. Lacunar infarction and small vessel disease: pathology and pathophysiology. *J Stroke.* January 2015;17(1):2–6.
2. Mok V, Kim JS. Prevention and management of cerebral small vessel disease. *J Stroke.* May 2015;17(2):111–122.
3. Norrving B. Lacunar infarcts: no black holes in the brain are benign. *Pract Neurol.* August 2008;8(4):222–228.
4. Pantoni L, Fierini F, Poggesi A. Thrombolysis in acute stroke patients with cerebral small vessel disease. *Cerebrovasc Dis.* 2014;37(1):5–13.

1.5 Watershed Strokes

Case History

A 76-year-old man with hypertension and diabetes underwent a coronary bypass artery graft that was complicated by severe blood loss. When he awoke, he was unable to move his proximal right arm and would not speak unless he became upset.

Diagnosis: Watershed Stroke

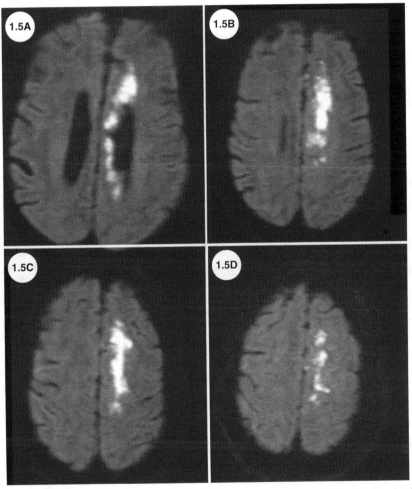

Images 1.5A–1.5D: Diffusion-weighted axial images demonstrate a subcortical, watershed infarction on the left.

Introduction

- A watershed stroke affects the brain areas farthest from direct perfusion of the major cerebral arteries. They occur in the brain areas bordered by the ACA/MCA or MCA/PCA. They account for up to 10% of strokes.

- They occur when there is hypoperfusion of the brain from systemic hypotension, congestive heart failure, or a high-grade carotid stenosis. In patients without these risk factors, microemboli have been proposed as a possible mechanism.

■ There are two types of watershed strokes:

1. **Cortical or outer infarctions** occur in the border zones between the MCA/ACA or MCA/PCA. These are thought to be due primarily to microemboli.

2. **Internal or subcortical infarctions** occur in the white matter adjacent to the lateral ventricles, between the deep and the superficial vessels of the MCA, or between the superficial systems of the MCA and ACA. These are thought to be due to hypotension or severe carotid stenosis.

Clinical Presentation

■ Patients present with weakness of the proximal arm and leg, with preservation of strength in the hands and feet; colloquially, this is known as the "man in a barrel" presentation. Patients with left-sided strokes may develop akinetic mutism, a condition where patients can speak, but will only do so when sufficiently motivated. A neglect syndrome may be seen in right-sided strokes. For unclear reasons, seizures are more common in watershed strokes.

Radiographic Appearance and Diagnosis

■ As with any suspected stroke, CT scans are required to rule out hemorrhage, and diffusion-weighted imaging is the most sensitive modality to detect ischemia.

■ In internal watershed infarctions, there will be a ribbon of infarction in the parafalcine subcortical white matter.

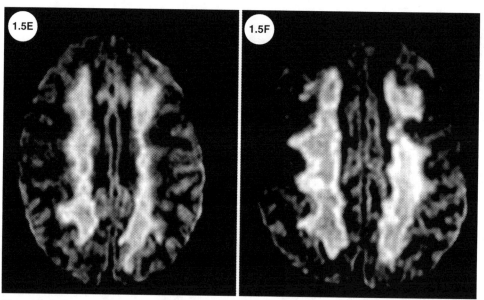

Images 1.5E and 1.5F: Diffusion-weighted axial images demonstrate restricted diffusion in the parafalcine subcortical white matter.

■ In cortical watershed infarctions, the infarction appears as wedge-shaped areas of abnormality in the border zones between the MCA and ACA or the MCA and PCA.

Treatment

■ Treatment is per ischemic stroke, with special attention given to evaluating the ICAs for stenosis.

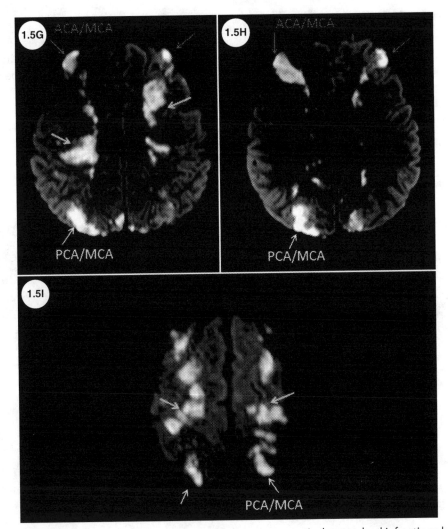

Images 1.5G–1.5I: Diffusion-weighted axial images demonstrate cortical watershed infarctions between the ACA and MCA (red arrows) bilaterally and the PCA and MCA (yellow arrows), as well as extensive subcortical, watershed infarctions (blue arrows).

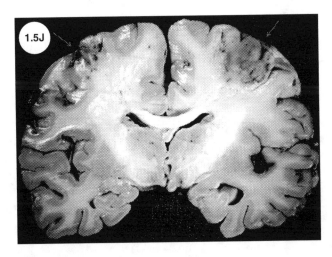

Image 1.5J: Gross pathology demonstrates recent bilateral watershed infarction, in the territories supplied by the distal branches of the anterior and middle cerebral arteries.

Reference

1. D'Amore C, Paciaroni M. Border-zone and watershed infarctions. *Front Neurol Neurosci.* 2012;30:181–184.

1.6 | Hypoxic/Ischemic Injury

Case History

A 76-year-old man was found down at home. On examination, he had a gag reflex and minimally reactive pupils, but no evidence of any other neurological function.

Diagnosis: Hypoxic-Ischemic Injury

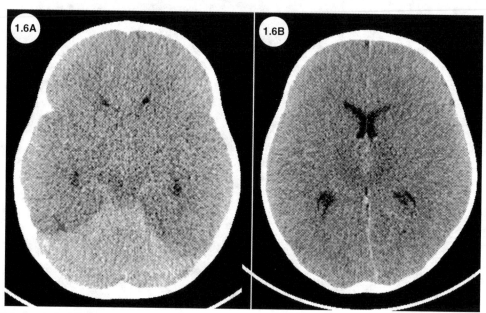

Images 1.6A and 1.6B: Axial CT images demonstrate global cerebral edema evidenced by the loss of distinction between the gray and white matter. There is sulcal effacement, bilateral uncal herniation, diffuse compression of the entire ventricular system, and complete effacement of the basal cisterns. Hyperdensity of the cerebellum (red arrow) is termed the "reversal sign."

Introduction

■ Hypoxic-ischemic injury occurs when there is either decreased perfusion to the brain, as in cardiac arrest, or decreased oxygenation, due to respiratory arrest, drowning, asphyxia, or carbon monoxide poisoning.

Clinical Presentation

■ These are typically devastating events where patients are left comatose or in a minimally conscious state. Less severely affected patients suffer from deficits in attention and memory. Patients present with a variety of movement disorders such as parkinsonism and dystonia.

Radiographic Appearance and Diagnosis

■ On CT, there is diffuse cortical edema with blurring of the gray–white junction. The relative hyperdensity of the cerebellum to the brain is termed the "reversal sign." This sign is associated with a very poor prognosis.

■ The putamen, caudate, globus pallidus, thalami, hippocampi, and substantia nigra are particularly vulnerable to hypoxic-ischemic injury. T2-weighted images demonstrate hyperintensity of these structures, and over time they become hypodense on CT. Hippocampal abnormalities are a poor prognostic factor.

■ Other findings include cortical laminar necrosis and infarctions in the watershed distribution. These are best seen on DWIs and are the earliest abnormalities to be seen on neuroimaging.

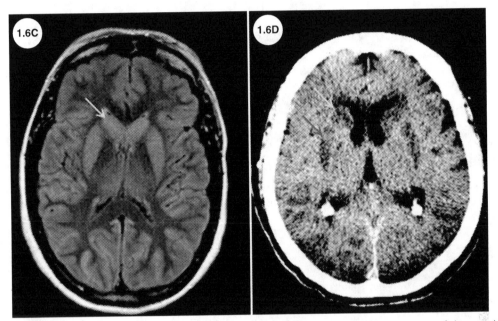

Images 1.6C and 1.6D: Axial FLAIR image and CT show hyperintensity and hypodensity of the caudate head (yellow arrow) and putamen (red arrow).

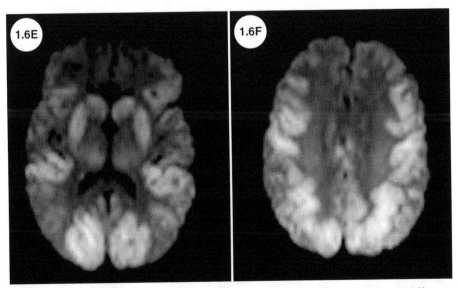

Images 1.6E and 1.6F: Axial diffusion weighted images (DWIs) demonstrate restricted diffusion of the basal ganglia and cortical ribbon. (*continued*)

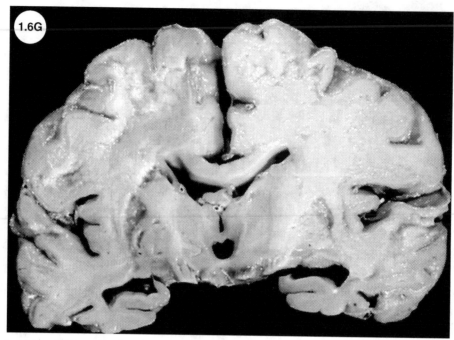

Image 1.6G: (*continued*) Gross pathology demonstrates thinning of the majority of the cortical ribbon and atrophy of the deep gray structures.

Treatment

■ Induced hypothermia has led to improved outcomes in patients whose cardiac function can be restored in a short amount of time and is now the standard of care for patients who suffered from cardiac arrest.

References

1. Arrich J, Holzer M, Havel C, Müllner M, Herkner H. Hypothermia for neuroprotection in adults after cardiopulmonary resuscitation. *Cochrane Database Syst Rev*. September 2012;9:CD004128.
2. Greer DM, Scripko PD, Wu O, et al. Hippocampal magnetic resonance imaging abnormalities in cardiac arrest are associated with poor outcome. *J Stroke Cerebrovasc Dis*. October 2013;22(7):899–905.
3. Greer D, Scripko P, Bartscher J, et al. Clinical MRI interpretation for outcome prediction in cardiac arrest. *Neurocrit Care*. October 2012;17(2):240–244.

1.7 Sinus Venous Thrombosis

Case History

A 34-year-old woman presented with an acute onset of left-side weakness and lethargy. She had a severe headache for the past week, but had not sought medical attention. In addition to her weakness, fundoscopic examination revealed papilledema.

Diagnosis: Sinus Venous Thrombosis

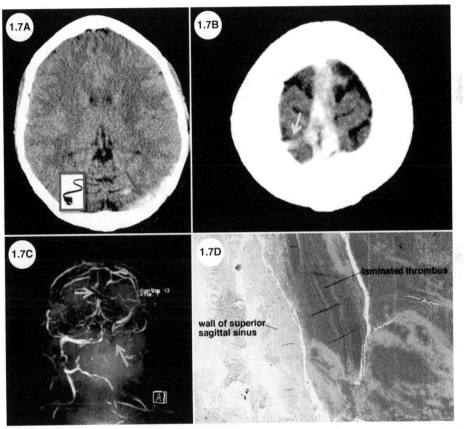

Images 1.7A and 1.7B: Axial CT images demonstrate hyperdensity in the left transverse sinus (red arrow), the superior sagittal sinus, and a cortical vein (yellow arrow). **Image 1.7C:** An MR venogram from the same patient reveals extensive thrombosis (absence of flow) in the left transverse sinus (blue arrow) and superior sagittal sinus (green arrow). **Image 1.7D:** Pathological specimen of a thrombosed superior sagittal sinus.

Introduction

■ The venous drainage of the brain is shown in **Table 1.7.1.** Cortical veins drain from the surface of the brain into the named venous sinuses. These include the superior sagittal sinus, the inferior sagittal sinus, the straight sinus, the vein of Galen, the occipital sinus, the transverse sinuses, the petrosal sinuses, and the sigmoid sinus. All of these eventually drain into the internal jugular vein. The confluence of sinuses is not an actual sinus, but rather is a reference point where the straight sinus, superior sagittal sinus, and transverse sinuses meet.

Table 1.7.1 Venous Drainage of the Brain

Sinus	Drains to
Inferior sagittal sinus	Straight sinus
Superior sagittal sinus	Right transverse sinus
Straight sinus	Left transverse sinus
Occipital sinus	Confluence of sinuses
Sphenoparietal sinus/superior ophthalmic vein	Cavernous sinuses
Cavernous sinuses	Superior and inferior petrosal sinuses
Superior petrosal sinus	Transverse sinuses
Transverse sinuses	Sigmoid sinus
Inferior petrosal sinus	Sigmoid sinus
Sigmoid sinuses	Internal jugular vein

■ Sinus venous thrombosis (SVT) occurs when there is an occlusion of the venous system, often leading to cerebral infarction. There can be both occlusions of the deep venous system (inferior sagittal and straight sinus, and vein of Galen), as shown in the original case, and the superficial venous system (superior sagittal and transverse sinus).

■ Risk factors for SVT include various hypercoagulable states, pregnancy/postpartum, otitis and mastoiditis, malignancy, and medications. The combination of oral contraceptives and smoking is a particular risk factor.

Clinical Presentation

■ Patients present with headaches and other signs of increased ICP. In severe cases, patients may be obtunded or comatose. Seizures occur in 40% of patients. Infarction occurs in approximately 50% of cases of SVT. There is generally a more indolent presentation as compared to arterial infarcts, and infarction may occur days to weeks after clot formation. Unlike arterial infarctions, there are no specific patterns of injury with SVT, but focal neurological deficits occur depending on the part of the brain that is affected. Infarctions of the deep venous system may lead to bilateral thalamic infarcts, which produces a confusional state and a decreased level of consciousness. This may be the only manifestation of such strokes.

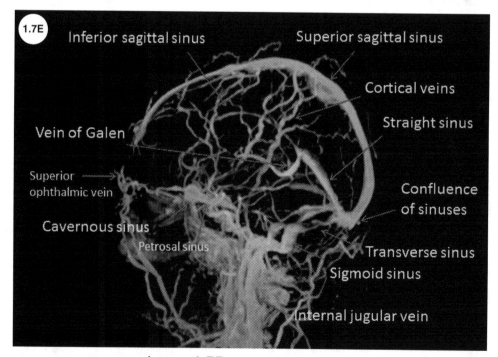

Image 1.7E: Normal MR venogram.

Radiographic Appearance and Diagnosis

■ Thrombosed veins may appear hyperdense on CT, a finding known as the "cord sign" when the transverse sinus is affected (**Image 1.7A**). An MR venogram can confirm the diagnosis in most cases.

■ Lack of contrast flow in the superior sagittal sinus on postcontrast images creates a triangular filling defect termed the "empty-delta sign."

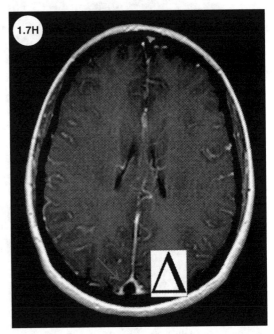

Image 1.7H: Postcontrast axial T1-weighted image demonstrates absence of flow in the superior sagittal sinus (red arrow), the "empty-delta sign."

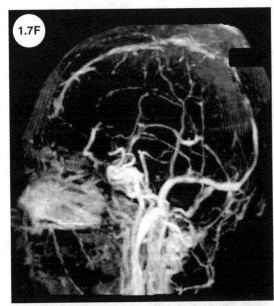

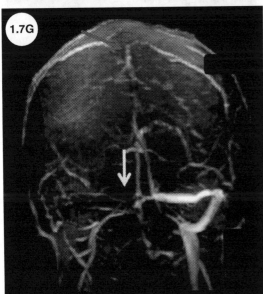

Images 1.7F and 1.7G: MR venogram demonstrates absence of flow in the superior sagittal sinus (red arrows) and transverse sinus (yellow arrow) on the left, consistent with clot within the lumen of the vein.

■ Restricted diffusion of any infarcted areas is seen within the brain parenchyma itself. The scans in **Images 1.7I–1.7L** demonstrate that the deep venous system may be affected as well.

■ In severe cases, hyperintensity is visible on T2-weighted images and frank hemorrhage may be seen.

■ Catheter angiography may be needed in equivocal cases. It is the most sensitive imaging modality and allows for the delivery of thrombolytics directly to the clot.

Treatment

■ The standard of care is immediate use of heparin even in the presence of hemorrhage. Patients are often treated with oral anticoagulation for several months, depending on the re-evaluation of the venous system. Neurointerventional

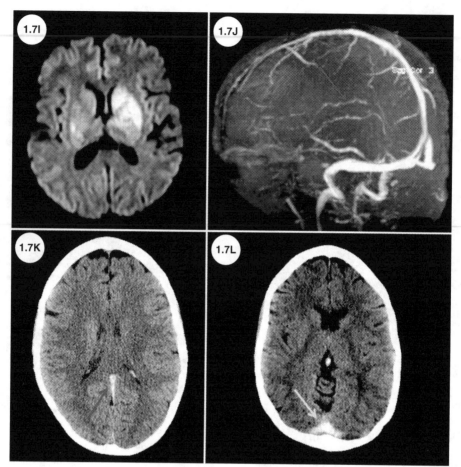

Image 1.7I: Diffusion-weighted axial image demonstrates a left basal ganglia and bithalamic infarcts. **Image 1.7J:** MR venogram demonstrates absence of flow in the deep venous system (red arrow). **Images 1.7K and 1.7L:** Axial CT images demonstrate hyperdensity of the inferior sagittal sinus (red arrow) and confluence of sinuses (yellow arrow).

procedures can be used to deliver thrombolytics directly to the clot in severe cases, and shunting of the ventricular system is required in patients with a persistently elevated ICP. Despite this, patients can become quite debilitated and die in severe cases.

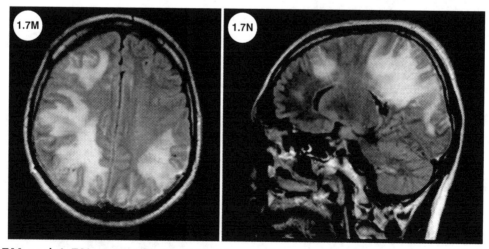

Images 1.7M and 1.7N: Axial and sagittal FLAIR images demonstrate severe, bilateral white matter disease in a patient with superior sagittal sinus thrombosis. (*continued*)

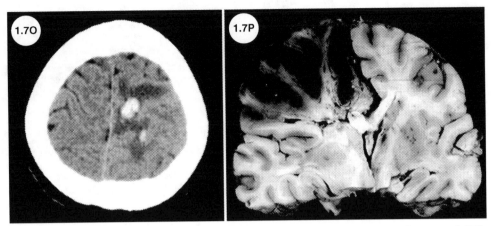

Image 1.7O: (*continued*) CT image demonstrates hemorrhage in the left frontal lobe. **Image 1.7P:** Gross pathology demonstrates hemorrhagic infarction in a patient with superior sagittal sinus thrombosis.

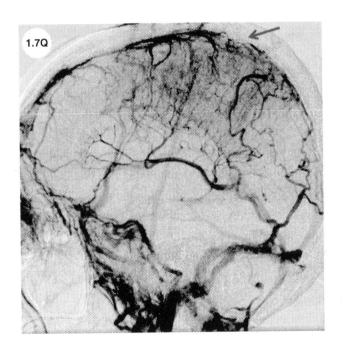

Image 1.7Q: Catheter angiogram demonstrates absence of flow in the superior sagittal sinus (red arrow) consistent with clot within the lumen of the vein in a patient with sinus venous thrombosis.

References

1. Stam J. Thrombosis of the cerebral veins and sinuses. *N Engl J Med*. April 2005;352(17):1791–1798.
2. Ferro JM, Canhão P. Cerebral venous sinus thrombosis: update on diagnosis and management. *Curr Cardiol Rep*. September 2014;16(9):523.
3. Kumral E, Polat F, Uzunköprü C, Callı C, Kitiş Ö. The clinical spectrum of intracerebral hematoma, hemorrhagic infarct, non-hemorrhagic infarct, and non-lesional venous stroke in patients with cerebral sinus-venous thrombosis. *Eur J Neurol*. April 2012;19(4):537–543.
4. Sagduyu A, Sirin H, Mulayim S, et al. Cerebral cortical and deep venous thrombosis without sinus thrombosis: clinical MRI correlates. *Acta Neurol Scand*. October 2006;114(4): 254–260.

1.8 | Cerebral Autosomal Dominant Arteriopathy With Subcortical Infarcts and Leukoencephalopathy

Case History

An otherwise healthy, 46-year-old woman presented with migraine headaches and two lacunar strokes.

Diagnosis: Cerebral Autosomal Dominant Arteriopathy With Subcortical Infarcts and Leukoencephalopathy

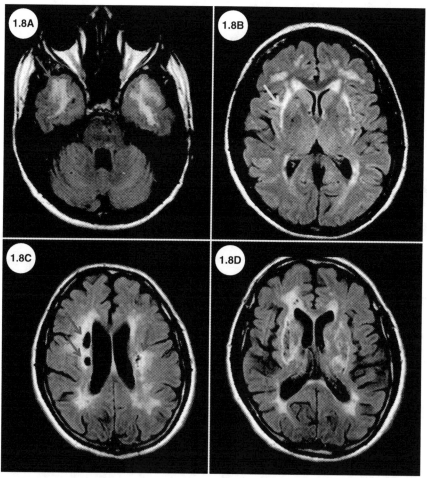

Images 1.8A–1.8D: Axial FLAIR images demonstrate extensive, symmetric white matter hyperintensities with multiple old lacunar infarctions (red arrows). In particular, there is hyperintensity in the white matter of the temporal poles (pink arrow) and the external capsule (yellow arrow).

Introduction

■ Cerebral autosomal dominant arteriopathy with subcortical infarcts and leukoencephalopathy (CADASIL) is the most common hereditary stroke disorder. The genetic mutation is located on the notch 3 gene on chromosome 19. It is an autosomal dominant inheritance disorder. There is degeneration of the smooth muscle cells in the microvasculature, most noticeably in the brain. Thickened blood vessels lead to impaired flow and ischemia.

■ The disease can present at any age, but most patients develop symptoms in mid-adulthood.

Clinical Presentation

■ Patients develop migraines and multiple lacunar strokes, usually in middle age and in the absence of other stroke risk factors. Visual or sensory disturbances are common during the migraines, and some patients have seizures. Psychiatric disturbances and personality changes are common. Eventually, patients become demented.

Radiographic Appearance and Diagnosis

■ MRI shows confluent white matter hyperintensities on T2-weighted and FLAIR images, with the vast majority having hyperintensities in the anterior temporal lobe and external capsule. Lesions in the thalamus, pons, and basal ganglia are common, and there is relative sparing of the occipital lobes and orbitofrontal cortex. Multiple old lacunar infarctions appear as cystic lesions in the basal ganglia and subcortical white matter. Microhemorrhages occur in about 50% of patients. Global cerebral atrophy is a late finding.

■ The arteriopathy is not limited to the CNS, and skin biopsies can be used to aid in the diagnosis.

■ The diagnosis is confirmed through genetic testing.

Treatment

■ There is no direct treatment. Antiplatelet agents are used with the hopes of preventing further infarcts. Minimization of other vascular risk factors such as smoking, hypertension, diabetes, and dyslipidemia is important. Almost all patients are demented by the age of 65 and few survive beyond 70 years of age.

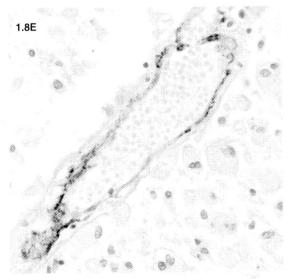

1.8E

Image 1.8E: Notch 3 immunohistochemical staining of small vessels shows a punctate staining of smooth muscle and pericytes with notch 3 (image credit nephron; https://commons.wikimedia.org/wiki/File:CADASIL_-_very_high_mag.jpg).

References

1. Chabriat H, Joutel A, Dichgans M, Tournier-Lasserve E, Bousser MG. Cadasil. *Lancet Neurol.* July 2009;8(7):643–653.
2. Rinnoci V, Nannucci S, Valenti R, et al. Cerebral hemorrhages in CADASIL: Report of four cases and a brief review. *J Neurol Sci.* July 2013;330(1–2):45–51.
3. Liem MK, Oberstein SA, van der Grond J, Ferrari MD, Haan J. CADASIL and migraine: A narrative review. *Cephalalgia.* November 2010;30(11):1284–1289.

1.9 Sickle Cell Disease

Case History

A 13-year-old child with sickle cell disease (SCD) presented with several small strokes and cognitive impairment.

Diagnosis: Sickle Cell Disease

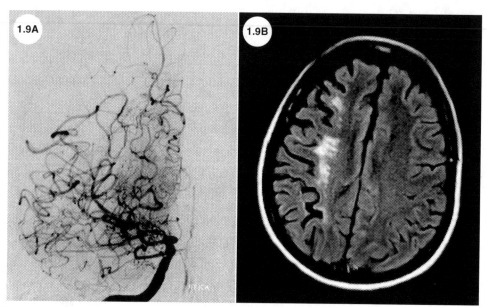

Image 1.9A: Catheter angiogram demonstrates significant luminal irregularities involving the right ICA bifurcation and the M1 segment of the right MCA, with a compensatory network of hypertrophied lenticulostriate arteries in a moyamoya-like pattern. **Image 1.9B:** Axial FLAIR image demonstrates multiple hyperintensities in the white matter on the right.

Introduction

■ **SCD** is an autosomal recessive hereditary disorder, found primarily in people of African descent, though it is also seen in people with Mediterranean or Middle Eastern heritage.

■ In SCD, the gene that codes for the beta chain of hemoglobin (HbS) is mutated, resulting in two abnormal beta chains. The abnormal hemoglobin sticks together, creating malformed, elongated (sickle-shaped) red blood cells. They are rigid, unable to flow smoothly through the microvasculature, resulting in widespread ischemia and infarction.

Clinical Presentation

■ Patients most often present in early childhood with abrupt, severe pain in the bones or abdominal visceral, often in the setting of infection or dehydration. The pain is due to microvascular blockage and subsequent ischemia.

■ Over time, multiple organs may be involved, including the lungs (acute chest syndrome, pneumonia), renal failure, abdominal pain, autosplenectomy, bone infarction and osteomyelitis, hemolytic anemia, and severe abdominal pain.

■ The most common neurological complications are both large- and small-vessel strokes and cognitive dysfunction. About 25% of patients suffer from a neurological complication of the disease.

Radiographic Appearance and Diagnosis

■ A wide variety of findings may be seen on neuroimaging, both of the brain and spine. Cerebral atrophy is the most common finding. Both large- and small-vessel strokes are often seen. A variety of vascular malformations occur, including moyamoya syndrome, tortuous intracranial arteries, and intracranial aneurysms.

- In the spine, microvascular endplate infarction causes central endplate depression, with sparing of the anterior and posterior margins. This creates a "Lincoln Log" or "H-shaped" appearance to the vertebral bodies. This finding is not specific to SCD, however, and may also be seen in Gaucher's disease.

- A peripheral smear will reveal the characteristic sickle-shaped red blood cells.

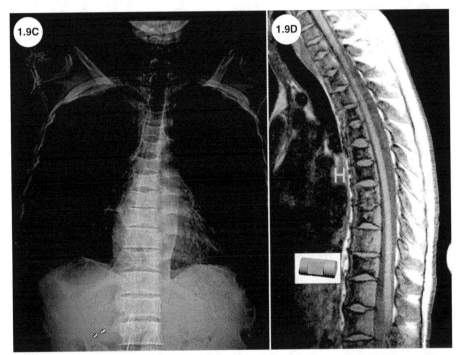

Images 1.9C and 1.9D: Anteroposterior radiograph and sagittal T1-weighted images of the spinal axes demonstrate the Lincoln Log sign and H-shaped vertebral bodies in a patient with sickle cell anemia.

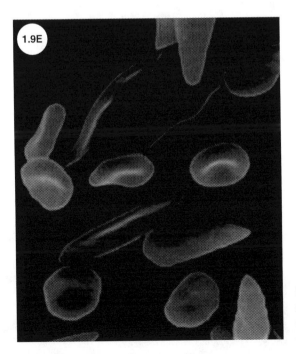

Image 1.9E: A peripheral smear demonstrating sickle-shaped red blood cells (image credit Drs. Noguchi, Rodgers, and Schechter of the National Institute of Diabetes and Digestive and Kidney Diseases [NIDDK]).

Treatment

■ Vaso-occlusive crises are treated with pain medications, oxygen, and hydration and analgesia. Hydroxyurea is used to minimize the severity of vaso-occlusive crises. Blood transfusions can be used to treat patients with symptomatic anemia. Screening children over the age of 2 with transcranial Doppler ultrasound and transfusing blood when there is a high stroke risk (>200 cm/sec) can reduce the risk of stroke by over 90%. Antiplatelet and antithrombotic agents have not been formally tested in stroke prevention. Bone marrow transplants are the only known cure.

References

1. Hansen GC, Gold RH. Central depression of multiple vertebral end-plates: a "pathognomonic" sign of sickle hemoglobinopathy in Gaucher's disease. *AJR Am J Roentgenol*. August 1977;129(2):343–344.
2. Lenchik L, Rogers LF, Delmas PD, Genant HK. Diagnosis of osteoporotic vertebral fractures: importance of recognition and description by radiologists. *AJR Am J Roentgenol*. October 2004;183(4):949–958.
3. Venkataraman A, Adams RJ. Neurologic complications of sickle cell disease. *Handb Clin Neurol*. 2014;120:1015–1025.
4. Gebreyohanns M, Adams RJ. Sickle cell disease: Primary stroke prevention. *CNS Spectr*. June 2004;9(6):445–449.

1.10 Spinal Cord Stroke

Case History

A 45-year-old man awoke with back pain and paraplegia. On exam, he had no movement of or sensation in his legs. However, his joint position sense was preserved. He was incontinent of urine.

Diagnosis: Anterior Spinal Artery Infarction

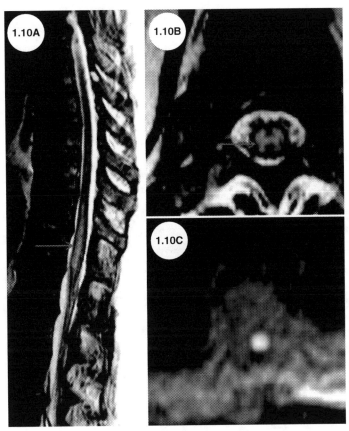

Images 1.10A and 1.10B: Sagittal and axial T2-weighted images demonstrate hyperintensity of the conus medullaris (red arrows). On axial imaging, the lesion is in the gray matter. **Image 1.10C:** Axial-diffusion-weighted image shows restricted diffusion in the center of the spinal cord.

Introduction

- The spinal cord receives its blood supply from a single anterior spinal artery (ASA) on the ventral surface of the cord and two paired posterior spinal arteries (PSAs) on the dorsal surface, though these often are not found below the mid-thoracic level. The ASA supplies the anterior two-thirds of the cervical and upper thoracic spinal cord, while the PSAs supply the dorsal columns.

- Rostrally, the spinal arteries arise from the vertebral arteries and from feeders known as segmental arteries. In the thoracic and lumbar area, the feeders to the spinal cord are known as radicular arteries that arise from the posterior aspect of aorta. One of the largest radicular arteries is the artery of Adamkiewicz, which arises from a left posterior intercostal artery and supplies the lower two-thirds of the spinal cord.

- The middle thoracic cord is a watershed area that is vulnerable to ischemic insults in the setting of systemic hypotension, abdominal surgeries, or pathology of the descending aorta, particularly near the artery of Adamkiewicz.

■ Punitive causes of ASA infarction are vasculitis, particularly systemic lupus erythematosus associated with antiphospholipid antibodies, advanced atherosclerosis, dissecting aneurysm (occludes or shears segmental spinal arteries at their origins), cholesterol embolism (after surgical procedures, angioplasty, or cardiopulmonary resuscitation [CPR]), fibrocartilaginous embolism, rupture of spinal arteriovenous malformation (AVM), cardioembolic disease, systemic hypotension, or surgical manipulation of the aorta. Often times, no cause is found.

Clinical Presentation

■ ASA infarction involves the anterior two-thirds of the spinal cord, with a variable vertical extent. It is characterized by quadriplegia or paraplegia and loss of pain and temperature below the lesion. Additional features include autonomic dysfunction and bowel and bladder retention or incontinence. Respiration can be compromised if the upper cervical cord is affected. Significant pain is common. Patients may present acutely with lower motor neuron signs, namely flaccidity and areflexia, due to spinal shock. Light touch and joint position sense are retained due to sparing of the dorsal columns.

■ Unlike cerebral infarctions in which symptom onset is nearly instantaneous, ASA infarctions may progress over 10 to 12 hours.

Radiographic Appearance and Diagnosis

■ On MRI, T2-weighted images show hyperintensities in the anterior two-thirds of the spinal cord. The gray matter is often affected preferentially. Restricted diffusion can be detected within hours and persists up to 1 week. There is minimal to no enhancement on postcontrast images. In hyperacute cases, an "owl eye" appearance can be seen, due to hyperintensity of the anterior horn cells, though this finding may be seen in other neurological disorders such as neuromyelitis optica.

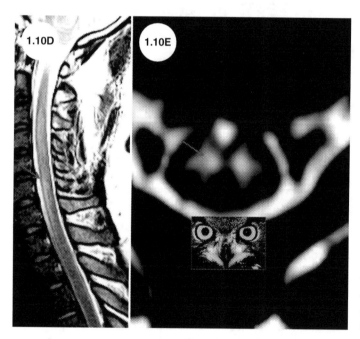

Images 1.10D and 1.10E: Sagittal and axial T2-weighted images demonstrate hyperintensity of the anterior horn cells, the "owl's eye" appearance on the axial image, in a patient with an anterior spinal artery infarction.

■ In certain cases, a spinal angiogram may be needed to document the occlusion and differentiate infarction from inflammatory or infectious myelopathies. However, in contrast to these myelopathies, cerebrospinal fluid (CSF) is normal in ASA infarction.

Treatment

■ There is no direct treatment, and supportive treatment involves care of bladder and bowel function along with active rehabilitation. Only half of patients regain the ability to walk independently.

References

1. Rigney L, Cappelen-Smith C, Sebire D, Beran RG, Cordato D. Nontraumatic spinal cord ischaemic syndrome. *J Clin Neurosci.* October 2015;22(10):1544–1549.

2. Gaeta TJ, LaPolla GA, Balentine JR. Anterior spinal artery infarction. *Ann Emerg Med.* July 1995;26(1):90–93.

1.11 Microvascular Disease

Case History

A 76-year-old man presented with subtle cognitive problems, which his wife had noticed over the past several years.

Diagnosis: Microvascular Disease

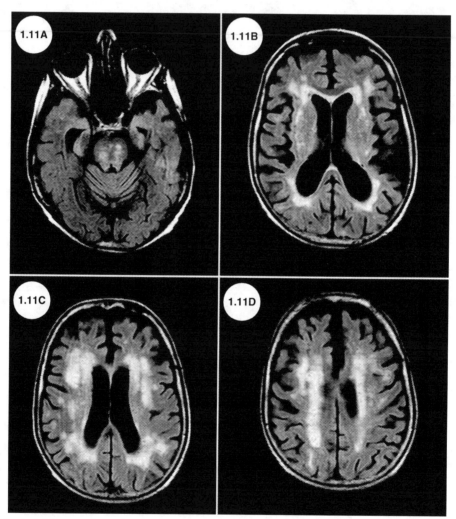

Images 1.11A–1.11D: Axial FLAIR images demonstrate symmetric confluent, hyperintense periventricular lesions as well as similar lesions in the center of the pons consistent with microvascular disease (MVD).

Introduction

■ Vascular dementia (VD), also known as multi-infarct dementia, is classically characterized by a gradual, step-wise decline in cognition. This pattern may be subtle or absent, however, as the infarctions may be clinically silent or the patient may recover function prior to his or her presentation. The term subcortical vascular dementia (Binswanger's disease) refers specifically to subcortical vascular dementia.

■ Differences in screening methods and diagnostic criteria lead to some variability in reports of prevalence and incidence. Estimations, however, suggest a prevalence of 1.2% to 4.2% of individuals over the age of 65.

■ MVD is a frequent cause of hyperintensities on FLAIR and T2-weighted images. It is most commonly seen in elderly patients with hypertension and other vascular risk factors such as smoking, diabetes, and dyslipidemia.

Clinical Presentation and Diagnosis

■ In older patients, some degree of MVD is a normal finding. Extensive disease may cause a subcortical dementia. Its characteristic features include:

- Focal motor signs
- Early gait disturbance, such as magnetic gait or parkinsonian gait
- History of unsteadiness or frequent falls
- Early unexplained urinary frequency, urgency, or incontinence
- Pseudobulbar palsy
- Personality changes, such as apathy and depression
- Cognitive impairment, particularly in executive function

Diagnosis and Radiographic Appearance

■ MVD appears as white matter hyperintensities on FLAIR and T2-weighted images. There is no mass effect or contrast enhancement. In many cases, the lesions of MVD may be difficult to distinguish from those of MS. White matter (WM) lesions due to MVD are much more common than in MS, especially in elderly patients, making the history and physical of paramount importance in evaluating patients. The lesions in MVD are scattered more throughout the white matter of the brain as opposed to the periventricular location most commonly seen in MS. Additionally, lesions are usually not seen in the corpus callosum or below the tentorium as in MS, though lesions are possible in these locations. In severe cases of MVD, the white matter lesions take on a confluent appearance.

Treatment

■ Individuals with mild cognitive impairment or evidence of mild cerebrovascular disease on imaging should be counseled on risk factor reduction. These include control of hypertension, diabetes management, and lifestyle and behavioral changes, such as healthy diet, smoking cessation, and exercise.

References

1. Román GC, Erkinjuntti T, Wallin A, Pantoni L, Chui HC. Subcortical ischaemic vascular dementia. *Lancet Neurol*. November 2002;1(7):426–436.
2. Biessels GJ. Diagnosis and treatment of vascular damage in dementia. *Biochim Biophys Acta*. November 22, 2015.

CHAPTER 2

HEMORRHAGE

2.1 Hypertensive Hemorrhage

Case History

A 54-year-old woman developed a headache and collapsed at home. She was unconscious on examination.

Diagnosis: Hypertensive Hemorrhage

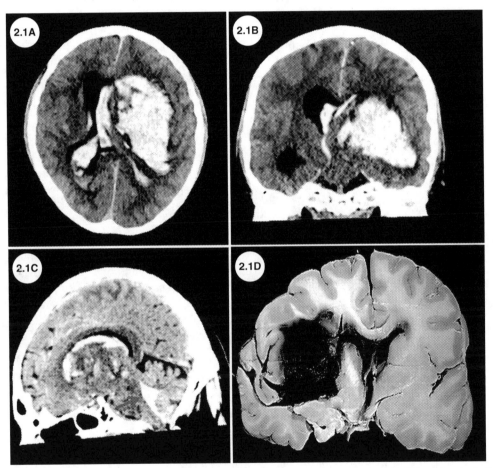

Images 2.1A–2.1C: Axial, coronal, and sagittal CT images demonstrate a massive, left basal ganglia hemorrhage with intraventricular extension involving the fourth ventricle (red arrow). **Image 2.1D:** Gross pathology of basal ganglia hemorrhage with intraventricular extension.

Introduction

▪ Intraparenchymal hemorrhage (IPH) comprises between 10% and 20% of strokes. The pathology is due to the rupture of small, penetrating arteries that have been weakened due to chronic hypertension (HTN), which is the biggest modifiable risk factor in IPH. Chronic HTN leads to lipohyalinosis in the small, penetrating arteries of the brain.

▪ Low serum cholesterol also increases the risk of IPH, particularly in patients with HTN. IPH is more common in Asians and African Americans. They are also more common in men than in women. This is likely due to increased rates of HTN in these populations.

Unless otherwise stated, all pathology images in this chapter are from the website http://medicine.stonybrookmedicine.edu/pathology/ neuropathology and are reproduced with permission of the author, Roberta J. Seidman, MD, Associate Professor. Unauthorized reproduction is prohibited.

The use of anticoagulation is the most common iatrogenic cause of IPH. The overall risk for IPH in a patient on warfarin is about 0.5% to 1.0% annually, and this is substantially increased in patients with an international normalized ratio (INR) greater than 2. The additional use of aspirin, HTN, advanced age, and the presence of cerebral amyloid angiopathy (CAA) increase the hemorrhage risk for patients on anticoagulant therapy. These are usually devastating hemorrhages and are often fatal.

Excessive alcohol consumption and smoking increase the risk, as does the use of sympathomimetic drugs such as cocaine or amphetamines. The substances may cause a vasculitis or produce acute rises in blood pressure (BP) leading to the rupture of preexisting vascular abnormalities.

Clinical Presentation

On clinical grounds alone, hypertensive IPH cannot reliably be distinguished from ischemic infarcts, though there may be some general differences. Unlike ischemic strokes, which tend to have an immediate onset, IPH progresses over 30 to 90 minutes. Hematoma expansion is unusual after 24 hours, and its occurrence portends a worse prognosis. IPH is more commonly associated with decreased levels of consciousness and headache as well as nausea and vomiting compared to ischemic strokes, due to the mass effect of a rapidly expanding hematoma and increased intracranial pressure (ICP). Finally, the clinical picture produced by intracerebral hemorrhages is somewhat more variable than those produced by ischemic events, as hemorrhages do not respect well-demarcated vascular territories.

Common locations for hypertensive IPH are the basal ganglia (in particular, the putamen), thalamus, pons, and cerebellum.

Basal ganglia: The basal ganglia, the putamen in particular, is the most common location for IPHs. Patients present with contralateral hemiplegia and sensory deficits. Larger hemorrhages may cause aphasias or neglect syndrome (depending on which side of the brain is involved), visual disturbances, and a decreased level of consciousness progressing to coma, especially if there is mass effect on the brainstem. Large hemorrhages may extend into the ventricular system causing a decreased level of consciousness, severe headache, and nausea and vomiting. Eventually, hydrocephalus may result leading to long-term cognitive impairment.

Thalamus: Thalamic hemorrhages present with contralateral sensory deficits and hemiplegia due to mass effect on the corticospinal tract as it runs through the posterior limb of the internal capsule. Aphasias or neglect syndrome may result. Larger thalamic hemorrhages may also extend into the ventricular system or produce mass effect on the upper brainstem causing disturbances of vertical gaze.

Pons: Pontine hemorrhages are devastating and often fatal events. They are due to the rupture of penetrating vessels that emerge from the basilar artery and travel into the

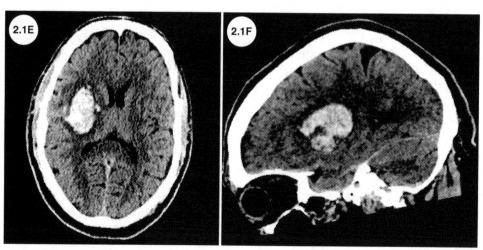

Images 2.1E–2.1G: Axial, sagittal, and coronal CT images demonstrate hemorrhage in the right putamen. *(continued)*

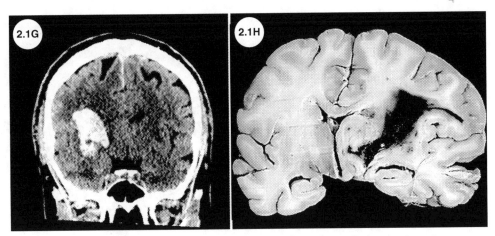

Image 2.1H: (*continued*) Gross pathology of basal ganglia hemorrhage.

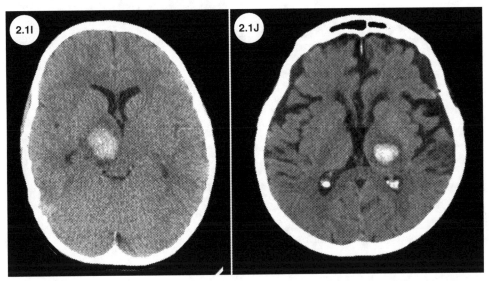

Images 2.1I and 2.1J: Axial CT images demonstrate hemorrhage in the right and left thalami in two different patients. Mass effect on the midbrain is obvious in Image 2.1I.

pons. Patients are quickly rendered quadriplegic with rigidity and decerebrate posturing. They are typically comatose and with minimal brainstem reflexes. The pupils are typically pinpoint. The overall prognosis is uniformly poor, especially once coma has developed. Most patients do not survive, and those who do rarely have meaningful recovery. In certain cases, if the initial hemorrhage is very small or is due to an underlying vascular disorder, some degree of recovery is possible.

- **Cerebellum:** Cerebellar hemorrhages comprise about 10% of all IPHs. They present with headache, ataxia, vertigo/dizziness, and vomiting. Patients may develop acute, lethal

obstructive hydrocephalus due to occlusion of the fourth ventricle.

Radiographic Appearance and Diagnosis

- CT scans are the imaging modality of choice for patients with a suspected IPH. They are 100% sensitive and specific for acute hypertensive hemorrhages.

- MRIs are used to evaluate for any underlying pathology that may have led to IPH. The appearance of a hemorrhage depends on the timing of the MRI and the sequence used (T1-weighted vs.

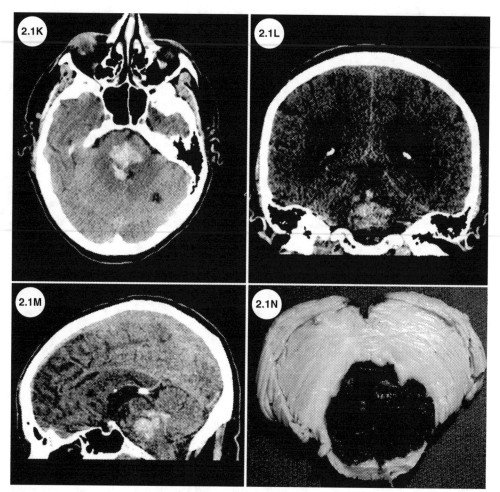

Images 2.1K–2.1M: Axial, coronal, and sagittal CT images demonstrate hemorrhage in the pons with extension into the fourth ventricle. **Image 2.1N:** Gross pathology of pontine hemorrhage.

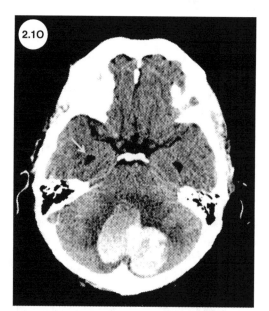

Image 2.1O: Axial CT image demonstrates hemorrhage in the cerebellum with extension into the fourth ventricle (red arrow). The yellow arrow shows the enlargement of the temporal horns of the lateral ventricle.

T2-weighted); see **Table 2.1.1**. This appearance reflects the underlying components of the hemorrhage. Gradient echo sequences of MRI are best for detecting degraded blood of older hemorrhages.

Table 2.1.1 The Appearance of Blood on MRIs

Time	T1WI	T2WI	Component
Hyperacute (0–1 day)	Isointense	Hyperintense	Oxyhemoglobin
Acute (1–3 days)	Isointense	Hypointense	Deoxyhemoglobin
Early subacute (4–7 days)	Hyperintense	Hypointense	Intracellular methemoglobin
Late subacute (>7 days)	Hyperintense	Hyperintense	Extracellular methemoglobin
Chronic (>2 weeks)	Hypointense	Hypointense	Hemosiderin/ferritin

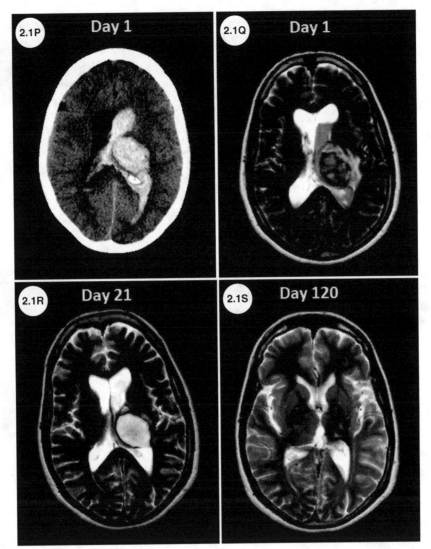

Image 2.1P: Axial CT image demonstrates a large hemorrhage in the left thalamus with intraventricular extension.
Images 2.1Q–2.1S: Axial T2-weighted images are shown on day 1, day 21, and day 120.

Treatment

- Patients should be admitted to a monitored setting with close monitoring of respiratory and circulatory status. Patients unable to safely protect their airways due to brainstem dysfunction or depressed levels of consciousness should have mechanical ventilation. The most common cause of decline in patients with IPH is early hematoma expansion, which occurs in about 40% of patients.

- There is no primary therapy of the hematoma itself with demonstrated improved outcomes. A trial of activated factor VIIa reduced the size of hematoma expansion, but failed to have an impact on patient outcome. Patients on anticoagulation should be given vitamin K and either fresh frozen plasma or recombinant factor VIIa. At present, there is no evidence to support the use of platelet transfusions in patients taking antiplatelet medications.

- Patients with large hematomas and poor neurological statuses benefit from placement of intraventricular monitors to measure ICP. Patients with elevated ICPs can have fluid drained from their intraventricular catheters. Other interventions to decrease brain edema, such as mannitol or hyperventilation, should be used in patients with impending herniation as a bridge to definitive treatment.

- The American Heart Association guidelines for treating elevated BP are as follows:

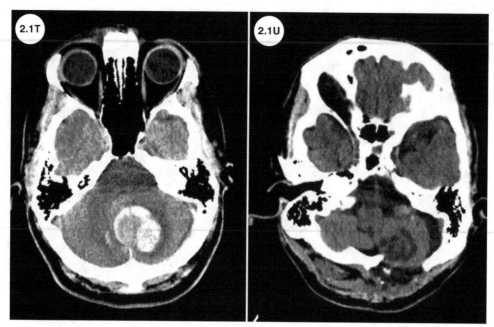

Image 2.1T: Axial CT image demonstrates cerebellar hemorrhage. **Image 2.1U:** Axial CT image after evacuation of the blood products.

- If systolic BP is greater than 200 mmHg or mean arterial pressure (MAP) is greater than 150 mmHg, then consider aggressive reduction of BP with continuous intravenous infusion with frequent BP (every 5 minutes) checks.

- If systolic BP is greater than 180 mmHg or MAP is greater than 130 mmHg and there is evidence or suspicion of elevated ICP, then consider monitoring of ICP and reducing BP using intermittent or continuous intravenous medications to maintain a cerebral perfusion pressure of 60-80 mmHg.

- If systolic BP is greater than 180 or MAP is greater than 130 mmHg and there is NO evidence or suspicion of elevated ICP, then consider modest reduction of BP (target MAP of 110 mmHg or target BP of 160/90 mmHg) with BP checks every 15 minutes.

- Careful attention to prevention of complications in critically ill patients such as infection, deep vein thrombosis, and electrolyte disturbances is essential. Antiepileptic medications are suggested only in those patients who have suffered seizures, which is more common in patients with lobar hemorrhages.

- "Fatal gastroenteritis" is the term given to nausea and vomiting due to unrecognized cerebellar pathology that eventually kills the patient. Relieving increased ICP by means of an external ventricular drain can be lifesaving. Hematomas larger than 3 cm in diameter are at most risk for neurological decline, and neurosurgical evacuation of the hematoma is required in such patients. Patients with smaller hematomas should be monitored closely both clinically and radiographically for hematoma expansion.

References

1. Elliott J, Smith M. The acute management of intracerebral hemorrhage: a clinical review. *Anesth Analg.* May 2010;110(5): 1419–1427.
2. Flower O, Smith M. The acute management of intracerebral hemorrhage. *Curr Opin Crit Care.* April 2011;17(2):106–114.
3. Manno EM. Update on intracerebral hemorrhage. *Continuum (Minneap Minn).* June 2012;18(3):598–610.
4. Adeoye O, Broderick JP. Advances in the management of intracerebral hemorrhage. *Nat Rev Neurol.* November 2010;6(11):593–601.
5. Hemphill JC 3rd, Greenberg SM, Anderson CS, et al. Guidelines for the management of spontaneous intracerebral hemorrhage: A guideline for healthcare professionals from the American Heart Association/American Stroke Association. *Stroke.* July 2015;46(7):2032–2060.

2.2 | Lobar Hemorrhages

Case History

A 75-year-old man developed a sudden onset headache and left homonymous hemianopsia.

Diagnosis: Lobar Hemorrhages Due to Amyloid Angiopathy

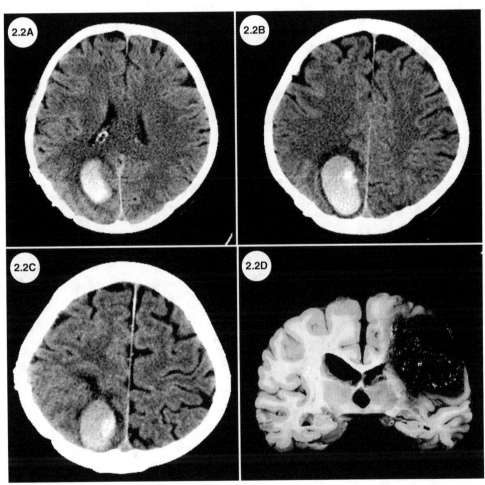

Images 2.2A–2.2C: Axial CT images demonstrate an acute hemorrhage in the right occipital lobe.
Image 2.2D: Gross pathology of a lobar hemorrhage.

Introduction

- Hemorrhages within the lobes of the brain adjacent to the cortex are called lobar hemorrhages.

They are most common in elderly, nonhypertensive patients and are associated with CAA. This occurs when there is an abnormal accumulation of beta-amyloid protein in the arterioles of the cortex and meninges. There are typically simultaneous hemorrhages or multiple hemorrhages of different ages. For unclear reasons, such hemorrhages are much more common in the parietal and occipital lobes. The basal ganglia, brainstem, and cerebellum are typically spared.

- The risk of lobar hemorrhage is increased in patients who have the e2 or e4 allele of the apolipoprotein E gene and is independent of the risk of HTN.

Clinical Presentation

- Patients present with a headache and rapid progression of focal neurological deficits, which depend on the location of the bleed. Patients may lose consciousness if there is mass effect on the brainstem or a rapid rise in ICP.

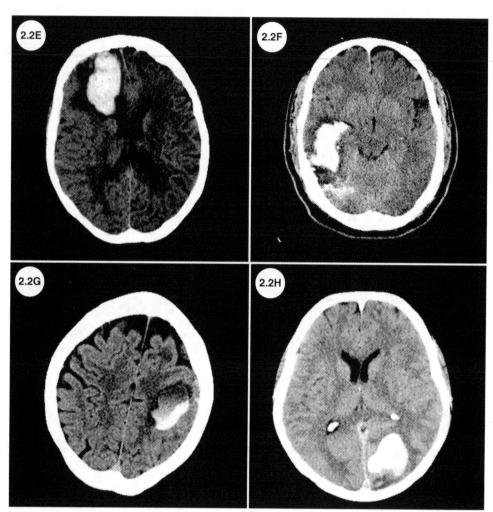

Images 2.2E–2.2H: Axial CT images demonstrate hemorrhage in the frontal, temporal lobes, parietal, and occipital lobes in four different patients.

Radiographic Appearance and Diagnosis

- CT scans are 100% sensitive for lobar hemorrhages.

- The diagnosis of CAA can only be definitively made with pathological examination of blood vessels, though a probable diagnosis can be made in the appropriate clinical setting with supportive evidence on imaging. The amyloid protein stains brightly with Congo red dye and demonstrates yellow-green birefringence under polarized light.

Treatment

- There is no definitive treatment, but antiplatelet agents and anticoagulation should be avoided. In certain cases, surgical evacuation of the hematoma may be considered especially if there is life-threatening mass effect, though there is little evidence to support this practice. Patients should be admitted to a monitored setting with close monitoring of respiratory and circulatory status.

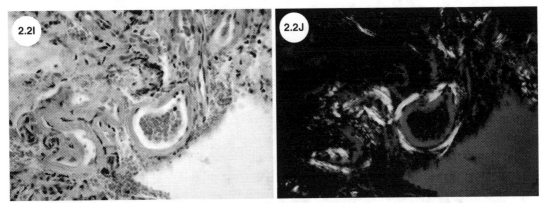

Images 2.2I and 2.2J: Histopathology of cerebral amyloid angiopathy showing deposition of amyloid (red) in hyalinized vessel walls on Congo red staining and birefringence in polarized light (image credit Marvin101).

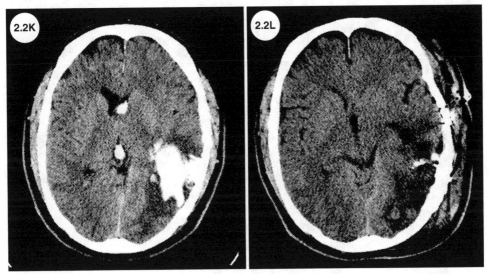

Images 2.2K and 2.2L: Axial CT images demonstrate hemorrhage in the left temporal lobe before and after evacuation of the blood.

References

1. Li XQ, Su DF, Chen HS, Fang Q. Clinical neuropathological analysis of 10 cases of cerebral amyloid angiopathy-related cerebral lobar hemorrhage. *J Korean Neurosurg Soc.* July 2015;58(1):30–35.
2. Mehndiratta P, Manjila S, Ostergard T, et al. Cerebral amyloid angiopathy-associated intracerebral hemorrhage: pathology and management. *Neurosurg Focus.* April 2012;32(4):E7.
3. Izumihara A, Suzuki M, Ishihara T. Recurrence and extension of lobar hemorrhage related to cerebral amyloid angiopathy: multivariate analysis of clinical risk factors. *Surg Neurol.* August 2005;64(2):160–164.
4. Thanvi B, Robinson T. Sporadic cerebral amyloid angiopathy—an important cause of cerebral haemorrhage in older people. *Age Ageing.* November 2006;35(6):565–571.

2.3   Amyloid Beta Related Angiitis

Case History

A 65-year-old otherwise healthy man developed progressive dementia.

Diagnosis: Amyloid Beta Related Angiitis

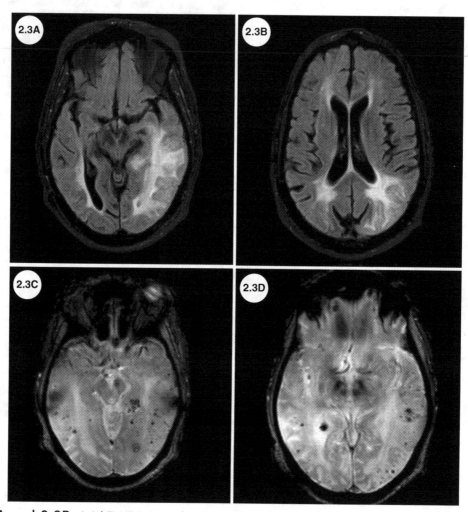

Images 2.3A and 2.3B: Axial FLAIR images demonstrate extensive white matter disease, mainly in the left temporal and bilateral occipital lobes. **Images 2.3C and 2.3D:** Axial gradient echo images demonstrate extensive punctate foci of old hemorrhage scattered throughout the brain parenchyma, though primarily in the occipital and temporal lobes.

Introduction

■   Amyloid beta related angiitis (ABRA) is characterized by transmural infiltration of vessel walls by lymphocytes and macrophages with the formation of granulomas and multinucleated giant cells in the background of CAA.

■   It is a vasculitis of small- and medium-sized leptomeningeal arteries and is thought to be an immune reaction to beta amyloid in blood vessel walls.

Clinical Presentation

■   Patients present with a combination of subacute dementia, seizures, focal neurological signs, and headaches. Patients present at a younger age than those with noninflammatory CAA.

Radiographic Appearance

■ Imaging reveals white matter hyperintensities, usually asymmetric, and microbleeds, best seen on gradient echo or T2-weighted MRI. The microbleeds are in a distribution distinct from the white matter lesions, and there is a correlation between the clinical course and the size of the lesions. The lesions shrink with improvement in symptoms and enlarge with recurrences. A brain biopsy is needed for definitive diagnosis.

Treatment

■ It is treated with immunosuppressants.

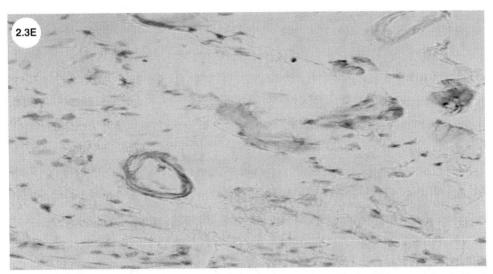

Image 2.3E: Congo red stain demonstrating amyloid deposits in blood vessel walls (image credit Dr. Seema Shroff, Fellow, New York University Langone Medical Center [NYULMC]).

References

1. Tschampa HJ, Niehusmann P, Marek M, Mueller CA, Kuchelmeister K, Urbach H. MRI in amyloid beta-related brain angiitis. *Neurology.* July 2009;73(3):247.

2. Danve A, Grafe M, Deodhar A. Amyloid beta-related angiitis—a case report and comprehensive review of literature of 94 cases. *Semin Arthritis Rheum.* August 2014;44(1):86–92.

2.4 | Hemorrhagic Conversion of Ischemic Stroke

Case History

A 71-year-old woman developed a seizure and obtundation after receiving tissue plasminogen activator (t-PA) for an ischemic stroke.

Diagnosis: Hemorrhagic Conversion of Ischemic Stroke

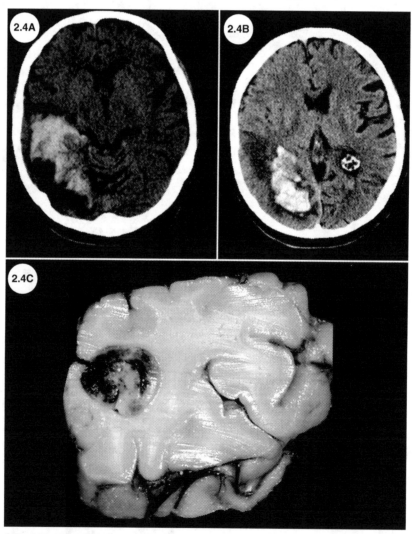

Images 2.4A and 2.4B: Axial CT images demonstrate a large hemorrhage within a right posterior cerebral artery infarct. **Image 2.4C:** Gross pathology demonstrates hemorrhagic infarction.

Introduction

- Ischemic stroke, especially after the administration of t-PA, is an important cause of IPH. The rate of symptomatic hemorrhage with the use of t-PA in ischemic hemorrhages is 6% and increases with deviations from the standard t-PA protocol, larger strokes, cortical strokes, strokes due to atrial fibrillation, advanced age, low platelet count, and hyperglycemia. Of these, large infarct size is the greatest risk factor.

- Two types of hemorrhages are seen after strokes: small petechial hemorrhages, called hemorrhagic infarctions, and larger hematomas into the ischemic bed, called parenchymal hematomas.

- Petechial hemorrhages are seen in about 50% of large cerebral infarcts, while larger parenchymal hematomas are less common. In patients who have received thrombolytic therapy, parenchymal hematomas usually occur in the first 24 hours. In untreated patients they occur within the first four days.

Clinical Presentation

- Petechial hemorrhages are asymptomatic and of no clinical consequence. They can be considered part of the natural evolution of large ischemic strokes due to reperfusion in the vascular bed of the infarct.

- Larger parenchymal hematomas can result in rapid, significant deterioration. The clinical presentation depends on the area into which the hemorrhage occurs as well as its size. Patients with parenchymal hematomas have worsened outcomes and mortality.

Radiographic Appearance

- CT scan is the imaging modality of choice for patients with a suspected hemorrhagic conversion. Petechial hemorrhages appear as small hyperdensities. They typically occur in the gray matter due to robust collateral circulation.

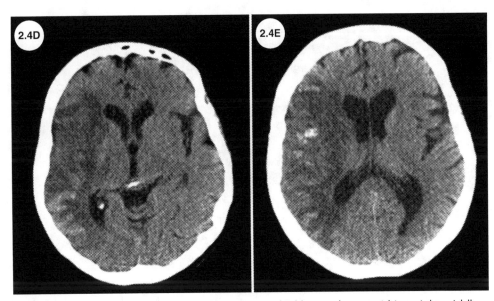

Images 2.4D and 2.4E: Axial CT scans demonstrate petechial hemorrhages within a right middle cerebral artery infarct.

- As seen in **Images 2.4A and 2.4B**, larger parenchymal hematomas may fill the entire ischemic deficit with mass effect on the surrounding brain tissue and secondary ischemia.

Treatment

- Proven treatment is limited to supportive measures and minimizing risk of further bleed or expansion.

References

1. Zhang J, Yang Y, Sun H, Xing Y. Hemorrhagic transformation after cerebral infarction: current concepts and challenges. *Ann Transl Med.* August 2014; 2(8):81.
2. Sussman ES, Connolly ES Jr. Hemorrhagic transformation: a review of the rate of hemorrhage in the major clinical trials of acute ischemic stroke. *Front Neurol.* June 2013;4:69.

2.5 | Hemorrhagic Tumor

Case History

A 76-year-old woman presented with a headache and deficits in her right visual field.

Diagnosis: Hemorrhagic Tumor

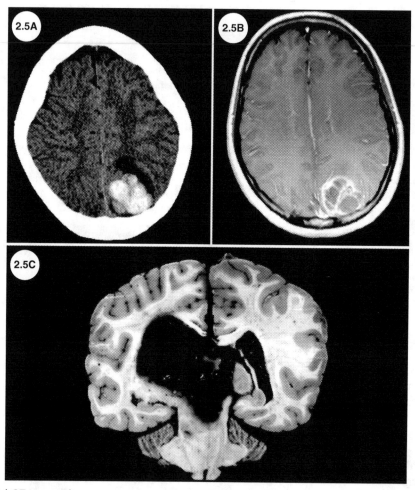

Image 2.5A: Axial CT image demonstrates hemorrhage in the left parietal lobe. **Image 2.5B:** Contrast-enhanced axial T1-weighted image demonstrates an underlying tumor. **Image 2.5C:** Gross pathology of a hemorrhagic tumor with extension into the ventricles (image credit www.wikidoc.org via Professor Peter Anderson, DVM, PhD, and published with permission © PEIR, University of Alabama at Birmingham, Department of Pathology).

Introduction

- High-grade primary brain neoplasms may hemorrhage into the necrotic center of the tumor, and this can be the presenting symptom of the tumor. Hemorrhage occurs in about 8% to 9% of glioblastomas and is the presenting symptom in about 2%. In children, medulloblastomas are commonly associated with hemorrhage. Lower grade neoplasms are much less likely to hemorrhage.

- Other primary central nervous system (CNS) neoplasms that are associated with hemorrhage include oligodendrogliomas, craniopharyngiomas, vestibular schwannomas, ependymomas, pituitary adenomas, and choroid plexus carcinomas.

■ Certain metastatic tumors are prone to hemorrhage. The tumors with the highest propensity to hemorrhage are melanoma, renal cell carcinoma, choriocarcinoma, and thyroid cancer. Hemorrhage is the presenting symptom in about half of these tumors. Because breast and lung cancers are much more common overall, hemorrhagic metastases are most likely due to these tumors.

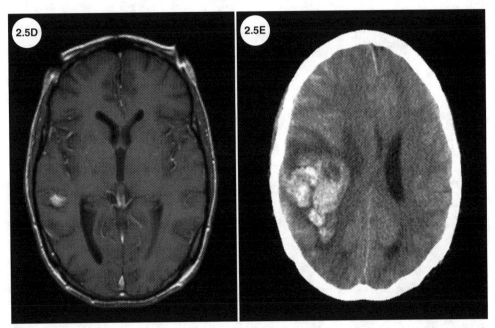

Image 2.5D: Contrast-enhanced axial T1-weighted image demonstrates a small enhancing lesion in the right temporal lobe in a patient with known melanoma. **Image 2.5E:** Axial CT image demonstrates a large, fatal hemorrhage in the same patient several weeks later.

Clinical Presentation

■ Patients develop headache and other symptoms of increased ICP due to the sudden increase in mass effect. Further symptoms depend on the area into which the hemorrhage occurs.

Radiographic Appearance

■ CT is the modality of choice for patients with a suspected hemorrhage. Oftentimes, the underlying tumor is obscured by blood products, and a biopsy or repeat MRI may be needed to find the tumor.

■ Within the supratentorial structures, hemorrhagic metastases may be indistinguishable from primary brain tumors. However, in the cerebellum the overwhelming majority of tumors are metastatic in adults.

Treatment

■ Treatment is directed toward the underlying tumor.

References

1. Lieu AS, Hwang SL, Howng SL, Chai CY. Brain tumors with hemorrhage. *J Formos Med Assoc.* May 1999;98(5):365–367.
2. Wakai S, Yamakawa K, Manaka S, Takakura K. Spontaneous intracranial hemorrhage caused by brain tumor: its incidence and clinical significance. *Neurosurgery.* 1982;10:437–444.

2.6 | Spinal Epidural Hematoma

Case History

A 46-year-old woman presented with the abrupt onset of a severe, stabbing pain in her neck and weakness of her arms and legs.

Diagnosis: Spinal Epidural Hematoma

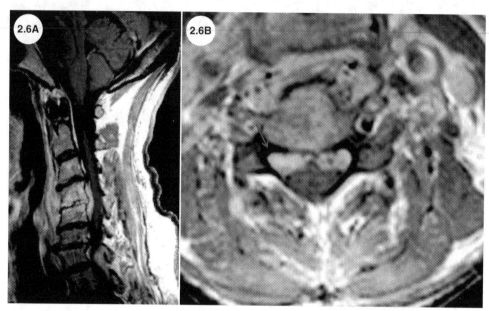

Images 2.6A and 2.6B: Sagittal and axial T1-weighted images of the cervical spine demonstrate an epidural hematoma (red arrows) with compression of the cervical spinal cord.

Introduction

■ A spontaneous spinal epidural hematoma (SEDH) is an accumulation of blood in the potential space between the dura and bone with the dorsal aspect of the thoracolumbar region most commonly involved. The epidural venous plexus is usually involved, although arterial sources of hemorrhage may also occur, and expansion is limited to a few vertebral levels.

■ Overall, it is a very rare condition. It most commonly presents in the fourth or fifth decade. They may occur spontaneously or in patients with impaired coagulation. In patients with impaired coagulation, a lumbar puncture may precipitate an epidural hematoma. Tumors and traumatic injuries are also predisposing factors.

Clinical Presentation

■ SEDHs are characterized by the acute onset of severe, stabbing pain, often in a radicular pattern, followed by signs of myelopathy depending on the location of the bleed and the speed at which it develops. There will be variable weakness and sensory loss below the level of the lesion.

Radiographic Appearance and Diagnosis

■ MRI best delineates the location and extent of SEDHs. It typically shows a well-circumscribed, biconvex hematoma in the epidural space. In the first 24 hours, the hematoma is isointense on T1-weighted images with a heterogeneous high signal on T2-weighted images. After 24 hours, the blood is hyperintense on T1-weighted images, and isointense to cerebrospinal fluid (CSF) on T2-weighted images.

Treatment

■ Prompt diagnosis and early surgical intervention (within 36–48 hours) with decompressive laminectomy and hematoma removal is the definitive treatment. This can prevent severe and permanent neurological injury in patients without preoperative deficits.

References

1. Ng WH, Lim CC, Ng PY, Tan KK. Spinal epidural hematoma: MRI-aided diagnosis. *J Clin Neuroscience*. 2002;9:92–94.
2. Liu Z, Jiao Q, Xu J, Wang X, Li S, You C. Spontaneous spinal epidural hematoma: analysis of 23 cases. *Surg Neurol*. March 2008;69(3):253–260.
3. Groen RJ. Non-operative treatment of spontaneous spinal epidural hematomas: a review of the literature and a comparison with operative cases. *Acta Neurochir (Wien)*. February 2004;146(2):103–110.

CHAPTER 3

VASCULAR MALFORMATIONS/ DISEASES OF BLOOD VESSELS

3.1 Subarachnoid Hemorrhage

Case History

A 45-year-old man developed a severe headache and collapsed.

Diagnosis: Subarachnoid Hemorrhage

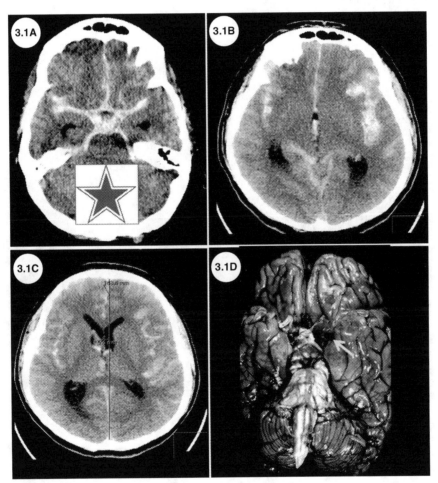

Images 3.1A–3.1C: Axial CT images demonstrate diffuse blood in the subarachnoid space. The "star sign" of subarachnoid hemorrhage is shown. **Image 3.1D:** Gross pathology of a subarachnoid hemorrhage with a ruptured aneurysm (yellow arrow) (image credit www.wikidoc.org via Professor Peter Anderson, DVM, PhD, and published with permission © PEIR, University of Alabama at Birmingham, Department of Pathology).

Introduction

- The most common cause of subarachnoid hemorrhage (SAH), other than trauma, is rupture of a berry aneurysm.

- Risk factors for developing an aneurysmal SAH include substance use (cocaine, amphetamines, cigarettes, alcohol), family history, hypertension, polycystic kidney disease, Marfan's syndrome, Ehlers–Danlos syndrome, and fibromuscular dysplasia.

- SAH accounts for about 5% of all strokes, and most patients are older adults.

Clinical Presentation

- SAH presents as a severe, abrupt headache. Patients classically complain of the "worst headache of my life." Many patients lose consciousness due to the sudden increase in intracranial pressure. Up to half of patients have a minor headache, referred to as a sentinel headache, in the weeks preceding frank rupture. This is presumably due to small amounts of blood leaking from the aneurysm.

- One of the most common grading systems for the severity of SAH is the Hunt and Hess scale. Other grading systems include the modified Hunt and Hess scale, the World Federation of Neurological Surgeons scale, and the Ogilvy and Carter scale.

- Hunt and Hess scale:

  - Grade 1: asymptomatic or mild headache and slight nuchal rigidity

  - Grade 2: moderate or severe headache, nuchal rigidity, no neurological deficit other than a cranial nerve palsy

  - Grade 3: drowsiness, confusion, mild focal neurological deficit

  - Grade 4: stupor with moderate to severe hemiparesis

  - Grade 5: coma, decerebrate posturing

Radiographic Appearance and Diagnosis

- A CT scan reveals the hemorrhage in over 95% of cases if done in the first 24 hours.

- The Fisher scale is used to grade the amount of blood on CT.

  - Grade 1: no blood detected

  - Grade 2: diffuse or thin layer of blood (less than 1 mm thick vertically)

  - Grade 3: clot and/or thick layer of blood (1 mm or more vertically)

  - Grade 4: intraventricular or intraparenchymal blood

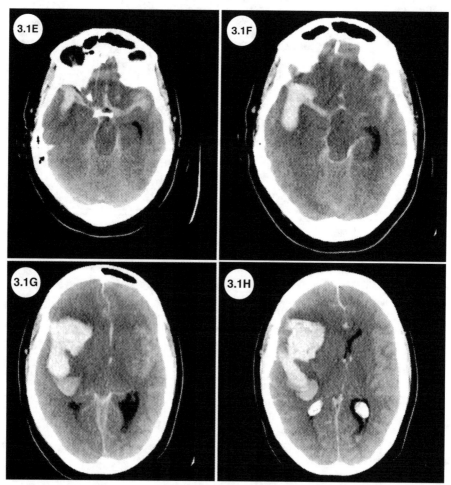

Images 3.1E–3.1H: Axial CT images demonstrate a grade 4 SAH. There is diffuse subarachnoid blood, as well as intraparenchymal blood in the right frontal and temporal lobes, with midline shift and herniation.

- As shown in **Image 3.1A**, the appearance of blood within the basal cisterns and Sylvian and interhemispheric fissure is called the "star sign."

- All patients who complain of a severe, sudden headache should have a lumbar puncture performed if the CT scan is normal. Cerebrospinal fluid (CSF) without an elevated red blood cell (RBC) count rules out SAH. A traumatic tap should have a declining number of RBCs in sequential tubes and will not show xanthochromia, which is the yellow tinge to CSF that occurs after 6 to 12 hours in patients with SAH due to breakdown of RBCs within the CSF.

Treatment

- Approximately 50% of cases are fatal, and survivors are often left with significant neurological deficits. All patients with SAH should be admitted to an intensive care unit and be monitored closely for signs of respiratory distress or neurological deterioration.

- Complications of SAH include rebleeding, vasospasm, hyponatremia, neurogenic cardiac dysfunction, and hydrocephalus.

Rebleeding

- The rerupture rate of an untreated aneurysm is about 30%, with the highest risk being in the first week. 50% of the patients who suffer a second bleed die as a result.

- Treatment of ruptured aneurysms is either neurosurgical clipping or endovascular coiling of the aneurysm. The International Study of Aneurysm Treatment showed a 23% relative reduction in mortality for patients treated with endovascular coiling compared to surgery. In patients who are doing well clinically, earlier repair of the aneurysm (within the first 3 days) is favored to prevent rebleeding. In patients who are medically unstable, the complications may be too great for early intervention. In these cases, intervention should be delayed until after 7 to 10 days to allow for swelling to resolve.

Vasospasm

- Vasospasm leading to ischemic stroke is a major complication of SAH. It occurs in 30% of patients, leading to stroke or death. The peak incidence is at days 7 to 10 after the bleed. It is rare before day 4 or after day 21. It is diagnosed by transcranial Doppler ultrasonography, which will show increased flow within the narrowed arteries, or computed tomography angiography (CTA).

- Medical treatment to prevent vasospasm involves induced hypertension, hypervolemia, and hemodilution. This is known as "Triple-H" therapy.

- Nimodipine, a calcium-channel blocker, has a neuroprotective effect, though it is not clear if this is by reducing vasospasm.

- In cases of refractory vasospasm, a calcium-channel blocker can be delivered directly to the affected arteries or a transluminal balloon angioplasty can be placed via angiography. Treated arteries are protected from recurrent spasms for 3 to 4 weeks.

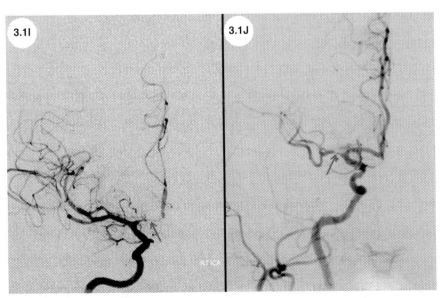

Images 3.1I and 3.1J: Angiograms demonstrate significant vasospasm (red arrows) of A1 segments of the anterior cerebral artery (3.1I) and M1 segment of the MCA (3.1J).

Hyponatremia

■ Hyponatremia is thought to occur as a result of the inappropriate secretion of vasopressin and is referred to as "cerebral salt wasting." It occurs between days 3 to 7 and should be treated with intravenous normal saline, sodium tablets, or in extreme cases, hypertonic saline. Treatment with free water restriction is contraindicated as it can cause cerebral ischemia.

Cardiac Dysfunction

■ T wave inversions and ST elevations on EKG are commonly found in cerebral insults that result in raised intracranial pressure, mimicking cardiac ischemia. Some patients suffer congestive heart failure from myocardial damage, thought to be due to a catecholamine surge. Cardiac function usually normalizes over the course of 3 to 4 weeks.

Hydrocephalus

■ Hydrocephalus is a common complication of SAH. It may occur acutely, presenting as obtundation or coma. In such cases, emergent ventricular drainage may be lifesaving. It can also occur after weeks to months due to obstruction of CSF reabsorption within the arachnoid granulations. It presents with the classic triad of a gait apraxia, dementia, and urinary incontinence. In such cases, ventricular shunting is needed.

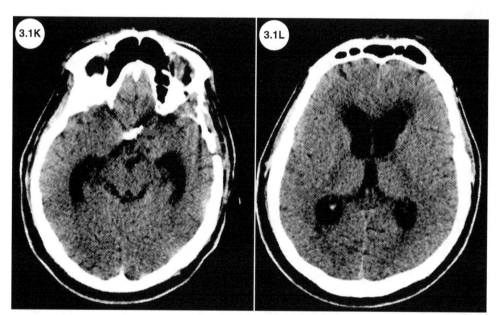

Images 3.1K and 3.1L: Axial CT scans demonstrate enlarged ventricles in a patient several months after a SAH. The aneurysm clip is visible (red arrow).

References

1. Suarez JI. Diagnosis and management of subarachnoid hemorrhage. *Continuum (Minneap Minn).* October 2015;21(5 Neurocritical Care):1263–1287.
2. Aisiku I, Abraham JA, Goldstein J, Thomas LE. An evidence-based approach to diagnosis and management of subarachnoid hemorrhage in the emergency department. *Emerg Med Pract.* October 2014;16(10):1–24.
3. Inagawa T. Risk factors for cerebral vasospasm following aneurysmal subarachnoid hemorrhage: a review of the literature. *World Neurosurg.* September 2015. pii: S1878-8750(15)01068-2.
4. Lo BW, Fukuda H, Nishimura Y, Farrokhyar F, Thabane L, Levine MA. Systematic review of clinical prediction tools and prognostic factors in aneurysmal subarachnoid hemorrhage. *Surg Neurol Int.* August 2015;6:135.

3.2 Aneurysms

Case History

A 56-year-old man presented with an enlarging right pupil.

Diagnosis: Berry Aneurysm

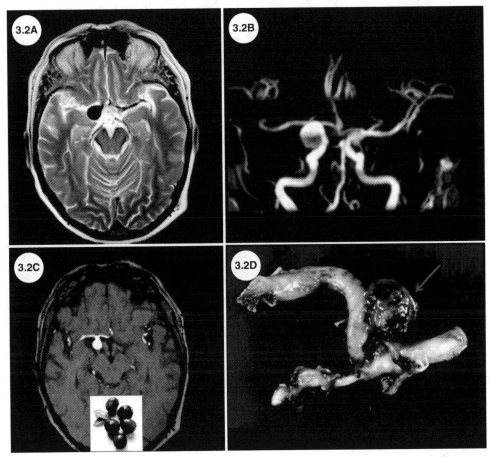

Images 3.2A–3.2C: Axial T2-weighted, MR angiogram maximum intensity projection (MIP) and postcontrast axial T1-weighted images demonstrate a berry aneurysm of the right posterior communicating artery. **Image 3.2D:** Gross image of berry aneurysm at the junction internal carotid and middle cerebral arteries (image credit www.wikidoc.org via Professor Peter Anderson, DVM, PhD, and published with permission © PEIR, University of Alabama at Birmingham, Department of Pathology).

Introduction

■ An aneurysm is an abnormal dilation of an artery due to weakness of the vessel wall. Saccular, or berry, aneurysms have a distinct neck and dome, whereas with fusiform aneurysms there is a uniform dilation of the artery.

■ About 2% of adults harbor an intracranial aneurysm and there are about 30,000 ruptured aneurysms per year in the United States.

■ Ninety percent of aneurysms arise from the anterior circulation. The remaining 10% are in the posterior circulation, most commonly at the tip of the basilar artery. They are most commonly found in the circle of Willis at the branching points of the major arteries. The most common locations are the junction of the anterior communicating artery and the anterior cerebral artery (ACA), the junction of the posterior communicating artery and the internal carotid artery (ICA), the bifurcation of the middle cerebral artery (MCA), and the tip of the basilar artery.

Most common sites of intracranial saccular aneurysms

incidence
<1%

10%

20%

30%

artery involved (incidence)

pericallosal artery (4%)

anterior communicating artery (30%)

lateral carotid artery bifurcation (8%)

middle cerebral artery (20%)

posterior communicating artery (25%)

basilar tip (7%)

posterior inferior cerebellar artery (3%)

Illustration 3.2.1: The most common sites of intracranial saccular aneurysms (image credit Nicholas Zaorsky, MD).

Clinical Presentation

■ Aneurysms usually present due to rupture and resultant subarachnoid hemorrhage or due to mass effect on adjacent structures. An oculomotor nerve palsy, particularly if the pupil is involved first, is concerning for an aneurysm of the posterior communicating artery.

■ Larger aneurysms are more prone to rupture. Aneurysms less than 10 mm have an annual rupture rate of about 0.1%, whereas those greater than 10 mm have an annual rupture rate of about 1%. Giant aneurysms over 25 mm have an annual rupture rate of about 6%, though they often present prior to rupture due to mass effect on adjacent brain structures.

■ Fusiform aneurysms of the basilar artery present most commonly with ischemic symptoms or compression of the brainstem and cranial nerves.

■ Many aneurysms are clinically silent and found incidentally on imaging done for other reasons.

Radiographic Appearance and Diagnosis

■ Many are hyperdense on CT scans due to thrombosed blood within the aneurysm. In patients who have had a subarachnoid hemorrhage, a conventional angiogram may be needed as the aneurysm can be obscured by the hemorrhage. Examples of giant aneurysms are shown on CT and angiograms in **Images 3.2E to 3.2W**.

■ On MRI, aneurysms are typically hypointense on T1-weighted images and hyperintense on T2-weighted images, though the appearance may vary somewhat depending on the degree of thrombosis. Large aneurysms can be detected on

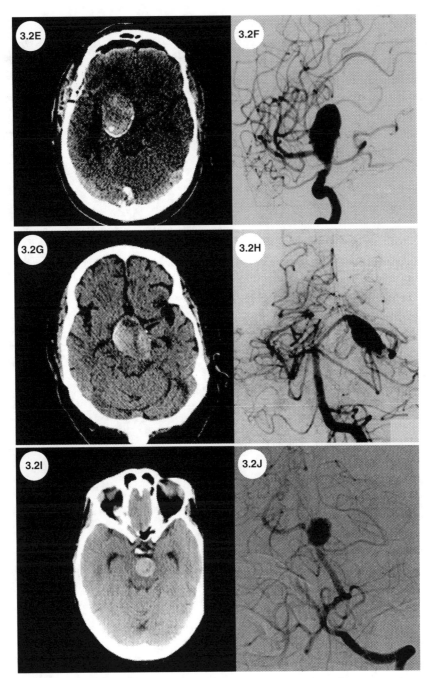

Images 3.2E and 3.2F: Axial CT image and catheter angiogram demonstrate a giant aneurysm of the right ICA. **Images 3.2G and 3.2H:** Axial CT image demonstrates a large suprasellar, hyperdense mass and an angiogram demonstrates a giant, mostly thrombosed fusiform aneurysm involving the P2 segment of the left PCA. **Images 3.2I and 3.2J:** Axial CT image demonstrates a large hyperdense mass in the interpeduncular fossa. Cerebral angiogram reveals a giant aneurysm at the tip of the basilar artery.

almost all imaging modalities, though catheter angiography is considered the gold standard. An aneurysm of the bifurcation of the MCA is shown on magnetic resonance angiography (MRA), catheter angiography, and CTA (note the conventional left–right orientation is reversed on CTAs).

- In about 10% to 30% of all cases there are multiple intracranial aneurysms. In the majority of such cases, only two aneurysms are seen.

- In contrast to saccular aneurysms, fusiform (spindle-shaped) aneurysms are characterized by uniform dilation of an artery.

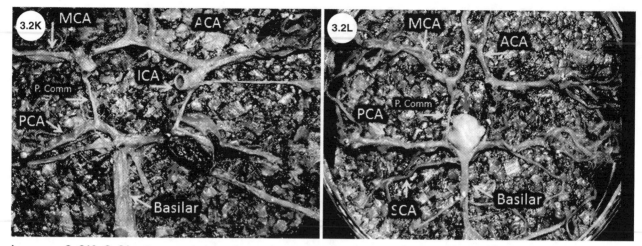

Images 3.2K–3.2L: Gross pathology demonstrates a large aneurysm at the junction of the posterior cerebral and posterior communicating arteries (3.2K) and at the tip of the basilar artery (3.2L).

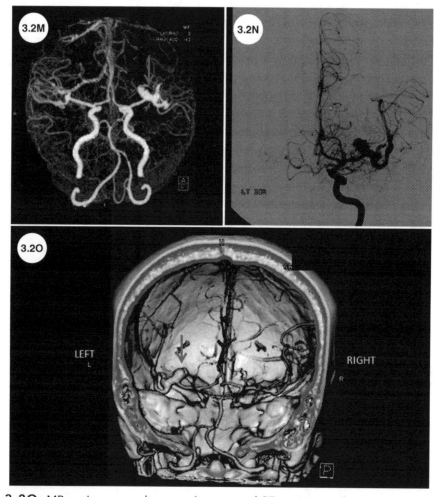

Images 3.2M–3.2O: MR angiogram, catheter angiogram, and CT angiogram demonstrate an aneurysm at the bifurcation of the left MCA (red arrows).

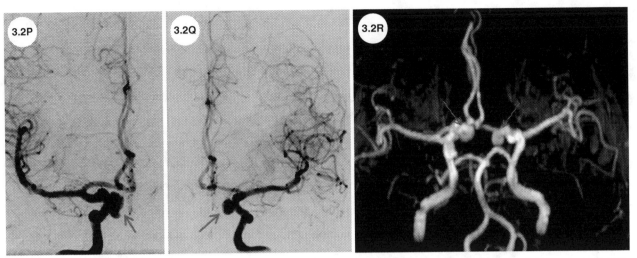

Images 3.2P and 3.2Q: Catheter angiogram demonstrates bilateral ICA aneurysms (red arrows). **Image 3.2R:** MR angiogram of the same patient.

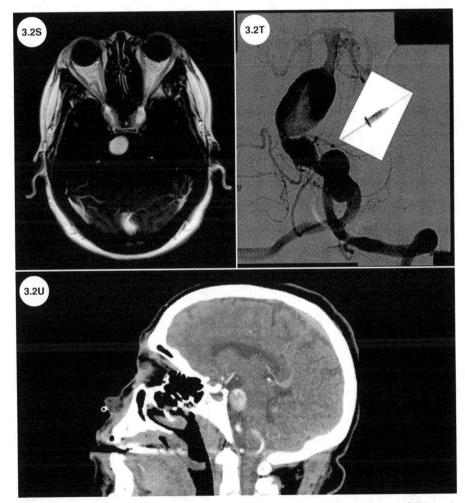

Images 3.2S–3.2U: Postcontrast axial T1-weighted image, catheter angiogram, and sagittal CT angiogram image demonstrate a fusiform aneurysm of the bilateral distal vertebral and basilar arteries.

Treatment

- Symptomatic aneurysms can be treated with endovascular coiling or neurosurgical clipping of the aneurysmal neck.

- Whether or not to treat intracranial aneurysms found incidentally is controversial. The decision should be based on the size and location of the aneurysm, the age and medical condition of the patient, and the surgeon's experience.

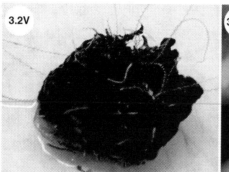 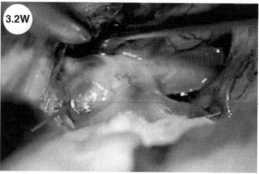

Image 3.2V: A resected MCA aneurysm filled with multiple coils (image credit Marvin 101). **Image 3.2W:** Intraoperative picture demonstrates clipping of an aneurysm of the anterior communicating artery (red arrow).

Aneurysms smaller than 10 mm in diameter have a lower rupture rate.

References

1. Unruptured intracranial aneurysms—risk of rupture and risks of surgical intervention. International Study of Unruptured Intracranial Aneurysms Investigators. *N Engl J Med.* December 1998;339(24):1725–1733.
2. Juvela S, Poussa K, Lehto H, Porras M. Natural history of unruptured intracranial aneurysms: a long-term follow-up study. *Stroke.* September 2013;44(9):2414–2421.
3. Brown RD Jr, Broderick JP. Unruptured intracranial aneurysms: epidemiology, natural history, management options, and familial screening. *Lancet Neurol.* April 2014;13(4):393–404.
4. Graziano F, Iacopino DG, Ulm AJ. Insights on a giant aneurysm treated endovascularly. *J Neurol Surg A Cent Eur Neurosurg.* July 2016;77(4):367–371.
5. Qureshi AI, Janardhan V, Hanel RA, Lanzino G. Comparison of endovascular and surgical treatments for intracranial aneurysms: an evidence-based review. *Lancet Neurol.* September 2007;6(9):816–825.
6. Serrone JC, Gozal YM, Grossman AW, et al. Vertebrobasilar fusiform aneurysms. *Neurosurg Clin N Am.* July 2014;25(3):471–484.

3.3 | Dissections

Case History

A 23-year-old woman developed neck pain and dizziness, vertigo, dysarthria, abnormal facial sensation, and a Horner's syndrome after strenuous exercise.

Diagnosis: Dissection

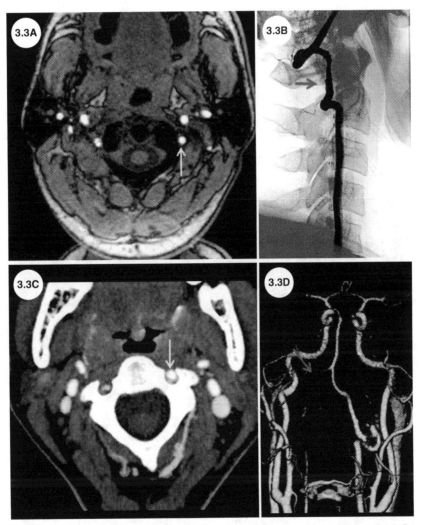

Image 3.3A: MR angiogram demonstrates attenuation of flow with an intramural hematoma flow in the right vertebral artery (red arrow) in a patient with a vertebral artery dissection. The normal left vertebral artery (yellow arrow) is shown for comparison. **Image 3.3B:** Conventional angiogram demonstrates severe narrowing of the arterial lumen at that level. **Images 3.3C and 3.3D:** CT angiogram demonstrates complete left distal extracranial and proximal intracranial vertebral artery occlusion (red arrow).

Introduction

■ A dissection of a vessel occurs when there is a tear in the tunica intima such that blood flows between the layers of the blood vessel wall, rather than within the lumen. Both the vertebral artery (VA) and ICA are vulnerable.

■ Dissections are primarily diseases of young people, and are the most common cause of ischemic stroke in this age group.

■ Both VA and ICA dissections can occur spontaneously, especially in patients with connective tissue disorders. They may occur after trauma to the neck. Chiropractic manipulation is a well-known risk factor for VA dissections.

Clinical Presentation

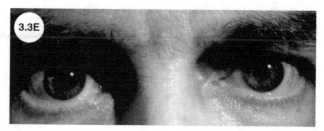

Image 3.3E: A Horner's syndrome is shown on the left. There is miosis and slight ptosis.

■ Dissections present with neck pain, retroorbital pain for ICA dissections, and cerebral ischemia. The dissection serves as a nidus for clot formation, and emboli dislodge leading to infarction. Infarctions may also occur via hypoperfusion to distal brain areas, though collateral blood flow often minimizes injury via this mechanism.

■ VA dissections present with neck pain and infarctions in the posterior circulation. VA dissection is a common cause of the lateral medullary (Wallenberg) syndrome.

■ ICA dissections, like VA dissections, are often accompanied by a Horner's syndrome, as sympathetic nerve fibers run along the carotid artery.

■ Dysphagia and dysarthria can also be seen due to mass effect on the glossopharyngeal and vagus nerves, which run adjacent to the carotid.

Radiographic Appearance and Diagnosis

■ CT angiograms, MR angiograms, and conventional angiography all have a role in the diagnosis of dissections. A hematoma can often be seen within the vessel wall.

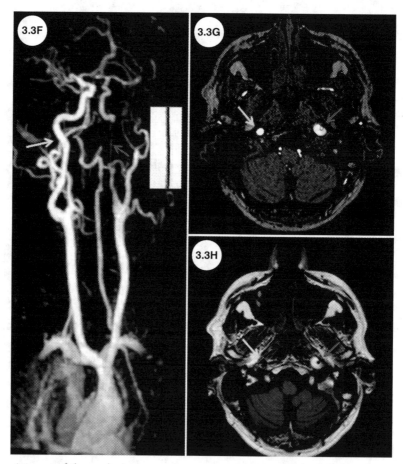

Image 3.3F: MR angiogram of the neck demonstrates severe narrowing of the left internal carotid artery (red arrow). This is known as the "string sign." **Image 3.3G:** MR angiogram source images demonstrate an intramural hematoma (red arrow) within the lumen of the artery. **Image 3.3H:** Axial T1-weighted image demonstrates the hyperintensity of the hematoma. In each image, the yellow arrow shows the unaffected carotid artery.

Treatment

▪ Dissections are treated with either anticoagulation or antiplatelet agents. There does not seem to be good data supporting one approach over the other. In patients with recurrent ischemia, neurointerventional procedures can be used. These include angioplasty and stent implantation.

References

1. Redekop GJ. Extracranial carotid and vertebral artery dissection: A review. *Can J Neurol Sci.* May 2008;35(2):146–152.
2. Jensen MB, Chacon MR, Aleu A. Cervicocerebral arterial dissection. *Neurologist.* January 2008;14(1):5–6.
3. Kadkhodayan Y, Jeck DT, Moran CJ, Derdeyn CP, Cross DT 3rd. Angioplasty and stenting in carotid dissection with or without associated pseudoaneurysm. *AJNR Am J Neuroradiol.* October 2005;26(9):2328–2335.

3.4 | Central Nervous System Vasculitis

Case History

A 47-year-old developed headaches and multiple small strokes.

Diagnosis: CNS Vasculitis

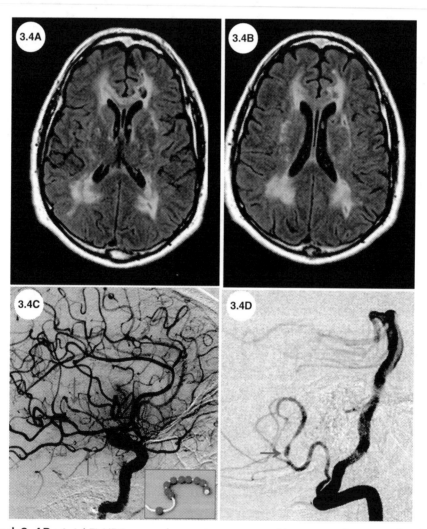

Images 3.4A and 3.4B: Axial FLAIR images demonstrate severe white matter disease and multiple hypodensities consistent with remote infarction. **Images 3.4C and 3.4D:** Catheter angiogram demonstrates the typical "beads on a string" pattern (red arrows) of CNS vasculitis.

Introduction

■ Primary diseases of the blood vessels, such as polyarteritis nodosa, Kawasaki disease, granulomatosis with polyangiitis, and Takayasu's arteritis, can affect the intracranial vessels leading to cerebral ischemia, most commonly in the posterior circulation of the eye. Isolated or primary central nervous system (CNS) angiitis is a rare condition, affecting 1 to 2 per million people.

- Vessels of all sizes, including capillaries, arterioles/venules, and arteries/veins, can be affected.

- CNS vasculitis can also be seen in conjunction with systemic rheumatologic diseases such as Behçet disease, Sjogren's syndrome, systemic lupus erythematosus, and rheumatoid arthritis.

- Substances of abuse, namely cocaine, 3,4-methylenedioxymethamphetamine (*MDMA* or ecstasy), and amphetamines, may cause a vasculitis, as can infectious diseases, namely tuberculosis, syphilis, *varicella zoster virus* (VZV), and *herpes simplex virus* (HSV).

- It may also be seen in the setting of malignancies such as lymphomas and leukemias.

Clinical Presentation

- Ischemic stroke is the most common CNS presentation. However, patients may suffer from a wide range of clinical presentations including hemorrhages, meningitis, and cognitive dysfunction. Involvement of the extracranial vessels leads to headaches, visual loss, jaw claudication, and cranial tenderness. Systemic symptoms such as fever, weight loss, and malaise are common.

Radiographic Appearance and Diagnosis

- On MRI, there will be symmetric, periventricular white matter hyperintensities on T2-weighted images along with evidence of small infarcts of varying ages. These findings are not specific for vasculitis, however.

- Angiography is the most sensitive imaging technique and will show irregular focal segmental stenoses of the affected vessels. This pattern is referred to as "beads on a string." In infectious vasculitis, the vasculature of the basal cisterns is most commonly affected, though syphilis may affect the distal branches of the MCA. A normal angiogram does not rule out vasculitis, and a meningeal biopsy may be needed to definitively make the diagnosis.

- Depending on the cause, serum markers of inflammation such as the erythrocyte sedimentation rate (ESR) and C-reactive protein are generally elevated, especially in patients with temporal arteritis. In patients with primary CNS angiitis, mild lymphocytic pleocytosis and mildly elevated total protein are expected in the CSF.

Treatment

- Steroids are used acutely to reduce inflammation. Many patients need long-term immunosuppression.

References

1. Amara AW, Bashir K, Palmer CA, Walker HC. Challenges in diagnosis of isolated central nervous system vasculitis. *Brain Behav.* September 2011; 1(1):57–61.
2. Berlit P, Kraemer M. Cerebral vasculitis in adults: what are the steps in order to establish the diagnosis? Red flags and pitfalls. *Clin Exp Immunol.* March 2014;175(3):419–424.
3. Lucke M, Hajj-Ali RA. Advances in primary angiitis of the central nervous system. *Curr Cardiol Rep.* 2014;16(10):533.

3.5 | Moyamoya Disease

Case History

A 12-year-old girl presented with multiple ischemic strokes over the course of several years.

Diagnosis: Moyamoya Disease

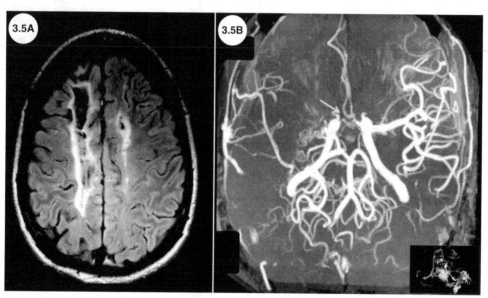

Image 3.5A: Axial FLAIR image demonstrates old, bifrontal, and parietal watershed territory infarctions.
Image 3.5B: MR angiogram demonstrates complete occlusion of the proximal right MCA with collateral flow through massively dilated right lenticulostriate vessels (red arrows). This appears as a "puff of smoke." There is also severe stenosis of both ACAs (yellow arrow).

Introduction

- Moyamoya disease ("smoke" in Japanese) is a progressive, occlusive arteriopathy that affects the terminal part of the ICA and the proximal segments of the ACA and MCA. The posterior cerebral arteries (PCAs) are affected in almost half of the patients. The vascular occlusions are typically slowly progressive, and collateral circulation develops via several different sources to supply the ischemic tissue. Most commonly, collaterals arise from the perforating arteries of the basal ganglia as well as from branches of the external carotid artery.

- It is most commonly an idiopathic disorder, but has been associated with radiation therapy, sickle cell disease, neurofibromatosis 1, Down syndrome, and chronic infections.

- There is a bimodal age of distribution, with most cases occurring in children under age 4, and a second peak occurring between the ages of 30 and 40. It is more common in people of Asian descent and is twice as common in women. About 10% of cases are familial.

Clinical Presentation

- In children, it presents with ischemic strokes or seizures, while in adults, intracranial hemorrhage is more common. Watershed strokes are particularly common and focal neurological deficits and global cognitive dysfunction result.

Radiographic Appearance and Diagnosis

- Affected vessels are stenotic, and a network of collateral circulation arises from the deep, penetrating arteries (lenticulostriate, thalamoperforating) and from surface vessels (leptomeningeal and dural arteries). With infusion of contrast,

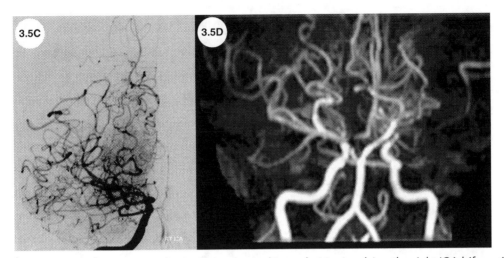

Image 3.5C: Catheter angiogram reveals significant luminal irregularities involving the right ICA bifurcation and the M1 segment of the right MCA with a compensatory network of hypertrophied lenticulostriate arteries in a patient with moyamoya. **Image 3.5D:** MR angiogram demonstrates severe stenoses of the bilateral ACAs and MCAs with hypertrophied lenticulostriate arteries.

this leads to the characteristic "puff of smoke" appearance on catheter angiogram.

- Multiple flow voids are often seen in the basal ganglia.

- Slow flow in extensive leptomeningeal collaterals may result in prominent enhancement and hyperintensity on FLAIR images. This is called the "ivy" sign as the brain appears to be covered in ivy.

Treatment

- Surgery to bypass the occluded vessels is the most common treatment. Connecting the external carotid artery or superficial temporal artery to the MCA is another common intervention. Encephaloduroarteriosynangiosis, a procedure where a scalp artery distribution is transposed onto the region of cortex normally fed by the MCA, is performed as well.

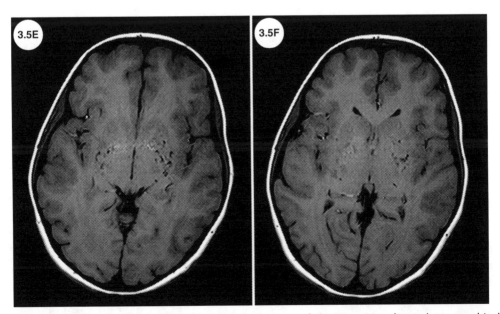

Images 3.5E and 3.5F: Axial T1-weighted images demonstrate hypointensities due to hypertrophied vessels (red arrows) throughout the basal ganglia.

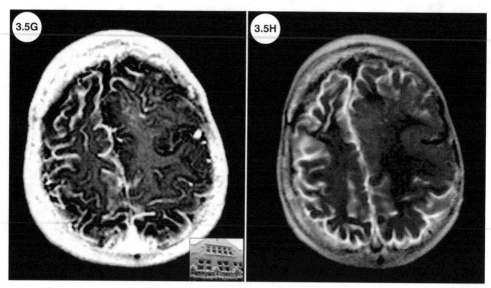

Images 3.5G and 3.5H: Postcontrast axial T1-weighted and FLAIR images demonstrate extensive meningeal enhancement and hyperintensity.

References

1. Yoon HK, Shin HJ, Chang YW. "Ivy sign" in childhood moyamoya disease: depiction on FLAIR and contrast-enhanced T1-weighted MR images. *Radiology.* May 2002;223(2): 384–389.

2. Hertza J, Loughan A, Perna R, Davis AS, Segraves K, Tiberi NL. Moyamoya disease: a review of the literature. *Appl Neuropsychol Adult.* 2014;21(1):21–27.

3. Thines L, Petyt G, Aguettaz P, et al. Surgical management of Moyamoya disease and syndrome: current concepts and personal experience. *Rev Neurol (Paris).* 2015 Jan;171(1):31–44.

3.6 | Arteriovenous Malformations

Case History

A 39-year-old man was found down on the street. His friends said that he complained of a headache and vomited before losing consciousness. He had a seizure 1 month ago but did not seek medical evaluation.

Diagnosis: Arteriovenous Malformation

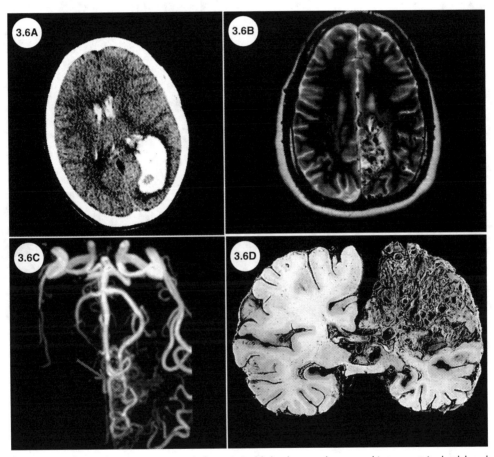

Image 3.6A: Axial CT image demonstrates a left occipital lobe hemorrhage and intraventricular blood. **Images 3.6B and 3.6C:** Axial T2-weighted image demonstrates flow voids in the left occipital lobe typical for an AVM, and MR angiogram demonstrates the AVM (red arrow). **Image 3.6D:** Gross pathology of AVM (image credit The Armed Forces Institute of Pathology).

Introduction

■ Arteriovenous malformations (AVMs) are collections of vessels composed of one or more enlarged feeding arteries that then drain into enlarged veins without an intervening capillary network. The veins then drain into the main venous system of the brain. They are considered congenital abnormalities, though they may enlarge over time.

■ There are two types of AVMs. Compact AVMs are sharply demarcated from the adjacent brain parenchyma with tightly woven vessels. In contrast, diffuse AVMs have neural tissue intermixed and lack clear borders.

- AVMs are the most common symptomatic vascular malformations in the CNS. The vast majority are solitary, and multiple AVMs are associated with hereditary syndromes such as **hereditary hemorrhagic telangiectasia.**

Clinical Presentation

- They can present with seizures, frank hemorrhage and severe headaches from rupture, neurological symptoms due to local mass effect, and symptoms of elevated intracranial pressure. Less commonly, patients develop slowly progressive neurological deficits.

- They are often clinically silent and found incidentally on scans done for other reasons.

- Spinal AVMs are uncommon, but are a potentially treatable cause of progressive myelopathy. They can be located anywhere in the spinal canal (intramedullary, intradural, dural, or extradural). They typically occur in middle-aged patients with progressive weakness, sensory deficits, and bladder incontinence. There may be periods of abrupt worsening if there is hemorrhage in the spinal cord. Abrupt worsening may also occur during exercise or changes in posture.

Radiographic Appearance

- On CT scans, engorged, hyperdense draining veins can be seen in large AVMs.

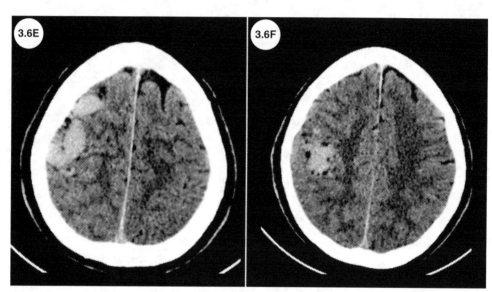

Images 3.6E and 3.6F: Axial CT images demonstrate enlarged, hyperdense vessels in the right frontal lobe due to an AVM.

- AVMs are better visualized on MRI. On T2-weighted images, the abnormal vessels appear as multiple dark flow voids within the brain parenchyma. The surrounding brain is often atrophic and gliotic, as blood supply is preferentially drained from the brain to the AVM. Increased flow may lead to aneurysms of both the arteries and the veins. There is avid enhancement with the administration of contrast.

- Catheter angiography provides the most detailed anatomical view. The feeding arteries, nidus of the AVM, and draining veins are best visualized on angiography. The AVM appears as a dense mass, and dilated draining veins can be seen in the arterial phase. The appearance has been likened to a "bag of worms."

- Less than 15% of AVMs are located infratentorially. With spinal AVMs, an MRI may reveal the diagnosis. As within the brain, the abnormal vessels appear as multiple dark flow voids. There is often intrinsic hyperintensity of the spinal cord. Spinal angiograms best reveal the anatomy of the lesion.

Treatment

- Symptomatic AVMs are treated with a combination of open surgical ligation or resection, endovascular embolization, and radiation. Compact AVMs are more amenable to surgical resection compared to diffuse AVMs.

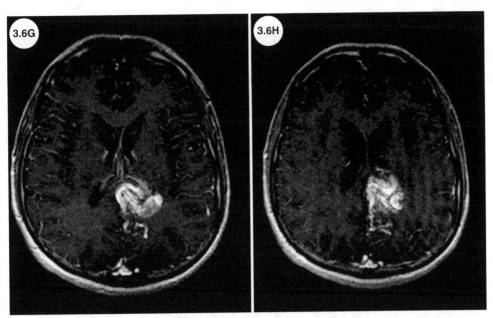

Images 3.6G and 3.6H: Postcontrast axial T1-weighted images demonstrate contrast within the vessels of an AVM.

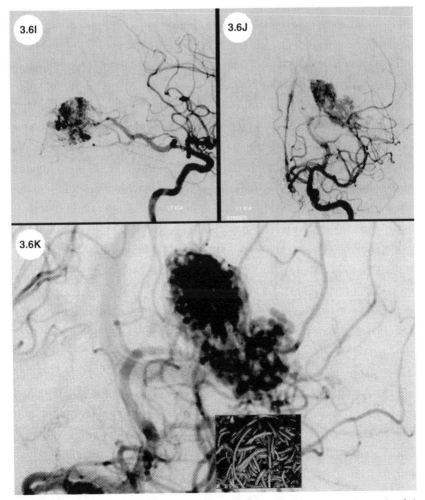

Images 3.6I–3.6K: Catheter angiogram demonstrates an AVM originating from a branch of the MCA. The "bag of worms" appearance is shown.

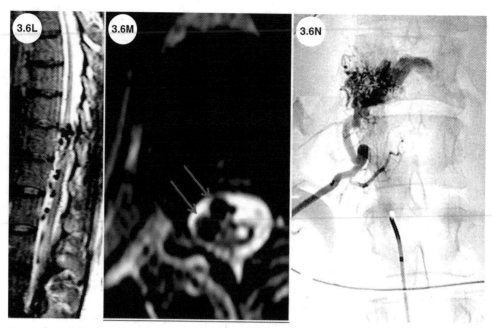

Images 3.6L and 3.6M: Sagittal and axial T2-weighted images demonstrate multiple flow voids in the lumbar spine due to an AVM. **Image 3.6N:** The AVM is visualized on spinal angiogram.

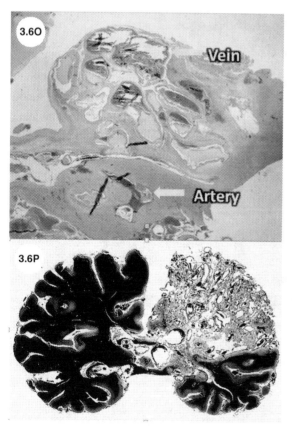

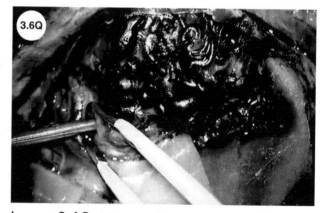

Image 3.6Q: Intraoperative picture of an AVM resection.

Images 3.6O and 3.6P: Hematoxylin and eosin (H&E) stain and brain section demonstrate the findings of an AVM.

- Ruptured AVMs have an annual rebleeding risk of approximately 5%. Unruptured AVMs have a much lower bleeding risk of approximately 2% to 3% annually. Older patients have an increased risk of rupture. The ARUBA trial found that conservative management of unruptured AVMs was superior to interventional approaches over a 33-month period, though there were multiple criticisms of the study design and interpretation.

References

1. Mohr JP, Parides MK, Stapf C, et al. Medical management with or without interventional therapy for unruptured brain arteriovenous malformations (ARUBA): a multi-centre, non-blinded, randomised trial. *Lancet*. February 2014;383(9917):614–621.

2. Kim H, Al-Shahi Salman R, McCulloch CE, Stapf C, Young WL, MARS Coinvestigators. Untreated brain arteriovenous malfor-mation: patient-level meta-analysis of hemorrhage predictors. *Neurology*. August 2014;83(7):590–597.

3. Cohen-Gadol A, Conger A, Kulwin C, Lawton M. Diagnosis and evaluation of intracranial arteriovenous malformations. *Surg Neurol Int*. 2015;6:76.

4. Lawton MT, Kim H, McCulloch CE, Mikhak B, Young WL. A Supplementary grading scale for selecting patients with brain arteriovenous malformations for surgery. *Neurosurgery*. April 2010;66(4):702–713.

3.7 Capillary Telangiectasia

Case History

Two patients had MRIs performed for headaches. Incidental findings were noted.

Diagnosis: Capillary Telangiectasia

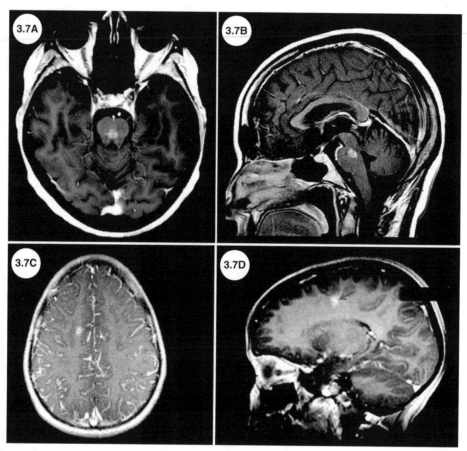

Images 3.7A and 3.7B: Postcontrast axial and sagittal T1-weighted images demonstrate a capillary telangiectasia in the pons (red arrows). **Images 3.7C and 3.7D:** Postcontrast axial and sagittal T1-weighted images demonstrate a capillary telangiectasia (red arrows) in the right frontal lobe.

Introduction

■ There are four types of vascular malformations of the CNS: capillary telangiectasias, arteriovenous malformations, cavernous angiomas, and developmental venous anomalies (DVAs). Capillary telangiectasias are formed by a network of dilated capillaries. The surrounding brain tissue is normal.

Clinical Presentation

■ They are rarely of clinical significance and are most often incidental findings on imaging done for other reasons. They are thought to hemorrhage rarely, though a definitive causal relationship is difficult to establish.

Radiographic Appearance

■ They are best visualized on postcontrast T1-weighted images where there is variable enhancement after the administration of contrast. They may appear as slightly hyperdense on T2-weighted images, though these scans are often normal. There is no mass effect.

■ They are most commonly located in the pons, but can be seen anywhere in the brain, cerebellum, and spinal cord.

Treatment

■ No treatment or follow-up is required.

References

1. Gross BA, Puri AS, Popp AJ, Du R. Cerebral capillary telangiectasias: a meta-analysis and review of the literature. *Neurosurg Rev.* April 2013;36(2):187–193.
2. Gelal F, Karakaş L, Sarsilmaz A, Yücel K, Dündar C, Apaydin M. Capillary telangiectasia of the brain: imaging with various magnetic resonance techniques. *JBR-BTR.* July–August 2014;97(4):233–238.

3.8 Cerebral Cavernous Malformations

Case History

A 58-year-old man presented with a seizure.

Diagnosis: Cerebral Cavernous Malformation

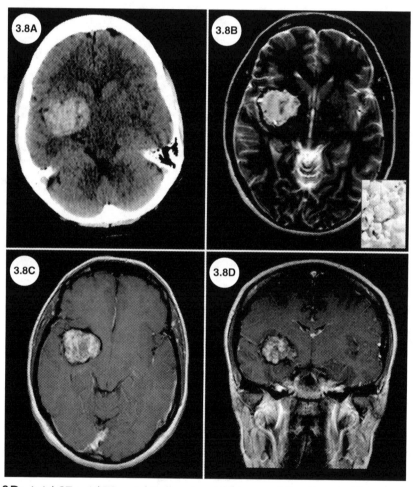

Images 3.8A–3.8D: Axial CT, axial T2-weighted, and postcontrast axial and coronal T1-weighted images demonstrate a mass in the right basal ganglia. It is hyperdense, hyperintense, and enhances with contrast, demonstrating a "popcorn-like" appearance consistent with a cavernoma.

Introduction

■ Cerebral cavernous malformations (CCMs), also known as cavernomas, are characterized by abnormally enlarged capillary cavities. They are without involvement of brain parenchyma, in contrast to arteriovenous malformations.

Clinical Presentation

■ They are clinically silent in about 75% of patients, but can cause headaches, seizures, or focal neurological deficits if they bleed. CCMs may present with an acute hemorrhage or symptoms may be progressive if there is slow enlargement of the

CCM due to repeated internal bleeding. Most patients present in middle age.

- Spinal cord cavernomas can present acutely in the setting of hemorrhage. Patients may develop sudden onset of severe back pain, paresis, numbness with a discrete sensory level, hyperreflexia, and urinary/fecal incontinence. A more progressive presentation, with the slow development of chronic myelopathy due to microhemorrhages or cavernoma enlargement causing mass effect on the adjacent neural structures, occurs as well.

- About 25% of patients have multiple CCMs. Certain patients may have innumerable cavernomas due to genetic mutations in one of three genes: *CCM1, CCM2,* or *CCM3.* In such cases, CCMs can increase in number and size over time. Multiple CCMs may also form after therapeutic radiation.

Radiographic Appearance and Diagnosis

- They are generally hyperdense on CT due to pooling of blood, but smaller CCMs are not seen on CT.

- On MRI, the most characteristic feature is blood products of different ages. On T2-weighted images there is characteristically an area of hyperintensity representing methemoglobin surrounded by a hypointense ring of hemosiderin. Their appearance is described as resembling "popcorn." They do not enhance with the administration of contrast, nor are they seen on conventional angiography.

- Most CCMs are located superficially in subcortical white matter, adjacent to the cerebral cortex, where they frequently cause seizures. However, they may be anywhere in the CNS, including the cerebellum, brainstem (most commonly the pons), and spinal cord.

- In patients with familial CCM mutations, gradient echo or T2* images are much more sensitive than T1-weighted or T2-weighted images in detecting the sometimes innumerable cavernomas.

Treatment

- They can be treated surgically if there are repeated bleeds or they cause medication-refractory epilepsy. Surgical resection is curative, though not

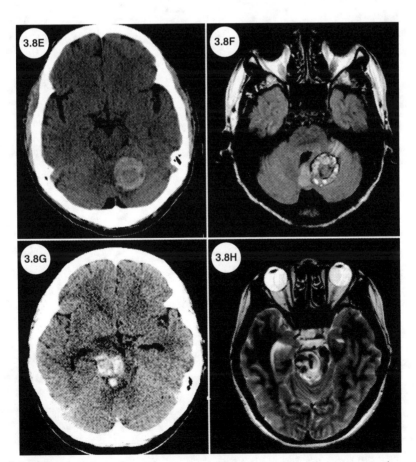

Images 3.8E and 3.8F: Axial CT and FLAIR images demonstrate a large cavernoma in the cerebellum. **Images 3.8G and 3.8H:** Axial CT and T2-weighted images demonstrate a pontine cavernoma.

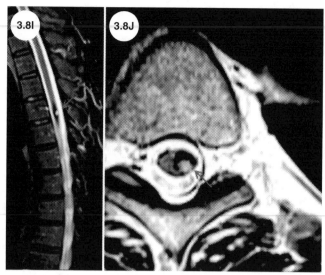

Images 3.8I and 3.8J: Sagittal and axial T2-weighted images of the thoracic spine demonstrate a cavernoma with a hypointense rim due to recent bleeding.

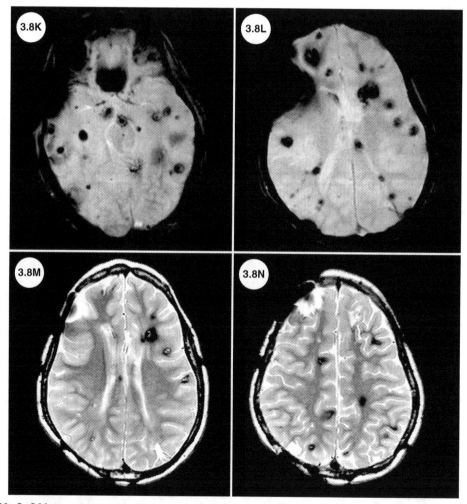

Images 3.8K–3.8N: Axial gradient echo images demonstrate blood products associated with multiple cavernomas. Multiple cavernomas are also visible on the T2-weighted images.

all CCMs are surgically accessible, such as those in the spine and brainstem.

References

1. Toulgoat F, Lasjaunias P. Vascular malformations of the brain. *Handb Clin Neurol*. 2013;112:1043–1051.

2. Hegde AN, Mohan S, Lim CC. CNS cavernous haemangioma: "popcorn" in the brain and spinal cord. *Clin Radiol*. April 2012;67(4):380–388.

3.9 Developmental Venous Anomalies

Case History

A 34-year-old woman had an MRI done for headaches. An incidental finding was noted.

Diagnosis: Developmental Venous Anomalies

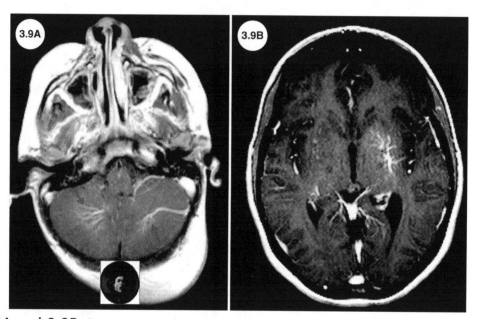

Images 3.9A and 3.9B: Postcontrast axial T1-weighted images demonstrate multiple developmental venous anomalies in the cerebellum and the basal ganglia (red arrows). The "caput medusae" sign is shown.

Introduction

■ Developmental venous anomalies (DVAs), also called venous angiomas, are the most common type of cerebral vascular malformations. They are composed of enlarged collections of veins that drain into a large vein.

■ Most are located in the frontal and parietal lobes where they drain into the frontal horns of the lateral ventricles. The cerebellum is the second most common location, and DVAs there drain into the fourth ventricle.

Clinical Presentation

■ DVAs are almost always incidental findings, but in rare cases can present with venous thrombosis and bleeding. In about 20% of cases, they are associated with other vascular malformations, most commonly cavernous malformations.

Radiographic Appearance and Diagnosis

■ They are well visualized on postcontrast T1-weighted images. They appear as a collection of vessels that drain into a central vein. They resemble Medusa's head of snakes on radiologic imaging, which is thus referred to as the **"caput medusae" sign.** Susceptibility-weighted imaging at a magnetic strength of 7 T is the most sensitive technique to detect DVAs.

Treatment

■ Surgical resection is contraindicated as it can lead to venous infarction. However, knowledge of the presence of DVAs is important in considering surgical interventions on associated vascular malformations.

References

1. Töpper R, Jürgens E, Reul J, Thron A. Clinical significance of intracranial developmental venous anomalies. *J Neurol Neurosurg Psychiatry*. August 1999;67(2):234–238.
2. Ruíz DS, Yilmaz H, Gailloud P. Cerebral developmental venous anomalies: current concepts. *Ann Neurol*. September 2009;66(3):271–283. doi:10.1002/ana.21754.
3. Frischer JM, Göd S, Gruber A, et al. Susceptibility-weighted imaging at 7 T: Improved diagnosis of cerebral cavernous malformations and associated developmental venous anomalies. *Neuroimage Clin*. September 2012;1(1):116–120.

3.10 Dolichoectasia of Vertebrobasilar Artery

Case History

A 65-year-old man presented with palsies of his right facial and trigeminal nerves.

Diagnosis: Dolichoectasia of the Basilar Artery

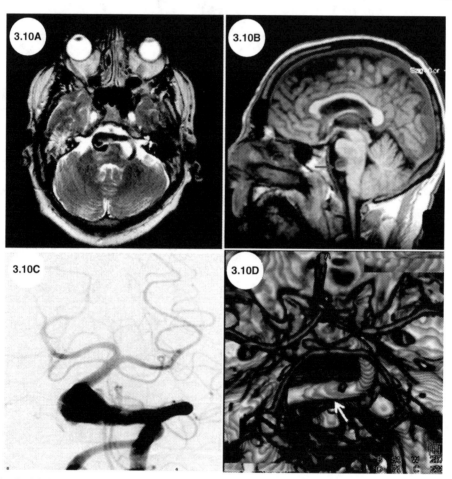

Images 3.10A–3.10D: Axial T2-weighted, sagittal T1-weighted, catheter angiogram, and CT angiogram demonstrate a markedly dolichoectatic fusiform basilar artery with a right-sided aneurysm (red and white arrows).

Introduction

■ Dolichoectasia refers to elongation and distension of an artery due to deterioration of its tunica intima and weakening of the vessel wall, usually due to longstanding hypertension. It also may occur in association with autosomal dominant polycystic kidney disease.

Clinical Presentation

■ The basilar artery is most commonly affected, and patients present with ischemia of the brainstem and cerebellum. Cranial nerve dysfunction, usually of the facial or trigeminal nerve, is common as well. The oculomotor, vestibulocochlear, and trochlear nerves may also be affected. Hemorrhagic stroke and subarachnoid hemorrhage are possible, though less common, manifestations. In some patients there is secondary hydrocephalus.

Radiographic Appearance and Diagnosis

■ The basilar artery is enlarged and tortuous with mass effect on the brainstem and cranial nerves.

By definition, the intraluminal diameter is greater than 4.5 mm. The ICA may be affected as well.

Treatment

■ There is currently no specific treatment beyond optimizing medical management of risk factors such as hypertension. Endovascular stenting is a possible future treatment.

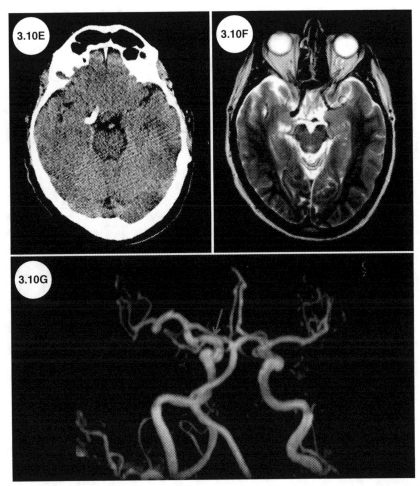

Image 3.10E: Axial CT image demonstrates marked calcification of the right ICA. **Images 3.10F and 3.10G:** Axial T2-weighted image and MR angiogram demonstrate dolichoectasia of the right MCA (red arrows). This was an incidental finding on a scan done for other reasons.

References

1. Passero SG, Rossi S. Natural history of vertebrobasilar dolichoectasia. *Neurology.* January 2008;70(1):66–72.
2. Wolfe T, Ubogu EE, Fernandes-Filho JA, Zaidat OO. Predictors of clinical outcome and mortality in vertebrobasilar dolichoectasia diagnosed by magnetic resonance angiography. *J Stroke Cerebrovasc Dis.* November–December 2008;17(6): 388–393.
3. Ubogu EE, Zaidat OO. Vertebrobasilar dolichoectasia diagnosed by magnetic resonance angiography and risk of stroke and death: a cohort study. *J Neurol Neurosurg Psychiatry.* January 2004;75(1):22–26.
4. Wolters FJ, Rinkel GJ, Vergouwen MD. Clinical course and treatment of vertebrobasilar dolichoectasia: a systematic review of the literature. *Neurol Res.* March 2013;35(2):131–137.
5. Yuan YJ, Xu K, Luo Q, Yu JL. Research progress on vertebrobasilar dolichoectasia. *Int J Med Sci.* August 2014;11(10):1039–1048.
6. Förster A, Ssozi J, Al-Zghloul M, Brockmann MA, Kerl HU, Groden C. A comparison of CT/CT angiography and MRI/MR angiography for imaging of vertebrobasilar dolichoectasia. *Clin Neuroradiol.* December 2014;24(4):347–353.

3.11 Fenestration of the Basilar Artery

Case History

A 56-year-old man presented with a brainstem stroke.

Diagnosis: Fenestration of the Basilar Artery

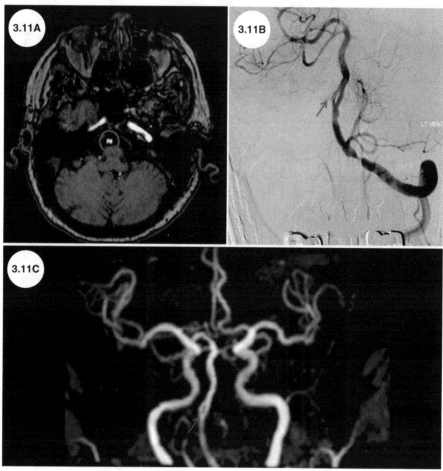

Images 3.11A–3.11C: Axial gradient echo, catheter angiogram, and MR angiogram demonstrate fenestration of the mid-basilar artery (red arrow and circle).

Introduction

- A fenestration is a congenital bifurcation of an artery into two unequal vascular channels. They can be found throughout the vasculature of the CNS, but are most common in the inferior portion of the basilar artery, just above the fusion of the vertebral arteries.

Clinical Presentation

- Fenestration of the basilar artery is most often an incidental finding. However, it may also be a risk for ischemia of the lower brainstem and cerebellum. There appears to be a slightly higher incidence of saccular aneurysms, possibly due to abnormal flow dynamics within the artery.

Radiographic Appearance and Diagnosis

■ Imaging of the cerebral vasculature reveals a division of the basilar artery into two unequal channels.

Treatment

■ No treatment is needed for incidentally detected fenestrations. Aneurysms may be treated with an endovascular approach or with surgical clipping.

References

1. van Rooij SB, Bechan RS, Peluso JP, Sluzewski M, van Rooij WJ. Fenestrations of intracranial arteries. *AJNR Am J Neuroradiol*. June 2015;36(6):1167–1170.
2. Tanaka M, Kikuchi Y, Ouchi T. Neuroradiological analysis of 23 cases of basilar artery fenestration based on 2280 cases of MR angiographies. *Interv Neuroradiol*. January 2006;12(Suppl. 1):39–44.
3. Sogawa K, Kikuchi Y, O'uchi T, Tanaka M, Inoue T. Fenestrations of the basilar artery demonstrated on magnetic resonance angiograms: an analysis of 212 cases. Interv Neuroradiol. December 2013;19(4):461–465.
4. Gao LY, Guo X, Zhou JJ, Zhang Q, Fu J, Chen WJ, Yang YJ. Basilar artery fenestration detected with CT angiography. *Eur Radiol*. October 2013;23(10):2861–2867.
5. Patel MA, Caplan JM, Yang W, Colby GP, Coon AL, Tamargo RJ, Huang J. Arterial fenestrations and their association with cerebral aneurysms. *Clin Neurosci*. December 2014;21(12):2184–2188.

3.12 | Persistent Trigeminal Artery

Case History

A 66-year-old man suffered a small lacunar infarction and was found to have a vascular anomaly.

Diagnosis: Persistent Trigeminal Artery

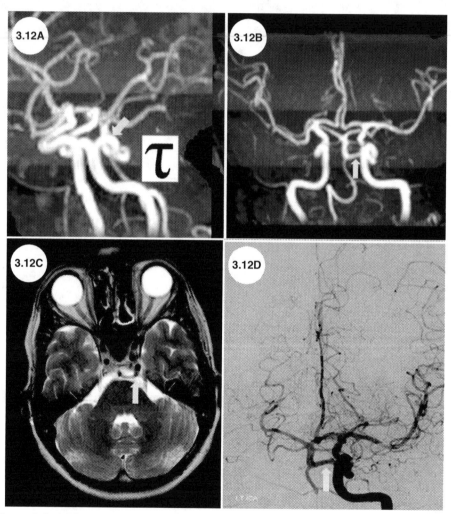

Images 3.12A and 3.12B: MR angiogram showing the left vertebral artery connecting to the left internal carotid artery via a persistent trigeminal artery (yellow arrow). The tau sign is seen on the sagittal view. **Images 3.12C and 3.12D:** Axial T2-weighted image and catheter angiogram, both showing the left vertebral artery connecting to the left internal carotid artery via a persistent trigeminal artery (yellow arrow).

Introduction

- There are three embryologic connections between the ICA and the vertebrobasilar system. These are known as the trigeminal, otic, and hypoglossal arteries. In fetal development, the trigeminal artery supplies the basilar artery prior to the development of other vessels of the posterior circulation.

- In adults, a persistent trigeminal artery is the most common remaining embryonic connection between the anterior and posterior circulations and is present in up to 1% of otherwise healthy adults.

Clinical Presentation

■ Though they are usually incidental findings, they may be associated with a higher rate of vascular malformations such as aneurysms and AVMs. Patients may also develop cranial nerve deficits or trigeminal neuralgia.

Radiographic Appearance and Diagnosis

■ Imaging of the cerebral vasculature will reveal a trigeminal artery arising from the ICA. On sagittal imaging it is called the **"tau sign" because of the resemblance to the Greek letter.** On conventional angiogram, the vertebrobasilar system will be seen with injection of the carotid artery.

Treatment

■ No treatment is necessary, but surgeons should be aware of this anatomic variation prior to performing procedures of the skull base.

References

1. Azab W, Delashaw J, Mohammed M. Persistent primitive trigeminal artery: a review. *Turk Neurosurg.* 2012;22(4):399–406.
2. Alcalá-Cerra G, Tubbs RS, Niño-Hernández LM. Anatomical features and clinical relevance of a persistent trigeminal artery. *Surg Neurol Int.* 2012;3:111.

3.13 Kissing Carotids

Case History

A 45-year-old female developed amenorrhea.

Diagnosis: Kissing Carotids

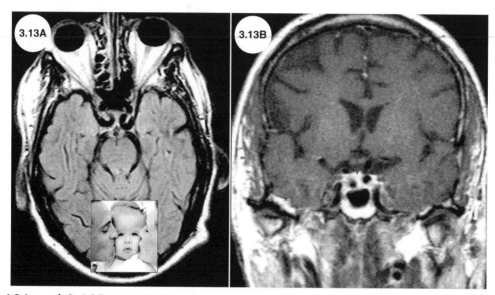

Images 3.13A and 3.13B: Axial FLAIR and postcontrast coronal T1-weighted images demonstrate the medial course of the cavernous segment of the internal carotid arteries bilaterally.

Introduction

- Different classification schemes exist to organize the segments of the ICA. The Bouthillier classification is presented in the following.

  1. Cervical segment (C1)
  2. Petrous segment (C2)
  3. Lacerum segment (C3)
  4. Cavernous segment (C4)
  5. Clinoid segment (C5)
  6. Ophthalmic (supraclinoid) segment (C6)
  7. Communicating (terminal) segment (C7)

- Carotid arteries that are deviated medially in the sella region are called "kissing carotids."

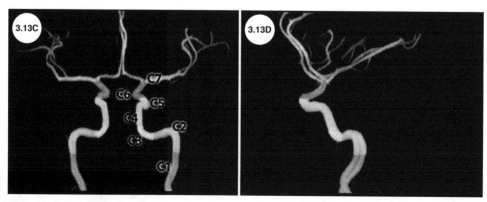

Images 3.13C and 3.13D: Illustration on normal angiogram of the segments of the ICA (image credit Behrang Amini).

Clinical Presentation

- They can compress the pituitary stalk, leading to pituitary dysfunction, but are most often incidental findings.

Radiographic Appearance

- Imaging of the cerebral vasculature will reveal elongated, medially deviated, and tortuous carotid arteries.

Treatment

- No treatment is necessary, but surgeons must be aware of them prior to performing transsphenoidal surgery on the pituitary gland.

References

1. Guo L, Qiu Y, Ge J, Zhang X. Kissing aneurysms of the internal carotid artery treated with surgical clipping. *Neurol India.* May–June 2012;60(3):353–355.
2. Gowdh NS, Gill FJ, Regan LA, Wilkie SW. Kissing carotid arteries: an unusual cause of prevertebral swelling. *BMJ Case Rep.* October 2014;2014. pii: bcr2014206099.
3. Okahara M, Kiyosue H, Mori H, Tanoue S, Sainou M, Nagatomi H. Anatomic variations of the cerebral arteries and their embryology: a pictorial review. *Eur Radiol.* October 2002;12(10):2548–2561.
4. Sahin M, Dilli A, Karbek B, et al. Unusual cause of primary amenorrhea due to kissing internal carotid arteries. *Pituitary.* June 2012;15(2):258–259.

3.14 | Absence of the Internal Carotid Arteries

Case History

A 56-year-old man presented with a sudden headache and was found to have a sub-arachnoid hemorrhage.

Diagnosis: Congenital Absence of the Internal Carotid Arteries

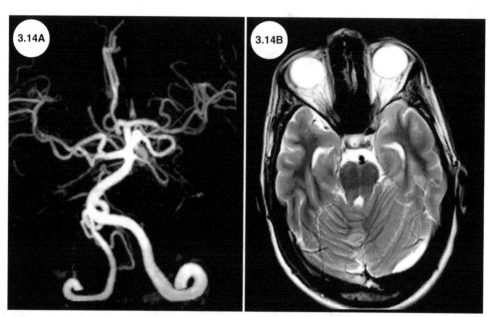

Images 3.14A and 3.14B: Coronal MR angiogram image and axial T2-weighted image demonstrate aberrant vasculature, with absence of the internal carotid arteries bilatearlly. There is enlargement of the posterior circulation, most notably the right vertebral artery.

Introduction

■ Congenital absence of an ICA is a very rare anomaly that occurs in about 1:10,000 individuals. Absence of these arteries bilaterally is even less common. Collateral flow to the anterior circulation is usually through the circle of Willis, from persistent embryonic vessels, or from transcranial collaterals originating from the external carotid artery.

Clinical Presentation

■ Absence of the ICA is often discovered on imaging done for other reasons, though there is an association with cerebral aneurysms. In a series of 158 patients with ICA aplasia/hypoplasia, aneurysms were found in 27.5% of the patients.

Radiographic Appearance and Diagnosis

■ On all imaging modalities, there will be absence of the internal carotid arteries. Collateral flow to the territories of the anterior circulation depends on the degree of hypoplasia or aplasia and the presence of collateral circulation.

Treatment

- There is no specific treatment. However, the finding is relevant for potential neurosurgical procedures and in the evaluation of patients with ischemic strokes.

References

1. Taşar M, Yetişer S, Taşar A, Uğurel S, Gönül E, Sağlam M. Congenital absence or hypoplasia of the carotid artery: radioclinical issues. *Am J Otolaryngol*. September–October 2004;25(5):339–349.
2. Lee JH, Oh CW, Lee SH, Han DH. Aplasia of the internal carotid artery. *Acta Neurochir (Wien)*. February 2003;145(2):117–125.
3. Zink WE, Komotar RJ, Meyers PM. Internal carotid aplasia/hypoplasia and intracranial saccular aneurysms: series of three new cases and systematic review of the literature. *J Neuroimaging*. April 2007;17(2):141–147.

3.15 | Carotid Paragangliomas

Case History

A 35-year-old woman presented with a painless neck mass and tongue weakness.

Diagnosis: Carotid Body Paragangliomas

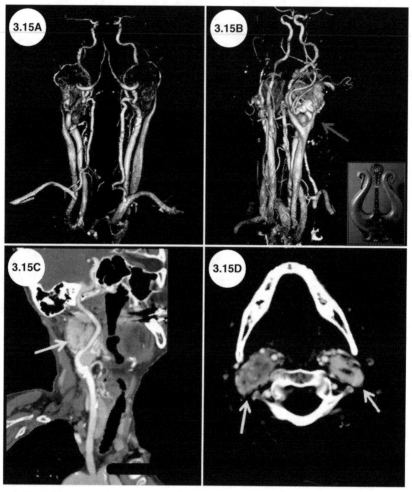

Images 3.15A and 3.15B: Three-dimensional and sagittal reformatted images from a CT angiogram demonstrate carotid body tumors. The splaying of the internal and external carotid artery, the "lyre" sign is shown (red arrow). **Images 3.15C and 3.15D:** Axial CT images demonstrate carotid body tumors (yellow arrows).

Introduction

- A paraganglioma is a rare neuroendocrine neoplasm, the vast majority of which are benign. They are a variation of glomus tumors, which arise from nonchromaffin paraganglion cells. They can develop in the abdomen, thorax, and neck, where they arise from the bifurcation of the internal and external carotid artery.

- Most are sporadic, but about 10% are familial, often associated with the neurocutaneous syndromes or multiple endocrine neoplasia.

- Patients typically present between the ages of 30 and 50 years.

Clinical Presentation

■ It typically presents with a painless mass in the neck, but also may present due to mass effect on the cranial nerves (9–12) that run in the carotid sheath. Rarely, they secrete catecholamines and present with endocrine dysfunction. The mass is mobile and can be moved horizontally, not laterally.

Radiographic Appearance and Diagnosis

■ CT scans with contrast provide excellent resolution of the tumors, which appear with the same density as soft tissue. The splaying of the internal and external carotid arteries by the tumor is called the **lyre sign**. They have mixed signal on MRI leading to the "salt and pepper" appearance.

Treatment

■ They are treated with surgical removal with excellent results. Large tumors may need radiotherapy if they are surgically inaccessible.

References

1. Wieneke JA, Smith A. Paraganglioma: carotid body tumor. *Head Heck Pathol.* December 2009;3(4):303–306.
2. Suárez C, Rodrigo JP, Mendenhall WM, et al. Carotid body paragangliomas: a systematic study on management with surgery and radiotherapy. *Eur Arch Otorhinolaryngol.* January 2014;271(1):23–34.

3.16 | Nonaneurysmal Perimesencephalic Subarachnoid Hemorrhage

Case History

A 65-year-old woman presented with a severe, acute headache.

Diagnosis: Perimesencephalic Subarachnoid Hemorrhage

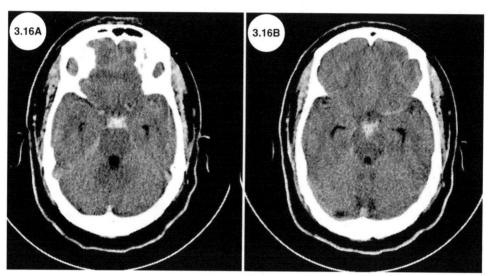

Images 3.16A and 3.16B: Axial CT images show acute blood in the interpeduncular fossa (red arrows).

Introduction

- Nonaneurysmal perimesencephalic subarachnoid hemorrhage is a benign disorder, thought to be due to a rupture of either a venous or arterial capillary.

Clinical Presentation

- They present in adults with a severe, acute headache. Alterations of consciousness may occur, but are much less common than with aneurysmal subarachnoid hemorrhage.

Radiographic Appearance and Diagnosis

- Head CT is the imaging modality of choice. Blood will be seen in the interpeduncular fossa, which is located anterior to the pons and midbrain. In larger hemorrhages, blood may be seen in the basal and suprasellar cisterns as well as the Sylvian and interhemispheric fissures.

- Angiography is required to rule out an aneurysm though the source is rarely identified.

Treatment

- The prognosis for such bleeds is good.

References

1. Rinkel GJ, Wijdicks EF, Vermeulen M, et al. Nonaneurysmal perimesencephalic subarachnoid hemorrhage: CT and MR patterns that differ from aneurysmal rupture. *AJNR Am J Neuroradiol*. September–October 1991;12(5):829–834.
2. Schwartz TH, Solomon RA. Perimesencephalic nonaneurysmal subarachnoid hemorrhage: review of the literature. *Neurosurgery*. September 1996;39(3):433–440.

3.17 | Posterior Reversible Encephalopathy Syndrome

Case History

A 65-year-old man presented with confusion and cortical blindness. His blood pressure in the emergency room (ER) was 231/180.

Diagnosis: Posterior Reversible Encephalopathy Syndrome

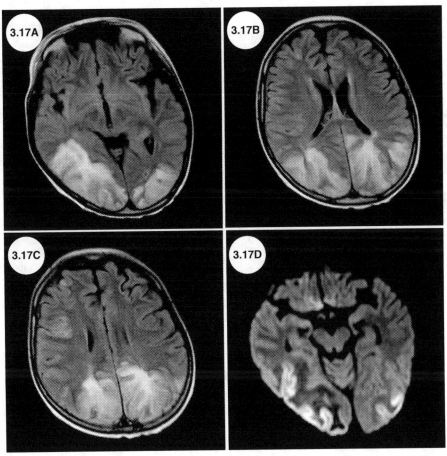

Images 3.17A–3.17D: Axial FLAIR and diffusion-weighted images demonstrate edema and gyral swelling in the occipital and posterior temporal lobes in a patient with PRES. There is hyperintensity on the diffusion-weighted images as well.

Introduction

■ Posterior reversible encephalopathy syndrome (PRES) occurs in the setting of rapid, severe increases in blood pressure, such as eclampsia, or due to the use of certain immunosuppressants such as tacrolimus or cyclosporine. It can also occur in association with autoimmune disorders such as systemic lupus erythematosus.

■ The pathophysiology is related to disordered cerebral autoregulation, primarily of the vasculature in the posterior regions of the brain.

Clinical Presentation

■ It presents with a combination of visual loss, seizures, headaches, and altered mental status.

Radiographic Appearance

■ Edema and diffuse hyperintensity on T2-weighted images can be seen throughout the posterior circulation, primarily in the occipital

and posterior temporal lobes. The watershed zones and superior frontal sulcus may also be affected. Infarction occurs in about 20% of cases and hemorrhage occurs in about 10% of cases.

■ It is transient and should gradually resolve as the patient improves clinically.

Treatment

■ Patients with PRES should have aggressive lowering of their blood pressure or discontinuation of the responsible medication. It is typically reversible with normalization of blood pressure or the discontinuation of the responsible medication, though some patients are left with permanent visual deficits.

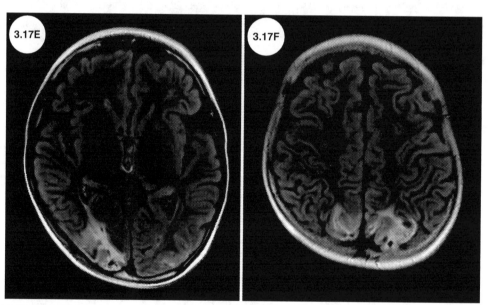

Images 3.17E and 3.17F: Axial FLAIR images from the same patient taken 3 weeks later demonstrate significant, though incomplete resolution of the white matter hyperintensities.

References

1. Thompson RJ, Sharp B, Pothof J, Hamedani A. Posterior reversible encephalopathy syndrome in the emergency department: case series and literature review. *West J Emerg Med.* January 2015;16(1):5–10.
2. Granata G, Greco A, Iannella G, Granata M, Manno A, Savastano E, Magliulo G. Posterior reversible encephalopathy syndrome—

Insight into pathogenesis, clinical variants and treatment approaches. *Autoimmun Rev.* September 2015;14(9):830–836.
3. Lamy C, Oppenheim C, Mas JL. Posterior reversible encephalopathy syndrome. *Handb Clin Neurol.* 2014;121:1687–701.
4. Lamy C, Oppenheim C, Méder JF, Mas JL. Neuroimaging in posterior reversible encephalopathy syndrome. *J Neuroimaging.* April 2004;14(2):89–96.

CHAPTER 4
NEOPLASTIC DISEASES

4.1 Glioblastoma

Case History

A 56-year-old man presented to the hospital with a seizure. He had been complaining of headaches for the past several months and becoming "slow" as per family. He also noticed that he was "bumping into things" for the past few months.

Diagnosis: Glioblastoma Multiforme

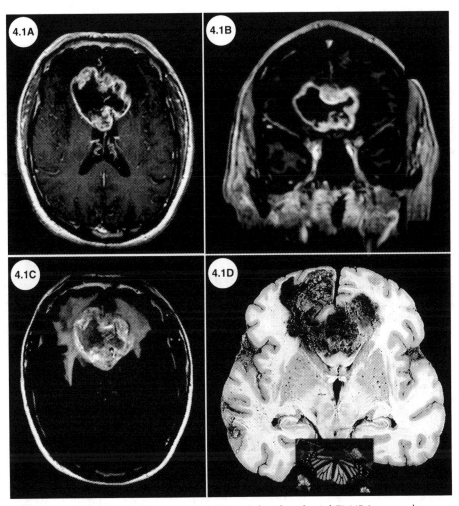

Images 4.1A–4.1C: Axial and sagittal postcontrast T1-weighted and axial FLAIR images demonstrate an enhancing mass spanning the splenium of the corpus callosum with mass effect and edema. The symmetrical appearance creates the characteristic "butterfly" appearance of high-grade gliomas. **Image 4.1D:** Gross pathology of a glioma (image credit The Armed Forces Institute of Pathology).

Introduction

■ Grade IV astrocytomas, glioblastomas, are the most common and most lethal type of astrocytoma, with a median survival of less than 1 year. They occur most often in people over the age of 50 and are slightly more common in men. They almost always arise in the cerebral hemispheres. Even though the tumor may appear as a discrete mass, neoplastic cells spread along white matter pathways and are invariably spread throughout the brain at the time of diagnosis. There are no known risk factors other than exposure to radiation or rare genetic traits such as Li–Fraumeni syndrome.

- Grades I/II constitute about 15% to 20% of tumors, grade III accounts for 30% to 35%, and the highest grade, IV, accounts for about 40% to 50% of tumors. **Table 4.1.1** details the WHO grading of central nervous system (CNS) tumors.

Table 4.1.1 WHO Grading of Glial Tumors

WHO Grade	Tumor Type	Average Life Span
I	Juvenile pilocytic astrocytomas, subependymal giant cell astrocytomas (most commonly associated with tuberous sclerosis), pleomorphic xanthoastrocytoma	These can be cured with complete resection and most often occur in children.
II	Diffuse or fibrillary astrocytomas, oligodendroglioma	7–8 years
III	Anaplastic astrocytoma, anaplastic oligodendroglioma	2–3 years
IV	Glioblastoma multiforme	9–12 months

Clinical Presentation

- Tumors of the CNS present with essentially four different symptoms:

  1. Progressive, focal neurological deficits
  2. Headaches that are characteristically worse in recumbency and are often associated with nausea, vomiting, and other symptoms of increased intracranial pressure (ICP)
  3. Seizures, if there is irritation of the cerebral cortex
  4. Gradual cognitive slowing and personality changes

- The symptoms experienced by each patient depend on the location of the tumor and its rate of growth (**Table 4.1.2**). Slowly growing tumors can grow quite large and have significant mass effect despite causing few symptoms. Occasionally, patients can present with the sudden onset of neurological symptoms. This is common if there is hemorrhage into the tumor, but it sometimes occurs without such a hemorrhage for unclear reasons. Patients with a CNS neoplasm who have symptoms of systemic disease, such as fever and weight loss, are more likely to have metastatic disease rather than a primary CNS neoplasm.

Table 4.1.2 Clinical Presentation of Glioblastomas

Tumor Location	Clinical Presentation
Anterior Frontal Lobe	- Weakness, primarily of the contralateral leg - Personality changes including disinhibition, poor judgment, cognitive slowing, and aphasia for left-sided lesions - Urinary incontinence due to disruption of the micturition inhibition center - Gaze preference if there is involvement of the frontal eye fields - Primitive reflexes such as grasp, suck, and snout reflex - Seizures
Posterior Frontal Lobe	- Contralateral weakness - Expressive aphasia for left-sided lesions, neglect for right-sided lesions - Seizures
Temporal Lobe	- Memory impairment - Wernicke-type aphasia for left-sided lesions - Contralateral superior quadrantanopia, neglect for right-sided lesions - Seizures
Occipital Lobe	- Contralateral homonymous hemianopia, visual hallucinations - Alexia without agraphia for left-sided tumors involving the corpus callosum - Seizures
Thalamus	- Contralateral sensory loss - Aphasias for left-sided lesions
Brainstem	- Headache and hydrocephalus if there is obstruction of the ventricular system - Cranial nerve deficits - Sensory and motor deficits
Cerebellum	- Ipsilateral limb ataxia for lateral tumors, truncal ataxia for midline tumors - Nausea and vomiting - Dizziness and vertigo - Headaches, often worse in the morning - Hydrocephalus if there is occlusion of the fourth ventricle

- Primary glioblastomas tend to arise de novo from glial cells, while secondary glioblastomas arise from lower grade tumors. The differentiating features are listed in **Table 4.1.3**.

- Mutations of isocitrate dehydrogenase (IDH1) are frequent in secondary glioblastomas (80%) and rare in primary glioblastomas (10%). Thus, IDH1 mutations are strong predictors of more favorable prognosis, and are highly selective molecular markers of secondary glioblastomas that complements clinical criteria for distinguishing it from primary glioblastomas. Additionally, O6-methylguanine-DNA methyltransferase

Table 4.1.3 Characteristics of Primary
and Secondary Glioblastomas

Primary Glioblastoma	Secondary Glioblastomas
Accounts for >90% of biopsied or resected cases	Comprises <5% of glioblastoma multiforme cases
Occurs in older patients (median age: 60 years)	Occurs in younger patients (median age: 45 years)
Develops de novo from glial cells ~5% can be multifocal	Develops from low-grade or anaplastic astrocytoma ~70% of lower grade gliomas develop into advanced disease within 5–10 years of diagnosis

(MGMT) is an important DNA repair enzyme that contributes to glioblastoma resistance to temozolomide. Methylation of MGMT has been reported to be a good prognostic factor for patients with glioblastomas.

Radiographic Appearance and Diagnosis

■ Glioblastomas generally appear as heterogeneously enhancing masses, with the nonenhancing areas representing areas of necrosis. There is mass effect and edema, best seen on T2-weighted images. As shown in **Images 4.1A–4.1C**, the tumor often crosses the corpus callosum creating a "butterfly" appearance. Ring-like enhancement, with a necrotic center, is common as well.

■ A biopsy is required to make the diagnosis. The typical pathology features include necrosis, vascular hyperplasia with plump endothelial cells, pseudopalisading cells around necrosis, and atypical mitotic figures as seen in **Images 4.1E–4.1H**.

Special Cases

Gliomatosis Cerebri and Multicentric Glioma

■ Gliomatosis cerebri refers to a type of malignant glioma that is characterized by extensive tumor infiltration without a discrete mass or areas of necrosis. Small areas of enhancement may be seen. There is no pathognomonic clinical presentation, but may present with headaches, seizures, personality change or dementia, or progressive weakness. This type of tumor commonly presents in people younger than 40. These tumors are treated with whole brain radiation and chemotherapy. With such treatment, there is a nearly 3-year life span. Gliomas may be multicentric in up to 5% of cases. These lesions may be very difficult to distinguish from metastatic disease or demyelination.

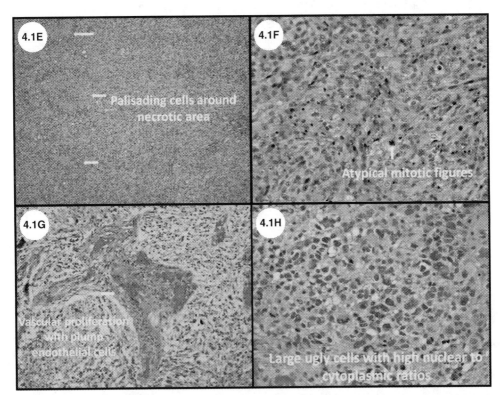

Images 4.1E–4.1H: Histological features of a glioblastoma are shown (image credit Kia Newman, MD).

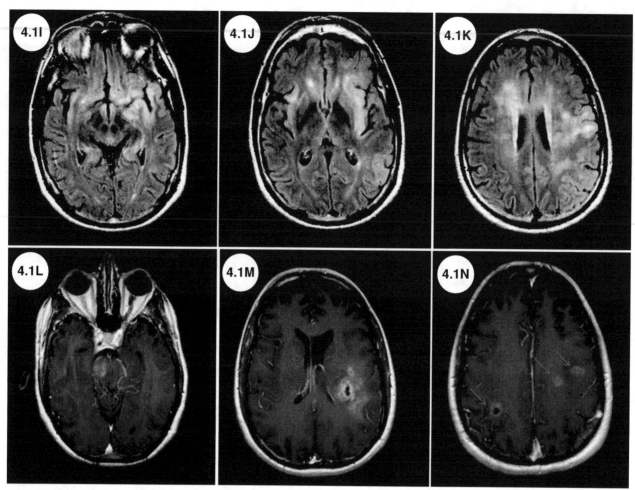

Images 4.1I–4.1K: Axial FLAIR images demonstrate numerous areas of hyperintensity in the bilateral cerebral hemispheres. On biopsy this was found to be gliomatosis cerebri. **Images 4.1L–4.1N:** Postcontrast axial T1-weighted images from a different patient demonstrate numerous areas of irregular contrast enhancement (red arrows) in the bilateral cerebral hemispheres. On biopsy, these were found to be a glioblastoma.

Brainstem Glioma

- Tumors of the brainstem present with:

  - Headache and hydrocephalus if there is obstruction of the ventricular system

  - Cranial nerve deficits ipsilateral to the lesion

  - Sensory and motor deficits contralateral to the lesion

- These tumors are not amenable to surgical resection.

Treatment

- Surgery aims to reduce the tumor burden (debulking/cytoreductive), thereby reducing symptoms and extending survival times. A cohort of 1,229 patients demonstrated that survival time is directly correlated with the degree of tumor removed. Patients who had surgical excision of abnormalities on fluid-attenuated inversion recovery (FLAIR) imaging tended to fair better than those in whom surgical excision was limited to total resection of the T1 contrast-enhancing tumor volume. However, complete removal is not possible, as tumor cells are widespread throughout the brain at the time of diagnosis, even in areas that are radiographically unremarkable. Additionally, tumors in the brainstem are not amenable to surgical resection.

- Most high-grade glioblastomas will eventually become resistant to treatment, but clinical picture can be confused with pseudoprogression, which is especially seen after chemoradiation when there is a slight increase in enhancement without tumor progression. There are techniques such as magnetic resonance spectroscopy (MRS), PET, and single photon emission computed tomography (SPECT) scans, which can help distinguish pseudoprogression from true recurrence.

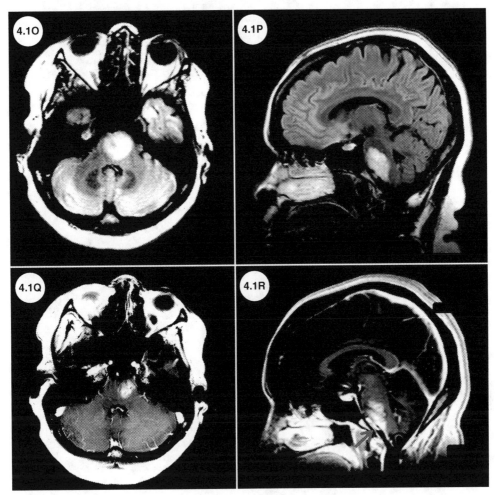

Images 4.1O–4.1R: Axial and sagittal FLAIR and postcontrast T1-weighted images demonstrate an enhancing, necrotic mass (red arrow) expanding the pons, mostly on the left.

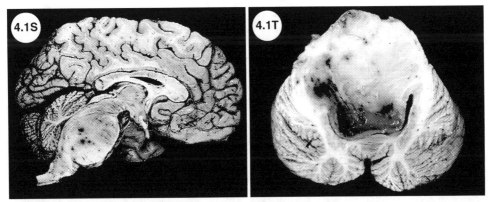

Images 4.1S and 4.1T: Gross pathology demonstrates a brainstem glioma (image 4.1S credit The Armed Forces Institute of Pathology. Image 4.1T credit www.wikidoc.org via Professor Peter Anderson, DVM, PhD, and published with permission © PEIR, University of Alabama at Birmingham, Department of Pathology).

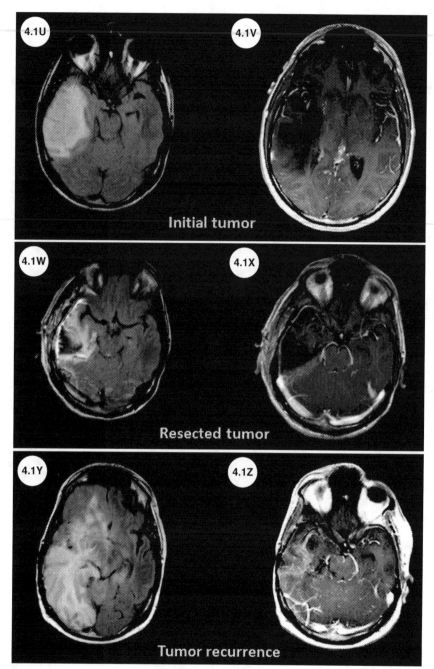

Images 4.1U and 4.1V: Axial FLAIR image and postcontrast axial T1-weighted images demonstrate a T2-hyperintense mass in the right temporal lobe without contrast enhancement. **Images 4.1W and 4.1X:** Axial FLAIR image and postcontrast T1-weighted images demonstrate postsurgical changes after resection of the mass, found to be an anaplastic glioma on histology. **Images 4.1Y and 4.1Z:** Axial FLAIR image and postcontrast T1-weighted images 2 years after the surgery demonstrate tumor recurrence with extensive FLAIR hyperintensity and contrast enhancement.

■ **Radiation therapy** has short-term side effects (hair loss, skin irritation, nausea, vomiting, fatigue, etc) and long-term sequelae (eg, neurological compromise and radiation-induced necrosis and vasculitis).

■ **Chemotherapy:**

– Temozolomide is an oral alkylating agent indicated for glioblastomas or recurrent anaplastic astrocytomas. In a trial of this medication in patients also treated with radiotherapy,

26.5% of patients treated with temozolomide were alive at 2 years, compared with 10.4% treated with radiotherapy alone.

- **Bevacizumab**: Tumors release the vascular endothelial growth factor (VEGF) protein, causing nearby blood vessels to sprout new vessels, a process called angiogenesis. These blood vessels feed the growth of the tumor. Bevacizumab is a therapeutic antibody that specifically binds to the VEGF protein, theoretically interfering blood supply of tumor, hence stopping the growth of cancer cells.

- Other second-line chemotherapy agents include procarbazine, carboplatin, and BCNU/CCNU.

■ Despite recent treatment advances, the prognosis for glioblastomas remains grim, as few patients survive beyond 2 years.

■ **Symptomatic therapy** includes the use of steroids to reduce vasogenic edema, antiemetics, antibiotics, and anticoagulants, as the incidence of venous thromboembolism is 20% to 30%. Despite advances in therapeutic anticoagulation, inferior vena cava filters continue to remain an important part of the therapeutic armamentarium. Anticonvulsants are used in patients who have had seizures, but there is no role for prophylactic treatment.

References

1. Omuro A, DeAngelis LM. Glioblastoma and other malignant gliomas: a clinical review. JAMA. November 2013;310(17):1842–1850.
2. Mukundan S, Holder C, Olson JJ. Neuroradiological assessment of newly diagnosed glioblastoma. *J Neurooncol.* September 2008;89(3):259–269.
3. Minniti G, Scaringi C, Baldoni A, et al. Health-related quality of life in elderly patients with newly diagnosed glioblastoma treated with short-course radiation therapy plus concomitant and adjuvant temozolomide. *Int J Radiat Oncol Biol Phys.* 2013;86:285.
4. Barnholtz-Sloan JS, Williams VL, Maldonado JL, et al. Patterns of care and outcomes among elderly individuals with primary malignant astrocytoma. *J Neurosurg.* 2008;108:642.
5. Malmstrom A, Gronberg BH, Marosi C, et al. Nordic clinical brain tumour study group (NCBTSG). Temozolomide versus standard 6-week radiotherapy versus hypofractionated radiotherapy in patients older than 60 years with glioblastoma: the Nordic randomised, phase 3 trial. *Lancet Oncol.* September 2012;13(9):916–926.
6. Stupp R, Hegi ME, Mason WP, et al. Effects of radiotherapy with concomitant and adjuvant temozolomide versus radiotherapy alone on survival in glioblastoma in a randomised phase III study: 5-year analysis of the EORTC-NCIC trial. *Lancet Oncol.* May 2009;10(5):459–466.
7. Stupp R, Mason WP, van den Bent MJ, et al. European Organisation for Research and Treatment of Cancer Brain Tumor and Radiotherapy groups; National Cancer Institute of Canada Clinical Trials Group. Radiotherapy plus concomitant and adjuvant temozolomide for glioblastoma. *N Engl J Med.* March 2005;352(10):987–996.
8. Li YM, Suki D, Hess K, Sawaya R. The influence of maximum safe resection of glioblastoma on survival in 1229 patients: Can we do better than gross-total resection? *J Neurosurg.* October 2015;124(4):977–988.

4.2 | Juvenile Pilocytic Astrocytoma

Case History

A 7-year-old child developed progressive headaches and ataxia.

Diagnosis: Juvenile Pilocytic Astrocytoma

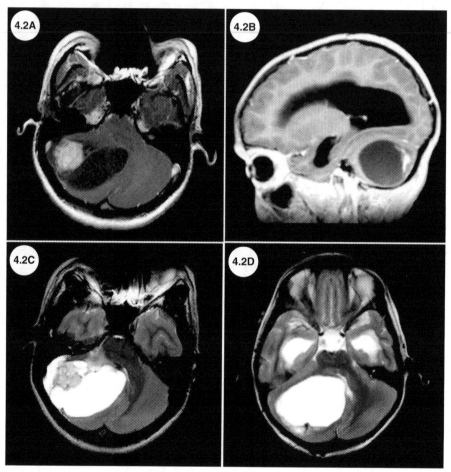

Images 4.2A–4.2D: Postcontrast axial and sagittal T1-weighted and axial T2-weighted images demonstrate predominantly cystic mass with a peripherally enhancing mural nodule in the right cerebellum. There is mass effect on the fourth ventricle and obstructive hydrocephalus (red arrows).

Introduction

▇ Astrocytomas are the most common type of intracranial neoplasms in children and young adults, comprising approximately half of such tumors. Of these, 75% are juvenile pilocytic astrocytomas (JPAs), which are benign, WHO grade I tumors.

Clinical Presentation

▇ JPAs typically occur in a cerebellar hemisphere where they present with symptoms of increased ICP and ataxia. In very rare cases, they may hemorrhage. They are second only to medulloblastomas in frequency in this location. Although

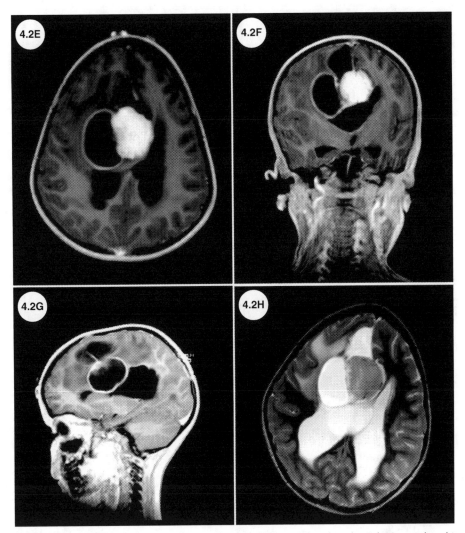

Images 4.2E–4.2H: Postcontrast axial, coronal, and sagittal T1-weighted and axial T2-weighted images demonstrate a complex cystic mass arising from the corpus callosum. There is both a ring-enhancing component and a solid-enhancing portion. There is mass effect on the right frontal lobe and hydrocephalus.

they occur in a cerebellar hemisphere over half of the time, they may occur anywhere in the CNS. Tumors outside of the cerebellum are more common in adults.

■ JPAs of the optic nerve, chiasm, and tract are common in neurofibromatosis type I.

■ JPAs may also occur in the spinal cord. They are most commonly found in the cervical cord where they present with central cord or hemicord syndromes and pain in the extremities.

Radiographic Appearance and Diagnosis

■ On MRI, JPAs are well-circumscribed lesions that commonly have a large cystic component with

an enhancing mural nodule. The cyst is typically isodense to cerebrospinal fluid (CSF) on all sequences, though cysts with a high protein content may by hyperintense to CSF on certain sequences. About 30% of cases have a more solid component or are completely solid. The major differential diagnostic consideration in such cases is hemangioblastomas.

■ On histology, intracytoplasmic inclusions known as Rosenthal fibers are characteristic for JPAs. They are beaded, elongated, or corkscrew-shaped.

Treatment

■ JPAs are usually amenable to surgical resection and have an excellent clinical outcome. The use of chemotherapy or radiation in the setting

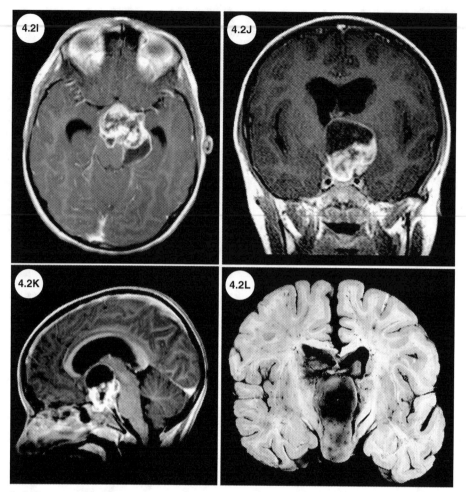

Images 4.2I–4.2K: Postcontrast axial, coronal, and sagittal T1-weighted images demonstrate a complex cystic mass arising from the optic chiasm in a patient with neurofibromatosis type I. **Image 4.2L:** Gross pathology of pilocytic astrocytoma of the hypothalamic region (image credit The Armed Forces Institute of Pathology).

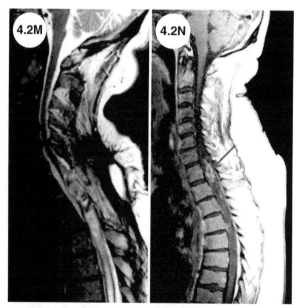

Images 4.2M and 4.2N: Sagittal T2-weighted and postcontrast T1-weighted images demonstrate a heterogeneously enhancing mass (red arrow) in the lower cervical spinal cord with a syrinx below. This was found to be a juvenile pilocytic astrocytoma.

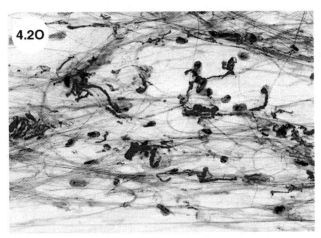

Image 4.2O: Hematoxylin and eosin (H&E) stain demonstrates Rosenthal fibers in a JPA (image credit The Armed Forces Institute of Pathology).

of incomplete tumor resection is controversial, given the young age of most patients. Spinal gliomas are not amenable to complete surgical resection, but surgery is needed to establish a diagnosis, and debulking of the tumor may delay progression of symptoms.

References

1. Bonfield CM, Steinbok P. Pediatric cerebellar astrocytoma: a review. *Childs Nerv Syst*. October 2015;31(10):1677–1685.
2. Chourmouzi D, Papadopoulou E, Konstantinidis M, et al. Manifestations of pilocytic astrocytoma: a pictorial review. *Insights Imaging*. June 2014;5(3):387–402.

4.3 | Oligodendroglioma

Case History

A 47-year-old man presented after a seizure. He was previously healthy and had slight left-sided weakness on neurological examination.

Diagnosis: Oligodendroglioma

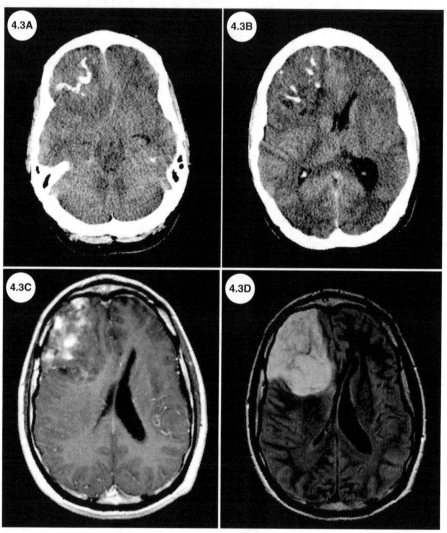

Images 4.3A–4.3D: Axial CT, postcontrast T-weighted, and FLAIR images demonstrate a mass in the right frontal lobe with areas of calcification. It demonstrates patchy enhancement and FLAIR hyperintensity, along with mass effect and compression of the lateral ventricle.

Introduction

■ Oligodendrocytes form the myelin sheath around axons in the CNS, allowing for a rapid increase in the speed of the action potential generated by neurons. A single oligodendrocyte can myelinate up to 50 axons.

■ Oligodendrogliomas are tumors that arise from oligodendrocytes. They account for 5% to 10% of primary CNS tumors in adults and occur more commonly in women. Patients usually present in their 40s and 50s.

- WHO classification:

  - **Oligodendroglioma (WHO grade II; low grade):** well differentiated, diffusely infiltrating, composed of cells resembling oligodendrocytes

  - **Anaplastic oligodendroglioma (WHO grade III; high grade):** malignant features such as the presence or absence of necrosis, vascular proliferation, increased number of mitoses, and increased nuclear atypia

Clinical Presentation

- Patients present with seizures, headache, cognitive dysfunction, or focal neurological abnormalities depending on the location of the tumor.

Radiographic Appearance and Diagnosis

- There is no radiographic feature that allows them to be reliably differentiated from other glial tumors. They are hypointense on T1-weighted images and hyperintense on T2-weighted images with mass effect. However, they are more likely to show calcification on CT scans and have less avid enhancement with the administration of contrast compared to glioblastomas. Only about 50% of them enhance, most commonly, heterogeneously.

- 85% are supratentorial, most commonly in the frontal lobes.

- Histologically, the cells are characterized by a "fried egg" appearance. Some have features of an astrocytoma as well, and are referred to as oligoastrocytomas. Tumors with a high astrocytic component have a worse prognosis.

- The most common molecular genetic abnormality is co-deletion of chromosomal arms 1p and 19q, with about 70% of cases showing this deletion. The high frequency of co-deletion is a "genetic signature" of oligodendrogliomas, and tumors with this co-deletion have a better prognosis and improved responsiveness to chemotherapy.

Treatment

- They are treated with a combination of surgical resection, adjuvant chemotherapy (Procarbazine, CCNU, vicristine [PCV] regimen or temozolomide), and radiation.

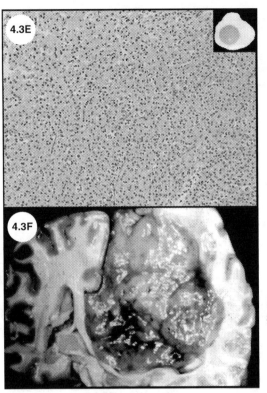

Image 4.3E: Histological specimen demonstrates the "fried egg" appearance of an oligodendroglioma.
Image 4.3F: Gross appearance of an oligodendroglioma (image credit www.wikidoc.org via Professor Peter Anderson, DVM, PhD, and published with permission © PEIR, University of Alabama at Birmingham, Department of Pathology).

- The natural history is a gradual progression from low-grade tumors to high-grade lesions with anaplastic features. Oligodendrogliomas have an improved clinical response compared to astrocytomas with a 5-year survival rate of 50% to 75%. Many patients may survive 10 years or longer. Predictors of poor outcome include older age, poor functional status, tumor size greater than 4 to 5 cm, tumor outside of frontal lobes, and lack of co-deletion of chromosomal arms 1p and 19q.

References

1. Roth P, Wick W, Weller M. Anaplastic oligodendroglioma: a new treatment paradigm and current controversies. *Curr Treat Options Oncol.* December 2013;14(4):505–513.
2. Jiang H, Zhang Z, Ren X, et al. 1p/19q-driven prognostic molecular classification for high-grade oligodendroglial tumors. *J Neurooncol.* 2014 Dec;120(3):607–614.
3. Bromberg JE, van den Bent MJ. Oligodendrogliomas: molecular biology and treatment. *Oncologist.* February 2009;14(2):155–163.
4. van den Bent MJ. Diagnosis and management of oligodendroglioma. *Semin Oncol.* October 2004;31(5):645–652.

4.4 | Primary Central Nervous System Lymphoma

Case History

A 45-year-old man presented with progressive right-sided numbness and weakness.

Diagnosis: Primary CNS Lymphoma

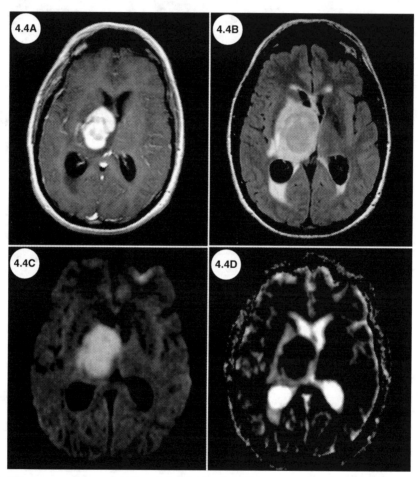

Images 4.4A–4.4D: Postcontrast axial T1-weighted, FLAIR, diffusion-weighted, and apparent diffusion coefficient images demonstrate an enhancing mass in the right thalamus with FLAIR hyperintensity and restricted diffusion.

Introduction

■ Primary CNS lymphoma (PCNSL) is the most common intracranial neoplasm in HIV-positive patients. About 5% of patients with AIDS will develop PCNSL, and the average CD4+ count at the time of diagnosis is 50/uL. In immunocompetent patients, it comprises 2% to 3% of all intracranial neoplasms, and the incidence has risen in the past several decades for unknown reasons.

■ Most are derived from B cells. The CNS contains no lymphoid tissue, and as such the cellular origin of these tumors is not clear, though lymphoid channels have been found in mice, running parallel to the venous sinuses.

■ It is highly associated with Epstein-Barr virus (EBV) in immunocompromised patients.

Clinical Presentation

■ They present with cognitive decline and focal neurological deficits. Headaches and seizures are also possible presentations. It may spread via the CSF as well as to the eyes and bones.

Radiographic Appearance and Diagnosis

■ They are usually subcortical in location, adjacent to the ependymal or subarachnoid surfaces. They are hypointense on T1-weighted images and have a variable appearance on T2-weighted images and they can be isointense, hypointense, and hyperintense to white matter. They enhance avidly and homogeneously with the administration of contrast. Higher grade tumors have more enhancement. A characteristic finding is avid restricted diffusion. There is less mass effect and edema than with other intracerebral tumors. They are usually hyperdense on T1-weighted images due to increased cellularity.

■ Intraventricular disease is possible, though uncommon, occurring in less than 10% of patients on presentation.

■ In contrast to immunocompetent patients, in immunosuppressed patients or those with AIDS, PCNSL typically presents as a ring-enhancing

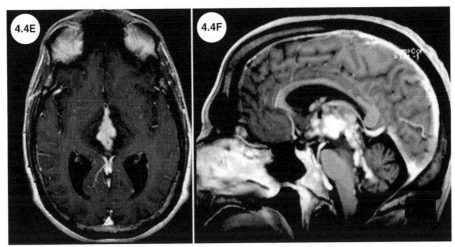

Images 4.4E and 4.4F: Postcontrast axial and sagittal T1-weighted images demonstrate an enhancing, lobulated tissue surrounding the ventricular system.

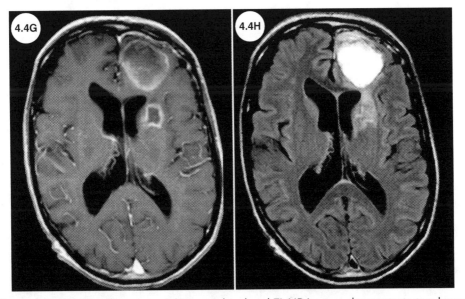

Images 4.4G and 4.4H: Postcontrast axial T1-weighted and FLAIR images demonstrate two hyperintense, ring-enhancing lesions in the left frontal lobe due to lymphoma in an HIV-positive patient.

mass. Multiple lesions are common as well. It may be indistinguishable from toxoplasmosis, and patients should be treated empirically for toxoplasmosis. A biopsy should be performed only if there is no clinical or radiographic response.

Treatment

- In immunocompetent patients there is often a positive response to chemotherapy (primarily with methotrexate) and radiation, but survival time is still only 3 to 4 years. In patients with HIV, the prognosis is dim with a survival time of only several months. There is no role for surgical resection.

- Treatment with glucocorticoids has a drastic effect on the radiographic appearance of the tumor as the tumor may shrink significantly and enhancement may disappear.

References

1. Patrick LB, Mohile NA. Advances in primary central nervous system lymphoma. *Curr Oncol Rep.* December 2015;17(12):60.
2. Hoang-Xuan K, Bessell E, Bromberg J, et al. Diagnosis and treatment of primary CNS lymphoma in immunocompetent patients: guidelines from the European Association for Neuro-Oncology. *Lancet Oncol.* July 2015;16(7):e322–e332.

4.5 | Dysembryoplastic Neuroepithelial Tumor

Case History

A 12-year-old girl presented with intractable partial seizures.

Diagnosis: Dysembryoplastic Neuroepithelial Tumor

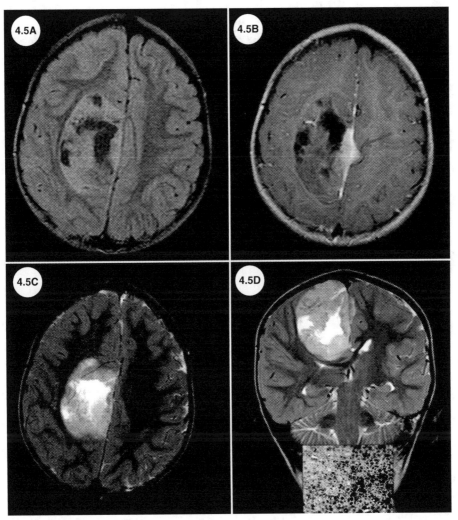

Images 4.5A–4.5D: Axial FLAIR, postcontrast axial T1-weighted, and axial and coronal T2-weighted images demonstrate a large mass, of mixed signal with "soap bubble" appearance in the R frontal lobe. On postcontrast images, there is slight enhancement of a mural nodule (red arrow).

Introduction

■ **Dysembryoplastic neuroepithelial tumors (DNETs)** are benign (WHO grade I) slow-growing tumors that arise most commonly from the cortex in the temporal lobe.

■ They are rare tumors and account for less than 1% of intracranial neoplasms.

Clinical Presentation

- **DNETs** present in children and teenagers with intractable partial epilepsy. Patients do not generally have progressive neurological deficits.

Radiographic Appearance and Diagnosis

- **DNETs** are hypointense on T1-weighted images and are hyperintense on T2-weighted images with a "soap bubble" appearance and up to 80% of cases present with cortical dysplasia. Enhancement, often a mural nodule, is seen in about 30% of cases. There is no edema and minimal mass effect associated with DNETs.

Treatment

- Surgical removal is indicated in patients with intractable seizures and is usually curative.

References

1. Zhang JG, Hu WZ, Zhao RJ, Kong LF. Dysembryoplastic neuroepithelial tumor: a clinical, neuroradiological, and pathological study of 15 cases. *J Child Neurol*. November 2014;29(11):1441–1447.
2. Shinoda J, Yokoyama K, Miwa K, et al. Epilepsy surgery of dysembryoplastic neuroepithelial tumors using advanced multitechnologies with combined neuroimaging and electrophysiological examinations. Epilepsy Behav Case Rep. July 2013;1:97–105.
3. Lee DY, Chung CK, Hwang YS, et al. Dysembryoplastic neuroepithelial tumor: radiological findings (including PET, SPECT, and MRS) and surgical strategy. J Neurooncol. April 2000;47(2):167–174.

4.6 | Ependymoma

Case History

A 4-year-old presented with a severe headache, nausea, vomiting, and blurry vision for the past several months. He had decreased visual acuity and papilledema on examination.

Diagnosis: Ependymoma

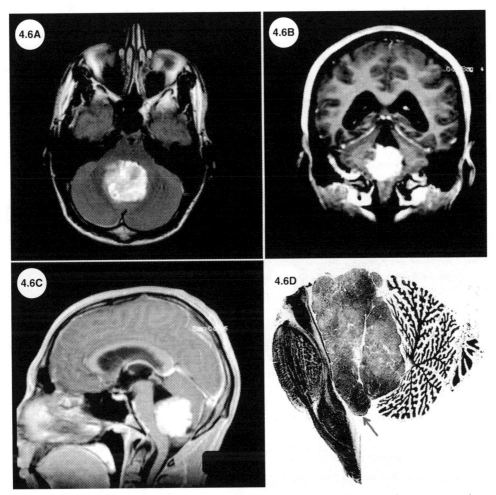

Images 4.6A–4.6C: Postcontrast axial, coronal, and sagittal T1-weighted images demonstrate a hyperintense, homogeneously enhancing mass arising from the floor of the fourth ventricle causing obstructive hydrocephalus.
Image 4.6D: Gross pathology of an ependymoma (image credit The Armed Forces Institute of Pathology).

Introduction

■ Ependymal cells line the walls of the ventricles in the CNS. The choroid plexus is formed by a network of ependymal cells and capillaries. Ependymal cells secrete and help circulate CSF throughout the ventricular system.

Ependymomas are tumors that arise from the ependymal cells.

■ These account for 2% to 9% of all intracranial tumors and about 12% of pediatric brain tumors. There is a bimodal age of distribution with ependymomas. Peaks occur in children aged 1 to 5 and adults aged 20 to 30.

- About 70% of these tumors occur infratentorially, usually from the fourth ventricle. They are the third most common posterior fossa tumor in children, behind juvenile pilocytic astrocytomas and medulloblastomas. Slightly less than half are supratentorial in location.

- The WHO assigns a grade to ependymomas based on the pleomorphism, mitotic count, cellularity, vascular proliferation and invasion and divides them into three different subtypes:

  1. **WHO grade I:** myxopapillary ependymoma, subependymoma
  2. **WHO grade II:** ependymoma (with cellular, papillary, and clear cell, tanycytic)
  3. **WHO grade III:** anaplastic ependymoma is a more aggressive, faster growing tumor

- In adults, they occur in the spinal canal. Spinal cord ependymomas are the most common intramedullary neoplasm, most often occurring in the cervical cord followed by the thoracic cord. **Spinal myxopapillary ependymomas** occur in the conus medullaris and filum terminale.

- The key histological features are perivascular pseudorosettes and ependymal rosettes. Electron microscopy is necessary to differentiate ependymoma from glioma if rosettes are not present.

- The gain of 1q25 and endothelial growth factor receptor (EGFR) overexpression in these tumors is associated with poor prognosis. In contrast, a better prognosis has been associated with the loss of the region 6q25.3 in patients with anaplastic ependymomas. The underexpression of nucleolin carries a favorable prognosis. They may be associated with neurofibromatosis type II.

Clinical Presentation

- **Intracranial ependymomas:** In children, they present primarily with enlarging head circumference and signs of increased ICP and hydrocephalus due to obstruction of the ventricular system. Additionally, the tumors often spread from the fourth ventricle to the spinal canal via the CSF, a pattern of metastasis termed drop metastases. Supratentorial ependymomas present with seizures, headaches, and focal neurological deficits related to their location. Infratentorial lesions can cause nausea, vomiting, ataxia, and nystagmus.

- **Spinal cord ependymomas:** These present with back pain, neck pain, and slowly progressive myelopathy.

- **Myxopapillary ependymomas:** These present with leg and/or back pain as well as cauda equina syndrome. They present in patients between the ages of 30 and 40 years.

Radiographic Appearance and Diagnosis

- **Intracranial ependymomas:** As seen in **Images 4.6A–4.6C**, ependymomas tend to fill the fourth ventricle and expand through the foramen of Luschka, Magendie, and the foramen magnum. They are heterogeneous, hyperintense on T2-weighted images and enhance avidly, but homogeneously with the administration of contrast. They can be difficult to distinguish from medulloblastomas, but calcification is present in nearly half of the ependymomas, making CTs a key part of the evaluation. Hemorrhage and cystic areas are more common as well.

- **Spinal cord ependymomas:** They are intramedullary tumors that expand the spinal cord. They are hyperintense on T2-weighted images with edema present in over 50% of the cases. About 25% of tumors are surrounded by a hypointense hemosiderin rim on T2-weighted images (the "cap" sign), though this is not entirely specific for ependymomas. There is avid enhancement with the administration of contrast. Histologically, most of these are clear-cell tumors.

- **Myxopapillary ependymomas:** They are intradural and extramedullary tumors. Larger tumors displace the nerve roots of the cauda equina, while smaller tumors engulf them. They are typically hyperintense on T2-weighted image, though may have surrounding hypointensity due to hemorrhage. There is avid and homogeneous enhancement with the addition of contrast.

Treatment

- Medical management includes steroids for treatment of peritumoral edema and anticonvulsants in patients with supratentorial ependymoma. Adjuvant therapy includes conventional radiation therapy, radiosurgery, or limited field fractionated external beam radiotherapy (LFFEBRT) and chemotherapy after gross total resection (GTR) of an intracranial WHO grade II ependymoma.

- Postoperative LFFEBRT is recommended for WHO grade II ependymomas, when subtotal resection is noted on postoperative MRI, and for grade III anaplastic ependymomas regardless of

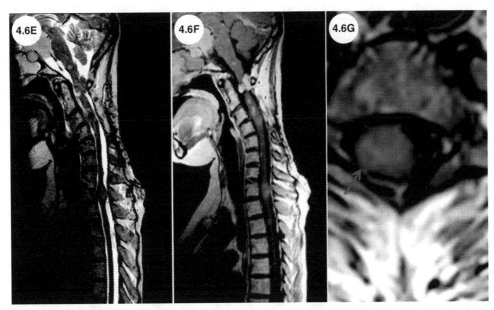

Images 4.6E–4.6G: Sagittal T2-weighted and postcontrast sagittal and axial T1-weighted images of the cervical spine demonstrate multiple homogeneously enhancing, intramedullary masses in the cervical spine in a patient with neurofibromatosis type II. The red arrow points to a dominant mass, which was found to be an ependymoma.

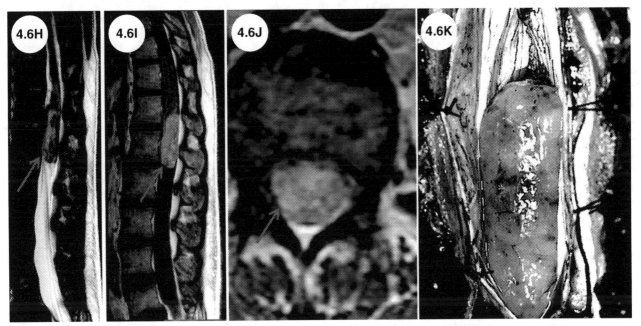

Images 4.6H–4.6J: Sagittal T2-weighted and postcontrast sagittal and axial T1-weighted images of the lumbar spine demonstrate a homogeneously enhancing mass (red arrows) in the lumbar spine compressing the cauda equina. **Image 4.6K:** Gross pathology of ependymoma (image credit The Armed Forces Institute of Pathology; Dr. E. Michael Scott).

extent of resection. Craniospinal radiation therapy is indicated regardless of grade or extent of resection if postoperative spinal MRI or lumbar puncture (LP) findings are positive.

- Children with posterior fossa lesions can be surgically accessed by a midline suboccipital approach; hydrocephalus can be managed with a perioperative external ventricular drain,

ventriculoperitoneal shunt, or, more rarely, third ventriculostomy.

- Filum terminale ependymoma should have gross total en bloc resection whenever possible.

- **Intracranial ependymomas:** Tumors that can be totally excised have an excellent prognosis, but due to their location this is often not possible. In

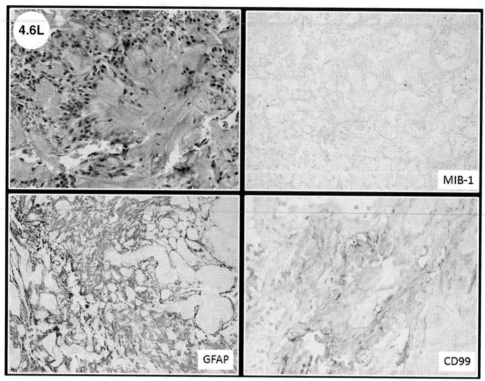

Image 4.6L: Myxopapillary ependymoma: H&E low power microscopic view shows relatively monomorphic cells arranged in perivascular pseudorosettes and abundant blue mucin. It is a slow-growing neoplasm (most commonly encountered at cauda equina) with a low MIB-1 proliferative index (top right). The glial tumor cells are immunoreactive for glial fibrillary acidic protein (GFAP) and sometimes CD99 (image courtesy of Dr. Seema Shroff, Fellow, Neuropathology, NYULMC).

these cases, adjuvant radiation therapy is given. The 5-year survival rate is up to 75%. Anaplastic ependymomas have a worse prognosis.

- **Spinal cord ependymomas:** They are generally benign tumors that grow slowly and do not infiltrate the cord, though they can rarely metastasize outside of the spinal cord. Complete surgical resection is possible in about 50% of cases and the 5-year survival rate approaches 90% and recurrence is uncommon. In cases of incomplete resection, the 5-year survival rate drops to 60%.

- **Myxopapillary ependymomas:** They can usually be excised completely with an excellent prognosis. Rarely, they may be spread throughout the CSF.

References

1. Cage TA, Clark AJ, Aranda D, et al. A systematic review of treatment outcomes in pediatric patients with intracranial ependymomas. *J Neurosurg Pediatr.* June 2013;11(6):673–681.
2. Joaquim AF, Ghizoni E, Tedeschi H. Myxopapillary ependymomas. *J Neurosurg Spine.* May 2014;20(5):598–599.
3. Benesch M, Weber-Mzell D, Gerber NU, et al. Ependymoma of the spinal cord in children and adolescents: a retrospective series from the HIT database. *J Neurosurg Pediatr.* August 2010;6(2):137–144.
4. Monoranu CM, Huang B, Zangen IL, et al. Correlation between 6q25.3 deletion status and survival in pediatric intracranial ependymomas. *Cancer Genet Cytogenet.* 2008;182:18–26.
5. Modena P, Lualdi E, Facchinetti F, et al. Identification of tumor-specific molecular signatures in intracranial ependymoma and association with clinical characteristics. *J Clin Oncol.* 2006;24:5223–5233.

4.7 Subependymoma

Case History

A 45-year-old man developed headaches. The following lesion was seen and was stable for many years.

Diagnosis: Subependymoma

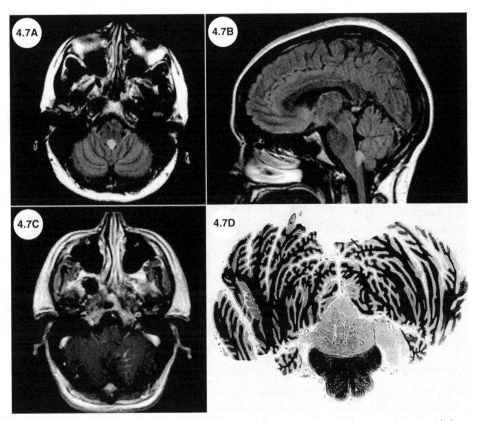

Images 4.7A and 4.7B: Axial and sagittal FLAIR images demonstrate a lesion consistent with low-grade neoplasm likely arising from the dorsal aspect of the medulla at the level of the pontomedullary junction.
Image 4.7C: Postcontrast axial T1-weighted image demonstrates that the lesions do not enhance. **Image 4.7D:** Gross pathology of subependymoma (image credit The Armed Forces Institute of Pathology).

Introduction

■ Subependymomas are benign, WHO grade I, slow-growing ependymal tumors.

■ They are most commonly found in the fourth ventricle and do not invade the brain or cerebellum. They can also arise in the lateral ventricles.

Clinical Presentation

■ They are often incidental findings, but can present in middle-aged patients with symptoms of increased ICP if they obstruct the ventricular system.

Radiographic Appearance and Diagnosis

■ MRI is the imaging modality of choice for visualizing these tumors. On T2-weighted images, they are hyperdense. Larger tumors may have a heterogeneous appearance. On T1-weighted images, they are hypointense or isointense to white matter. They rarely enhance with the administration of contrast.

Treatment

- Surgery is curative, but should be reserved only for symptomatic patients with hydrocephalus or in lesions that grow over time.

References

1. Bi Z, Ren X, Zhang J, Jia W. Clinical, radiological, and pathological features in 43 cases of intracranial subependymoma. *J Neurosurg*. January 2015;122(1):49–60.

2. Jain A, Amin AG, Jain P, et al. Subependymoma: clinical features and surgical outcomes. *Neurol Res*. September 2012;34(7):677–684.

4.8 | Medulloblastoma

Case History

A 9-year-old boy presented with severe headaches, gait unsteadiness, and blurry vision.

Diagnosis: Medulloblastoma

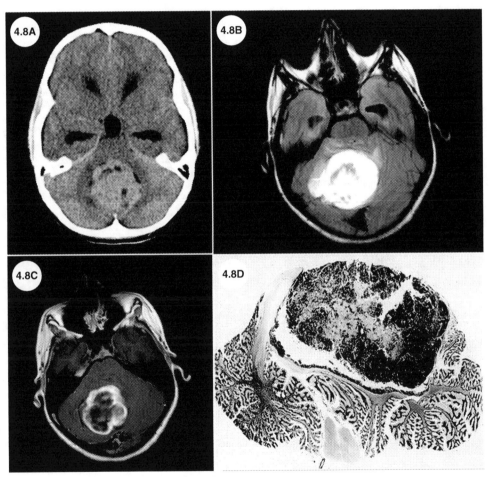

Images 4.8A–4.8C: Axial CT, FLAIR, and postcontrast T1-weighted images demonstrate a hyperintense and hyperdense midline cerebellar mass. It is growing within and expanding the fourth ventricle. There is evidence of secondary hydrocephalus. There is avid ring enhancement with central necrosis. **Image 4.8D:** Pathological demonstration of a medulloblastoma (image credit The Armed Forces Institute of Pathology).

Introduction

- Medulloblastomas are pediatric tumors that arise from the primitive neuroectoderm of the cerebellar vermis in the fourth ventricle.

- They comprise about 20% of all childhood brain tumors and 50% of cerebellar tumors. They occur more commonly in boys than girls with average age of diagnosis of 9 years. They account for less than 1% of tumors in adults.

Clinical Presentation

- They present with symptoms of increased ICP due to obstruction of the fourth ventricle or ataxia due to compression of the cerebellum. Symptoms emerge over the course of several weeks.

Radiographic Appearance and Diagnosis

- Medulloblastomas arise from the cerebellar vermis and project into the fourth ventricle. They are hyperdense on CT and 50% of cases have cystic necrosis. They are hyperintense on T2-weighted images and almost all have heterogeneous enhancement with contrast administration.

- They are most often confused with ependymomas. However, in contrast to ependymomas, which tend to grow within and enlarge the fourth ventricle, medulloblastomas compress the fourth ventricle, leading to hydrocephalus. Calcifications are present in about 10% of medulloblastomas, and in 50% of ependymomas. Occasionally, JPAs may arise from the midline of the cerebellum, but they more commonly arise from the cerebellar hemispheres.

Treatment

- Surgical resection is the mainstay of treatment, along with radiation and chemotherapy in select patients. They have the potential to spread through the CSF to other locations in the CNS. Imaging of the entire neuroaxis is important for this reason.

- In patients without metastases, favorable tumor markers, and in whom complete surgical resection is possible, the 5-year survival rate is about 80%. Survival drops to 20% in patients with metastases and incomplete surgical resection. Children younger than 3 years of age have a worse prognosis.

References

1. Gerber NU, Mynarek M, von Hoff K, Friedrich C, Resch A, Rutkowski S. Recent developments and current concepts in medulloblastoma. *Cancer Treat Rev.* April 2014;40(3):356–365.
2. Dhall G. Medulloblastoma. *J Child Neurol.* November 2009;24(11):1418–1430.
3. Martin AM, Raabe E, Eberhart C, Cohen KJ. Management of pediatric and adult patients with medulloblastoma. *Curr Treat Options Oncol.* December 2014;15(4):581–594.
4. Fruehwald-Pallamar J, Puchner SB, Rossi A, et al. Magnetic resonance imaging spectrum of medulloblastoma. *Neuroradiology.* June 2011;53(6):387–396.

4.9 | Ganglioglioma

Case History

A 12-year-old child presented with seizures.

Diagnosis: Ganglioglioma

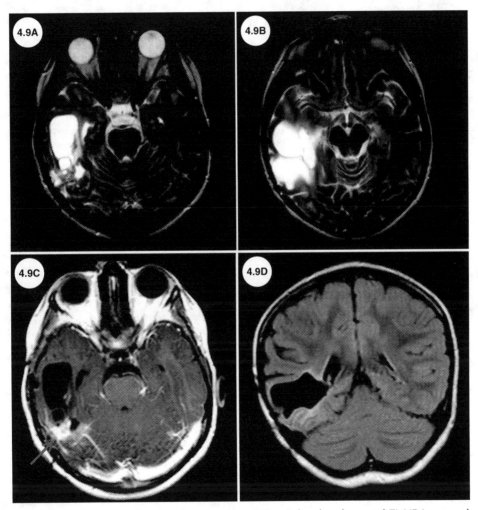

Images 4.9A–4.9D: Axial T2-weighted and postcontrast T1-weighted and coronal FLAIR images demonstrate a cystic mass in the right temporal lobe with a small enhancing nodule.

Introduction

■ Gangliogliomas are slow-growing tumors that most commonly occur in children and young adults. They are composed of a mixture of glial and neural elements. They are WHO grade I or II tumors, though they may undergo malignant transformation in rare cases. When the neural elements predominate, they are termed ganglioneuromas.

■ They account for 10% of primary CNS neoplasms in children.

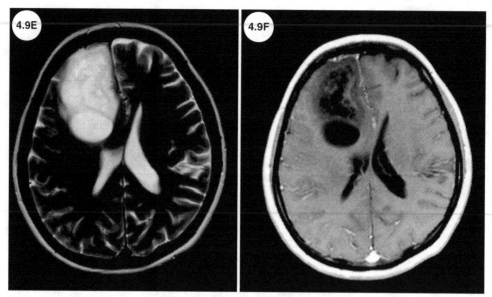

Images 4.9E and 4.9F: Axial T2-weighted and postcontrast T1-weighted images demonstrate a mass with a large cystic component in the right frontal lobe with minimal enhancement of the tumor wall (red arrow).

Clinical Presentation

■ They present with refractory seizures in children and young adults.

Radiographic Appearance and Diagnosis

■ They are generally cystic tumors with or without a solid component. They are isodense or hypointense on T1-weighted images and hyperintense on T2-weighted images. There is usually no peritumoral edema. There is a variable degree of enhancement with the administration of contrast and is present in about 50% of tumors. CT will reveal calcifications about 40% of the time, which helps differentiate these tumors from juvenile pilocytic astrocytomas and pleomorphic xanthoastrocytomas.

■ They are most commonly found in the temporal lobes, followed by the frontal, parietal, and occipital lobes. They may also be found near the hypothalamus and infratentorially.

Treatment

■ They are treated with surgery, and total resection is curative. Radiation and chemotherapy can be added in cases where the location of the tumor renders complete resection impossible or those with malignant histological features.

References

1. Karremann M, Pietsch T, Janssen G, Kramm CM, Wolff JE. Anaplastic ganglioglioma in children. *J Neurooncol.* April 2009;92(2):157–163.
2. Ogiwara H, Nordli DR, DiPatri AJ, Alden TD, Bowman RM, Tomita T. Pediatric epileptogenic gangliogliomas: seizure outcome and surgical results. *J Neurosurg Pediatr.* March 2010;5(3):271–276.
3. Hu WH, Ge M, Zhang K, Meng FG, Zhang JG. Seizure outcome with surgical management of epileptogenic ganglioglioma: a study of 55 patients. *Acta Neurochir (Wien).* May 2012;154(5):855–861.

4.10 | Hemangiopericytoma

Case History

A 45-year-old man presented with a seizure.

Diagnosis: Hemangiopericytoma

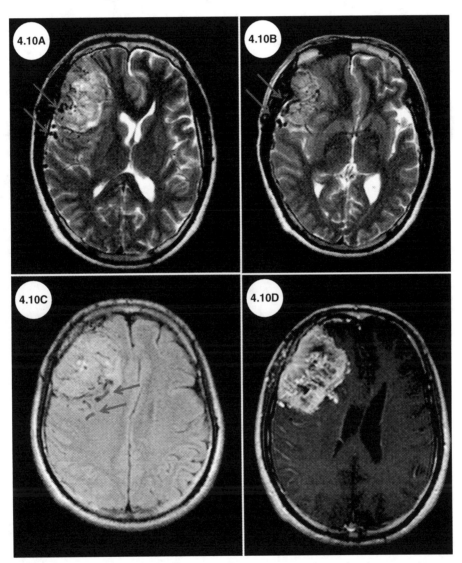

Images 4.10A–4.10D: Axial T2-weighted, FLAIR, and postcontrast T1-weighted images demonstrate an extraaxial mass in the right frontal lobe with mass effect. There are multiple flow voids (red arrows) due to blood vessels. There is prominent, but heterogeneous enhancement.

Introduction

- A hemangiopericytoma is an aggressive, extraaxial, meningeal WHO grade II tumor. They are highly vascularized mesenchymal neoplasms.

- More aggressive tumors, called anaplastic hemangiopericytomas, can metastasize outside the CNS and are WHO grade III.

- They are uncommon, accounting for less than 1% of all intracranial neoplasms.

Clinical Presentation

■ They present with headaches, seizures, and focal neurological deficits depending on the location of the tumor. They can be seen at any age, but are most common in patients aged 30 to 40 years.

Radiographic Appearance and Diagnosis

■ They are isointense to gray matter on T1-weighted images and isointense or hyperintense on T2-weighted images. Flow voids due to prominent vessels are commonly seen on T2-weighted images. There is avid, though heterogeneous enhancement with contrast administration. This contrasts with more homogeneous enhancement of meningiomas. Like meningiomas, hemangiopericytomas are adherent to the dura and a dural tail is often present.

■ In contrast to meningiomas, there is no calcification on CT, and though they may invade and erode the bone, there is no hyperostosis.

Treatment

■ They are treated with surgical resection, but commonly recur even with complete resection of the visible tumor mass. Chemotherapy and radiation are usually added for this reason. The median survival rate is 8 to 16 years and correlates with the degree of tumor resection.

References

1. Rutkowski MJ, Sughrue ME, Kane AJ, et al. Predictors of mortality following treatment of intracranial hemangiopericytoma. *J Neurosurg.* August 2010;113(2):333–339.
2. Rutkowski MJ, Jian BJ, Bloch O, et al. Intracranial hemangiopericytoma: clinical experience and treatment considerations in a modern series of 40 adult patients. *Cancer.* March 2012;118(6):1628–1636.
3. Melone AG, D'Elia A, Santoro F, et al. Intracranial hemangiopericytoma--our experience in 30 years: a series of 43 cases and review of the literature. *World Neurosurg.* March–April 2014;81(3–4):556–562.

4.11 | Pineoblastoma

Case History

An 11-year-old girl developed headaches and restricted upgaze.

Diagnosis: Pineoblastoma

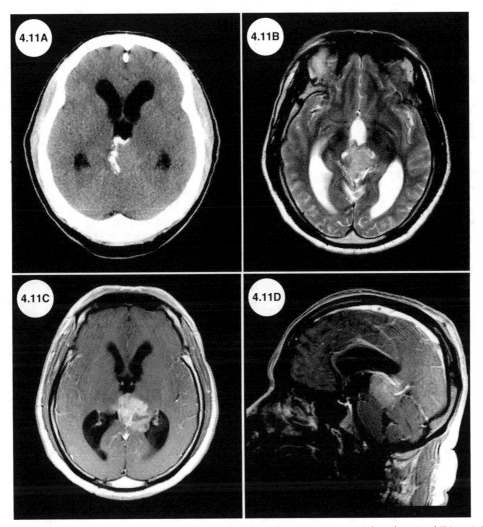

Images 4.11A–4.11D: Axial CT scan, axial T2-weighted, and postcontrast axial and sagittal T1-weighted images demonstrate a heterogeneously enhancing pineal mass with peripheral calcification.

Introduction

▓ Primary tumors of the pineal gland are known as pinealomas. The two forms are pineocytomas and pineoblastoma. Pineoblastomas are WHO grade IV tumors. They present before the age of 20, most commonly in children younger than 10.

Pineocytomas are less malignant tumors that do not occur in children.

▓ They comprise 15% to 20% of pineal region tumors. They occur equally in males and females, in contrast to germinomas, which are more common in males.

Clinical Presentation

■ Tumors of the pineal region present with the dorsal midbrain syndrome, disturbances in circadian rhythms, hydrocephalus, and headaches due to increased ICP.

■ Pineocytomas are often clinically silent until they affect the midbrain and cause visual symptoms (primarily paralysis of upgaze), though they can cause disruptions of circadian rhythms as well. Large tumors may directly invade surrounding brain tissue.

Radiographic Appearance and Diagnosis

■ Calcification around the periphery of the tumor is common. With germinomas, the calcification is more in the center of the tumor. On both T1-weighted and T2-weighted images, the tumor is isodense to the adjacent brain. Cystic areas are common. There is homogeneous enhancement with the addition of contrast. A biopsy is required to make the diagnosis.

■ Imaging of the entire neuroaxis to screen for metastases is required as they are found in nearly 50% of patients.

Treatment

■ Pineoblastomas are treated with surgical resection and radiation treatment to the entire brain and spinal cord to treat potential metastases. These tumors can spread throughout the subarachnoid space. The 5-year survival rate is only around 50%. Pineocytomas are treated with surgery alone. The 5-year survival rate is nearly 90%.

References

1. Farnia B, Allen PK, Brown PD, et al. Clinical outcomes and patterns of failure in pineoblastoma: a 30-year, single-institution retrospective review. *World Neurosurg.* December 2014;82(6):1232–1241.
2. Tate M, Sughrue ME, Rutkowski MJ, et al. The long-term postsurgical prognosis of patients with pineoblastoma. *Cancer.* January 2012;118(1):173–179.
3. Lee JY, Wakabayashi T, Yoshida J. Management and survival of pineoblastoma: an analysis of 34 adults from the brain tumor registry of Japan. *Neurol Med Chir (Tokyo).* March 2005;45(3):132–141.

4.12 | Germinoma of Pineal Gland

Case History

An 11-year-old boy developed headaches and "blurry vision" over the course of several months. On exam, the patient had difficulty looking upwards and his pupils did not react to accommodation, though they reacted to light.

Diagnosis: Pineal Germinoma

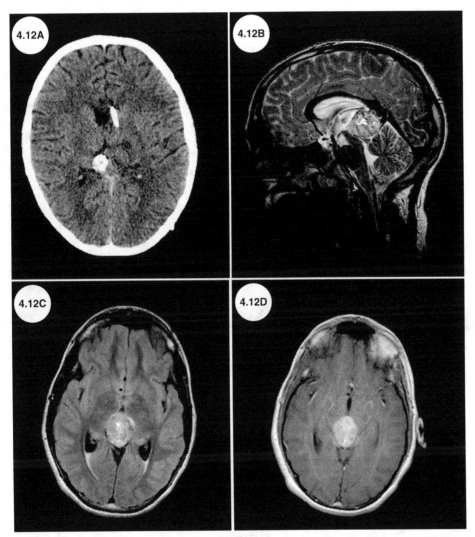

Images 4.12A–4.12D: Axial CT, sagittal T2-weighted, axial FLAIR, and postcontrast axial T1-weighted images demonstrate a partially, centrally calcified, homogeneously enhancing pineal mass. It has mixed signal intensity on T2-weighted image.

Introduction

■ The pineal gland is a midline endocrine gland that secretes melatonin, a hormone that regulates the sleep–wake cycle. It is stimulated by darkness and inhibited by light.

■ Pineal region neoplasms account for 1% of all CNS tumors. They can be subdivided into those that arise from the pineal gland itself (pineoblastomas and pineocytomas), and those of germ cell origin (germinomas, teratomas, embryonal carcinomas, and choriocarcinomas).

■ The majority of pineal tumors are of germ cell origin. Of these, germinomas comprise about 60% of all germ cell tumors and 40% of pineal regions masses overall. Germinomas are also frequently found in the suprasellar region and in the floor of the third ventricle.

■ Other germ cell tumors include teratomas, embryonal carcinomas, and choriocarcinomas. These are collectively referred to as nongerminous germ cell tumors. Teratomas are the next most frequent germ cell tumor.

Clinical Presentation

■ Tumors of the pineal region present with vertical gaze palsy, disturbances in circadian rhythms, hydrocephalus, and headaches due to increased ICP, if there is obstruction of the cerebral aqueduct,

and occasionally thrombosis of the vein of Galen, which courses over the pineal gland.

■ The dorsal midbrain syndrome (Parinaud's syndrome) is a combination of eye movement and pupil dysfunction. It is commonly seen due to pineal tumors. Its core features are:

▫ Severe restriction of upgaze with preservation of downward gaze. In the primary position, the eyes are often deviated downward and inward, due to an inability to abduct the eyes (the sun-setting sign).

▫ Accommodative paresis, where patients' pupils do not react to light, but constrict during accommodation. This is also termed pupillary light-near dissociation and when due to neurosyphilis, is referred to as Argyll Robertson pupils.

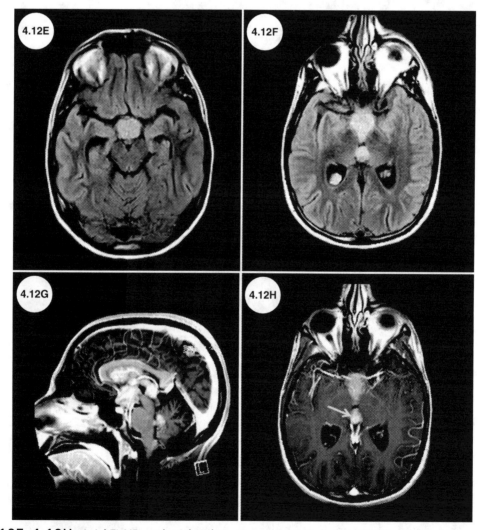

Images 4.12E–4.12H: Axial FLAIR, and axial and postcontrast sagittal and axial T1-weighted images demonstrate multifocal enhancing masses of the pituitary stalk (red arrows), pineal gland (yellow arrows), and within the ventricular system in a patient with a germinoma.

▨   Convergence–retraction nystagmus.

▨   Eyelid retraction (Collier's sign).

■ Involvement of the pituitary stalk leads most commonly to diabetes insipidus, hypopituitarism, and visual disturbances due to involvement of the optic chiasm.

■ Germinomas of the pineal region are more common in males and in people of Asian descent. They present in children between the ages of 10 and 13, with only 10% of patients presenting after the age of 20.

Radiographic Appearance and Diagnosis

■ On CT, germinomas are hyperdense due to increased cellularity. The center of the tumor frequently calcifies, which is always pathological in children under 6 and a normal finding in only 10% of children under the age of 12. On both T1-weighted and T2-weighted images, they are either isointense or hyperintense compared to the brain. Cystic components are seen in 50% of cases. They enhance avidly and homogeneously with the addition of contrast. Germinomas frequently occur in the pineal region and within the ventricular system as well.

■ In addition to its imaging characteristics, germinomas may have serum markers such as elevated human chorionic gonadotropin (HCG) and placental alkaline phosphatase. A biopsy is required to make the diagnosis.

■ Teratomas frequently contain bone, fat, calcium, and sebaceum leading to a pattern of irregular enhancement, with a cystic component, in contrast

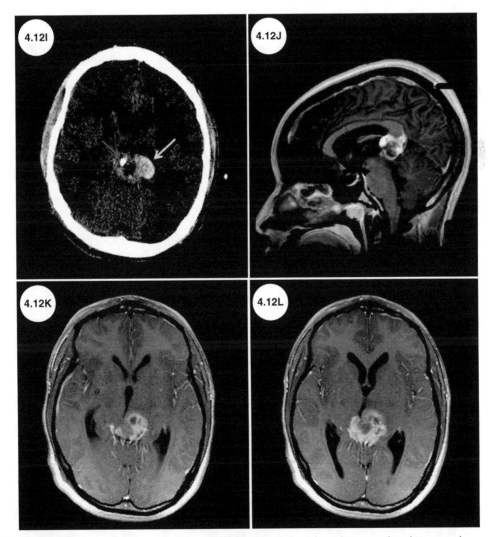

Images 4.12I–4.12L: Axial CT image and postcontrast sagittal and axial T1-weighted images demonstrate a hyperdense, centrally calcified (red arrow) and hemorrhagic (yellow arrow), homogeneously enhancing mass in the pineal region. This was found to be a choriocarcinoma on biopsy.

to germinomas, which enhance homogeneously. The serum commonly contains β-human chorionic gonadotropin (β-hCG) and alpha-fetoprotein.

■ Choriocarcinomas are commonly hemorrhagic, and the serum contains β-hCG and placental lactogen.

Treatment

■ Germinomas respond well to chemotherapy and radiotherapy, with surgery playing a secondary role. Up to 90% of tumors can be cured using radiotherapy. Spreading of tumor cells throughout the CSF is a frequent occurrence, though this does not influence the long-term prognosis.

■ Teratomas and choriocarcinomas have a worse prognosis compared to germinomas.

References

1. Salzman KL, Rojiani AM, Buatti J, et al. Primary intracranial germ cell tumors: clinicopathologic review of 32 cases. *Pediatr Pathol Lab Med.* September–October 1997;17(5): 713–727.
2. Westphal M, Emami P. Pineal lesions: a multidisciplinary challenge. *Adv Tech Stand Neurosurg.* 2015;42:79–102.
3. Dufour C, Guerrini-Rousseau L, Grill J. Central nervous system germ cell tumors: an update. *Curr Opin Oncol.* November 2014;26(6):622–626.
4. Echevarría ME, Fangusaro J, Goldman S. Pediatric central nervous system germ cell tumors: a review. *Oncologist.* June 2008;13(6):690–699.

4.13 | Central Neurocytoma

Case History

A 34-year-old woman presented with severe headaches for the past several months. They are accompanied by blurry vision and are much worse during mornings.

Diagnosis: Central Neurocytoma

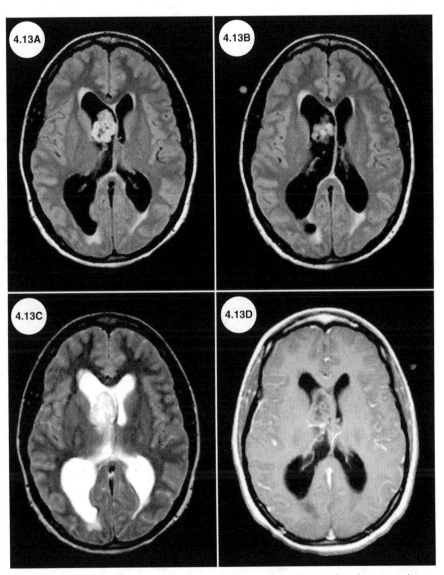

Images 4.13A–4.13D: Axial FLAIR, T2-weighted, and postcontrast T1-weighted images demonstrate a hyperintense, though cystic, moderately enhancing mass in the right frontal horn.

Introduction

■ Central neurocytomas typically develop in the lateral ventricles, next to the septum pellucidum in the region of the foramen of Monro.

■ They are generally benign, although aggressive variants do exist. For this reason, they are WHO grade II tumors.

■ They are rare and represent less than 0.5% of intracranial tumors.

Clinical Presentation

■ Patients present with signs of increased ICP, namely headache, nausea, vomiting, and blurry vision, especially when there is obstruction of the foramen of Monro.

■ Symptoms usually develop over the course of several months. Tumors extending outside the ventricular system may present with seizures. In rare cases, they may present with hemorrhage.

■ Patients typically present between the ages of 20 and 40. These tumors are more common in people of Asian descent.

Radiographic Appearance and Diagnosis

■ Tumors usually have both solid and cystic components. The solid component is typically isointense or hyperintense to gray matter on T2-weighted images. Flow voids may be seen. There is a variable degree of enhancement with the addition of contrast, ranging from intense enhancement to none at all. Punctate calcification is common and is best visualized on CT scan.

■ **Table 4.13.1** enlists other intraventricular tumors, which can be mistaken for central neurocytomas.

■ On histological examination, central neurocytomas have neuronal features characterized by monotonous bland cells with minimal cytoplasm, often an empty-appearing "halo" resembling oligodendroglioma, salt and pepper fine chromatin, embedded in eosinophilic fibrillar matrix with rare Homer Wright rosettes and ganglion cells. These tumors typically lack necrosis, infiltrating margin, endothelial proliferation, and

Table 4.13.1 Differential Diagnosis of Central Neurocytomas

Ependymoma
Subependymoma
Choroid plexus papilloma
Intraventricular meningioma
Intraventricular metastasis
Oligodendroglioma

mitotic figures but rarely may show necrosis and mitotic figures. The cells are positive for synaptophysin, Neu-N, and neuron specific enolase immunostains.

Treatment

■ Surgical resection is usually curative and a 5-year survival rate is over 80%. They recur 20% of the time and can be treated with adjuvant chemotherapy and radiotherapy.

References

1. Donoho D, Zada G. Imaging of central neurocytomas. *Neurosurg Clin N Am.* January 2015;26(1):11–19.
2. Patel DM, Schmidt RF, Liu JK. Update on the diagnosis, pathogenesis, and treatment strategies for central neurocytoma. *J Clin Neurosci.* September 2013;20(9):1193–1199.
3. Monaco EA 3rd, Niranjan A, Lunsford LD. The management of central neurocytoma: radiosurgery. *Neurosurg Clin N Am.* January 2015;26(1):37–44.
4. Garcia RM, Ivan ME, Oh T, Barani I, Parsa AT. Intraventricular neurocytomas: a systematic review of stereotactic radiosurgery and fractionated conventional radiotherapy for residual or recurrent tumors. *Clin Neurol Neurosurg.* February 2014;117:55–64.

4.14 Hypothalamic Hamartoma

Case History

A 5-year-old boy presented with gelastic seizures and behavioral problems.

Diagnosis: Hypothalamic Hamartoma

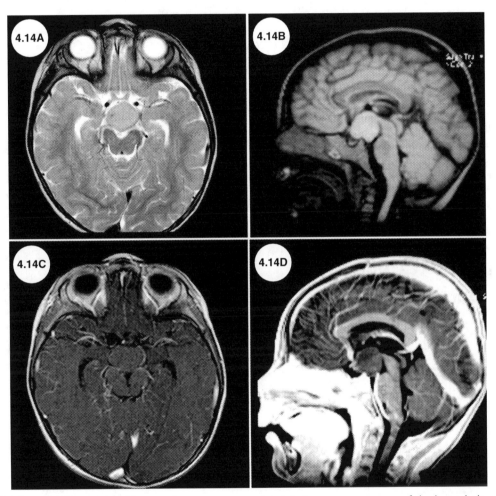

Image 4.14A: Axial T2-weighted image demonstrates a round, heterogeneous mass of the hypothalamus that is isointense to the gray matter. The optic tracts are splayed and the optic chiasm is anteriorly displaced. The floor of the third ventricle is elevated. The interpeduncular fossa shows displacement of the cerebral peduncles laterally without edema. **Images 4.14B–4.14D:** Sagittal and axial T1-weighted images with and without contrast demonstrate the mass elevating the floor of the third ventricle. The lesion does not enhance with the administration of contrast.

Introduction

■ Hypothalamic hamartomas (HH) are rare, benign lesions that are likely congenital in nature. They are composed of ganglion cells arranged singly and in clusters against a neurofibrillary background.

■ They arise from the tuber cinereum, which consists of neuronal tissue in an ectopic location. Most of these lesions occur in the hypothalamus. Other locations may be the subcortical cerebral cortex and periventricular region.

Clinical Presentation

■ The age of clinical presentation can vary from neonates to early childhood, though occasionally patients do not present until adulthood. There are two types of HH, sessile and pedunculated.

■ Sessile tumors have a broad-based attachment to the hypothalamus and are typically associated with gelastic seizures. Gelastic seizures are characterized by fits of uncontrolled laughter. They last less than 30 seconds, though they are often only a few seconds long, and consciousness may not be impaired. Note that gelastic seizures can also originate from temporal and mesial frontal regions. Other seizure types such as atonic, tonic, generalized tonic–clonic seizures, or focal onset seizures may also occur.

■ The pedunculated tumors are associated with precocious puberty, which results from the capacity of ganglion cells to secrete hypothalamic hormones in an aberrant fashion. They can also present with visual loss due to mass effect on the optic chiasm. Patients may have depression, behavioral abnormalities, and cognitive impairment.

Radiographic Appearance and Diagnosis

■ MRI is the imaging modality of choice to evaluate suspected HHs. On all imaging modalities, they are isodense to the cortex and do not enhance with the administration of contrast. They do not grow on serial imaging. These lesions may be quite large at presentation and may be associated with other congenital or neuronal migration abnormalities.

Treatment

■ Patients with precocious puberty can be treated with hormonal suppression therapy, such as leuprolide, a luteinizing hormone receptor agonist. This may also help control the seizures.

■ There are various surgical options: endoscopy, microsurgery, stereotactic radiosurgery (SRS), and stereotactic laser ablation. Many patients have been treated with multimodality staged strategy as there are pros and cons of different surgical techniques.

References

1. Pati S, Sollman M, Fife TD, Ng YT. Diagnosis and management of epilepsy associated with hypothalamic hamartoma: an evidence-based systematic review. *J Child Neurol.* July 2013;28(7):909–916.
2. Mittal S, Mittal M, Montes JL, Farmer JP, Andermann F. Hypothalamic hamartomas. Part 1. Clinical, neuroimaging, and neurophysiological characteristics. *Neurosurg Focus.* June 2013;34(6):E6.
3. Striano S, Santulli L, Ianniciello M, Ferretti M, Romanelli P, Striano P. The gelastic seizures-hypothalamic hamartoma syndrome: facts, hypotheses, and perspectives. *Epilepsy Behav.* May 2012;24(1):7–13.
4. Fenoglio KA, Wu J, Kim do Y, et al. Hypothalamic hamartoma: basic mechanisms of intrinsic epileptogenesis. *Semin Pediatr Neurol.* 2007;14(2):51–59.
5. Kameyama S, Shirozu H, Masuda H, Ito Y, Sonoda M, Akazawa K. MRI-guided stereotactic radiofrequency thermocoagulation for 100 hypothalamic hamartomas. *J Neurosurg.* May 2016;124(5):1503–1512.

4.15 | Clivus Chordoma

Case History

A 21-year-old female presented with dizziness and dysphagia over the course of several months. On exam, she had dysarthria and brisk reflexes in all four extremities.

Diagnosis: Clivus Chordoma

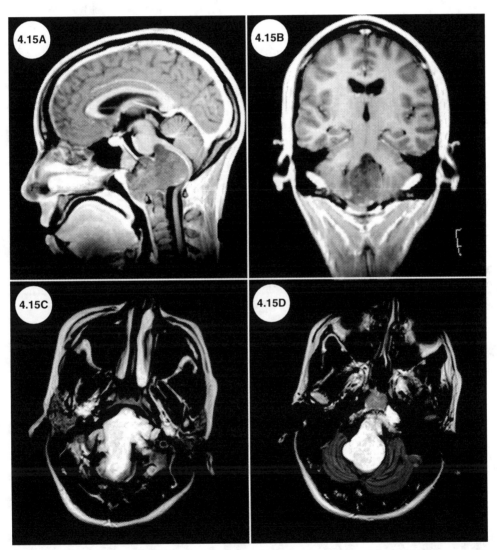

Images 4.15A–4.15D: Postcontrast sagittal and coronal T1-weighted and axial FLAIR images demonstrate an enormous, hyperintense mass arising from the clivus with significant mass effect on the medulla.

Introduction

- Chordomas are tumors that arise from remnants of the notochord, an embryologic structure that eventually forms part of the spinal column that did not appropriately form bone.

- They are considered benign tumors, though they are often locally invasive causing bone destruction. They can metastasize in about 10% of patients and are then called chondrosarcomas.

- Chordomas are slow-growing tumors that most commonly involve the midline of the axial skeleton. About 30% to 40% involve the base of the skull (clivus in the region of the spheno-occipital synchondrosis), approximately 49% involve the sacrum, and ~15% involve the vertebral column, usually the cervical spine.

■ They arise from the bone and are extraaxial tumors and represent less than 1% of intracranial tumors.

■ Chordomas: This neoplasm is composed of hepatoid trabeculae of epithelioid cells with eosinophilic and bubbly cytoplasm in a myxoid matrix. The bubbly cells are called **physaliphorous cells.**

■ **Ecchordosis physaliphora** are small, well-circumscribed gelatinous masses/lesions adherent to the brainstem, which behave like benign developmental remnants of notochord and histologically resembles a chordoma.

■ The other two chondroid CNS tumors are chordoid glioma of the third ventricle and chordoid meningioma.

■ There are three types of chordomas, which can be differentiated based on histological markers. These are:

1. **Conventional:** There is absence of cartilaginous or additional mesenchymal components. These are keratin positive, epithelial membrane antigen (EMA) positive, S100 positive, and carcinoembryonic antigen (CEA) negative.

2. **Chondroid:** They have chordomatous and chondromatous features, have a predilection for the spheno-occipital region, and account for 5% to 15% of all chordomas.

Chondrosarcoma would be S100 positive, keratin negative, and EMA negative.

3. **Dedifferentiated:** Sarcomatous transformation can occur in 2% to 8% of chordomas and are typically keratin positive, EMA positive, CEA positive, and usually S100 negative.

Clinical Presentation

■ Clival chordomas usually present in young adults (ages 20–40) with pain from bone destruction, cranial neuropathies (especially if there is involvement of the cavernous sinuses), and mass effect on the brainstem.

■ Sacrococcygeal chordomas present in older patients with back pain that is worse when seated. They may also present with cauda equina syndrome, which includes saddle anesthesia, and bladder and/or bowel dysfunction.

Radiographic Appearance and Diagnosis

■ Clivus chordomas are very hyperintense on T2-weighted images and isointense on T1-weighted images. They enhance heterogeneously with the administration of contrast. A classic finding is an indentation of the pons, called the "thumb sign."

■ Local bone destruction is best appreciated on CT. The tumor is typically isodense or slightly hyperdense. Areas of hemorrhage or calcification may be seen.

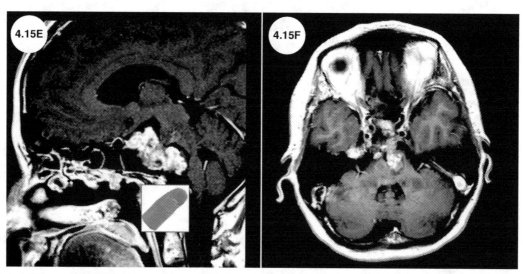

Images 4.15E and 4.15F: Postcontrast sagittal and axial T1-weighted images demonstrate a heterogeneously enhancing mass indenting the pons, the "thumb sign."

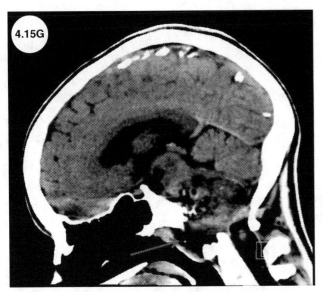

Image 4.15G: Reformatted sagittal CT image demonstrates destruction of the clivus (red arrow) in a patient with a clivus chordoma.

Treatment

■ The best results in the treatment of chordomas of the skull base are reported when using surgery and adjuvant high-dose proton therapy. The surgical techniques for margin-free, en bloc tumor resection have been proven to be effective in terms of local control and long-term prognosis for chordomas occurring in the thoracic and lumbar spine. They have a very high recurrence rate with slightly less than half of the patients surviving 10 years.

■ Chordomas are not sensitive to chemotherapy, similar to many other low-grade malignancies. Accordingly, chemotherapy response has been reported in patients with high-grade dedifferentiated chordomas, which represent less than 5% of all chordomas. Cytotoxic chemotherapy has virtually no role in this disease; however, molecularly targeted therapy is showing significant promise and is an area of great potential.

References

1. Neelakantan A, Rana AK. Benign and malignant diseases of the clivus. *Clin Radiol.* December 2014;69(12):1295–1303.
2. Radner G, Dross PE. Clivus chordoma. *Del Med J.* September 1997;69(9):467–469.
3. Géhanne C, Delpierre I, Damry N, Devroede B, Brihaye P, Christophe C. Skull base chordoma: CT and MRI features. *JBR-BTR.* November–December 2005;88(6):325–327.

4.16 Corpus Callosum Lipoma

Case History

A 23-year-old woman presented with a seizure.

Diagnosis: Pericallosal Lipoma

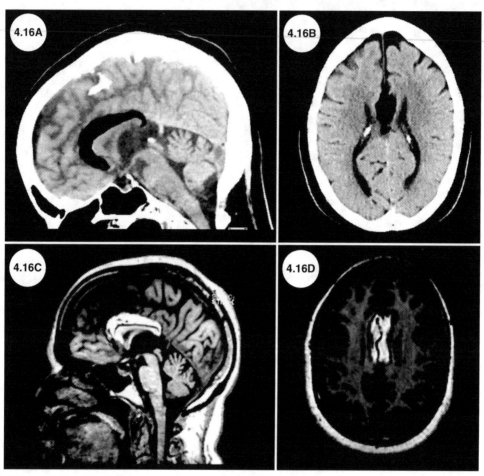

Images 4.16A and 4.16B: Sagittal and axial CT images demonstrate a hypodense mass consistent with a corpus callosum lipoma. **Images 4.16C and 4.16D:** Noncontrast sagittal and axial T1-weighted images demonstrate a pericallosal, hyperintense mass consistent with a corpus callosum lipoma.

Introduction

■ **Pericallosal lipomas** are congenital, adipose lesions of the interhemispheric fissure that trace the trajectory of the corpus callosum, which is often hypoplastic.

■ They are rare, accounting for less than 1% of all intracranial neoplasms.

Clinical Presentation

■ Seizures are the most common clinical manifestation. There is a wide range in their severity. In older adults, they are often incidental findings.

Radiographic Appearance and Diagnosis

■ The lesion follows fat on all sequences. On CTs, it is hypodense, though there may be some calcifications. On T1-weighted images, they are hyperintense, and there is no enhancement with the administration of contrast.

■ There are two distinct varieties: tubulonodular and curvilinear. Tubulonodular lipomas are thicker (>2 cm), located more anteriorly, and are round or lobulated. They are more common, and patients may have facial abnormalities. The corpus callosum is markedly dysmorphic. Curvilinear lipomas are thinner (<1 cm), located posteriorly, and follow the corpus callosum rather than replace it.

Treatment

■ Antiepileptic medication is the mainstay of treatment. There is no role for surgery.

References

1. Karakaş E, Doğan MS, Çullu N, Kocatürk M, et al. Intracranial lipomas: clinical and imaging findings. *Clin Ter.* 2014;165(2):e134–e138.
2. Loddenkemper T, Morris HH, Diehl B, Lachhwani DK. Intracranial lipomas and epilepsy. *J Neurol.* 2006;253:590–593.

| 4.17 | Meningioma |

Case History

A 65-year-old woman presented with personality changes, paranoia, and confusion over the course of several months. On exam, she had mild bilateral papilledema and weakness of her legs.

Diagnosis: Meningiomas

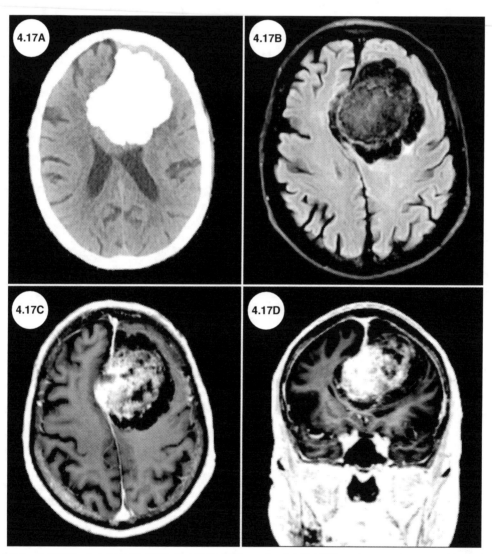

Images 4.17A–4.17D: Axial CT (4.17A), FLAIR (4.17B), and axial (4.17C) and coronal T1-weighted images (4.17D) post-Gd demonstrate a calcified extraaxial mass in the interhemispheric fissure, which is isointense to gray matter and demonstrates near homogeneous enhancement, consistent with a meningioma.

Introduction

- Meningiomas are slow-growing, generally benign tumors that comprise 20% of all primary CNS neoplasms. They are the most common benign, extraaxial, intracranial neoplasm and are second only to gliomas in frequency.

- They are believed to arise from cells of the arachnoid and they are firmly adherent to the dura. Only rarely do they invade the brain and surrounding bone.

- They occur most commonly in middle-aged women; multiple meningiomas may occur in patients with neurofibromatosis II. Prior irradiation, often for other cancers, is the only known environmental risk factor.

- There are a number of histological subtypes of meningiomas, the vast majority of which are WHO grade I tumors. Atypical meningiomas are WHO grade II, while anaplastic or malignant meningiomas are WHO grade III tumors that exhibit a high mitotic index (**Table 4.17.1**). Anaplastic meningiomas are very rare, accounting for less than 1% of tumors. The major difference between the 2007 and 2000 WHO grading versions is that brain invasion in an otherwise grade I meningioma is a criterion for classification as grade II.

Table 4.17.1 Subtypes and WHO Grading of Meningiomas

WHO Grading	Types
Grade I	Meningothelial, fibrous, transitional, psammomatous, angiomatous, microcystic, secretory, lymphoplasmacyte-rich, metaplastic
Grade II	Atypical, clear cell, chordoid
Grade III	Anaplastic, papillary, rhabdoid

Clinical Presentation

- They are extraaxial tumors that produce symptoms by compressing nervous tissue externally. They can present with headaches, seizures, and focal neurological findings depending on the location of the tumor.

- They can arise anywhere along the neuraxis. Over 95% are supratentorial in location. Locations include: the falx cerebri (25%), cerebral convexities (20%), cerebellopontine angle (CPA),

the sphenoid wing (20%), the suprasellar region (10%), the planum sphenoidale/olfactory groove (10%), the posterior fossa (CPA tentorium cerebelli 10%), intraventricular (2%), the orbit, and the spinal cord. Meningiomas are slow-growing tumors; these can be asymptomatic or symptomatic; symptoms may vary according to their location (**Table 4.17.2**).

Table 4.17.2 Common Locations and Symptomatology of Meningiomas

Location	Symptoms
Parasellar or subfrontal	Foster Kennedy syndrome
Intraventricular	Dizziness, headache or altered sensorium due to obstructive hydrocephalus
Convexity	Seizures, headache, neurological deficits
Falx and parasagittal	Personality changes, vision, headache, vision changes, arm or leg weakness
Olfactory groove	Anosmia, personality or vision changes
Intraorbital	Loss of vision
Cerebellopontine angle	Sensorineural hearing loss
Petroclival	Trigeminal neuralgia
Foramen magnum	Headache, difficulty walking
Spinal	Back pain, loss of sensation, paraparesis or paralysis of legs

- Although the vast majority are benign, even grade I meningiomas sometimes invade blood vessels and may metastasize, most commonly to the lungs.

Radiographic Appearance and Diagnosis

- On CT, they are hyperdense to the brain. They are highly calcified about 25% of the time. Edema is common and is hypodense on CT.

- Meningiomas only very rarely invade the brain, but often invade and remodel the skull. This remodeling or secondary excessive growth of bone is termed hyperostosis. This is best seen with CT scans. Some meningiomas are associated with cyst formation.

- On MRI, they are typically isointense to the brain T1-weighted image and isointense or hyperintense on T2-weighted image. They may be

(*text continues on page 169*)

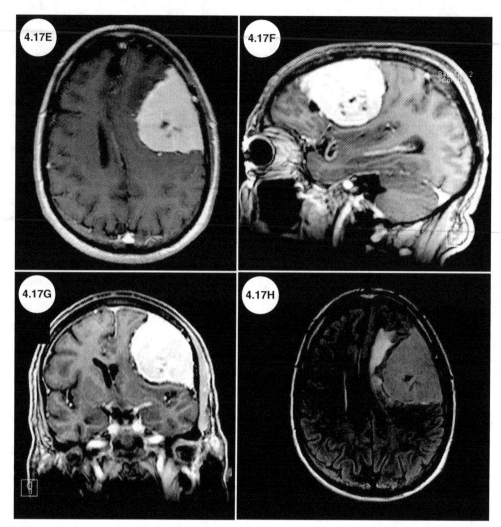

Images 4.17E–4.17G: Postcontrast axial, sagittal, and coronal T1-weighted images demonstrate a meningioma arising from the cerebral convexity on the left with mass effect. **Image 4.17H:** Axial FLAIR image demonstrates peritumoral edema.

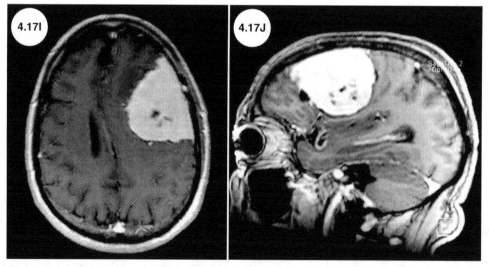

Images 4.17I–4.17K: Axial and coronal T2-weighted and postcontrast T1-weighted images demonstrate a large meningioma arising from the sphenoid wing with significant mass effect on the left temporal lobe and lateral ventricle. **Image 4.17L:** Gross pathology of a sphenoid wing meningioma. (*continued*)

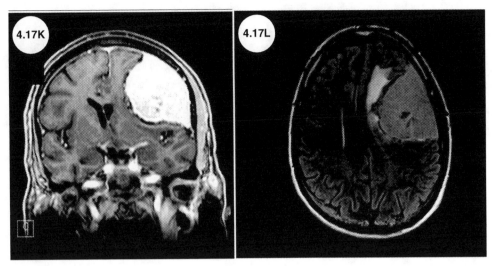

Images 4.17I–4.17K: (*continued*)

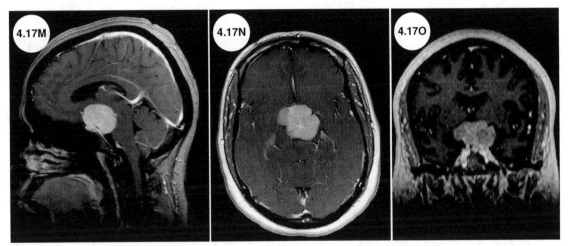

Images 4.17M–4.17O: Postcontrast sagittal, axial, and coronal T1-weighted images demonstrate a homogeneous enhancing mass in the suprasellar region.

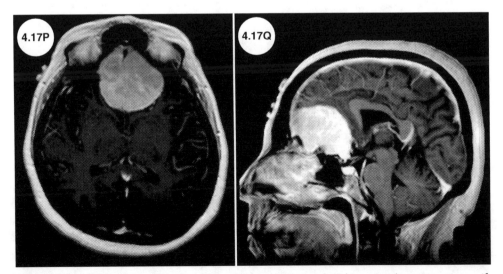

Images 4.17P and 4.17Q: Postcontrast axial and sagittal T1-weighted images demonstrate a uniformly enhancing meningioma arising from the planum sphenoidale.

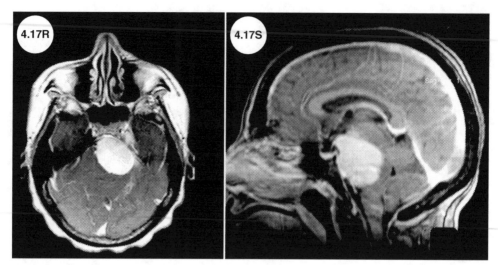

Images 4.17R and 4.17S: Postcontrast axial and sagittal T1-weighted images demonstrate a uniformly enhancing meningioma in the cerebellopontine angle.

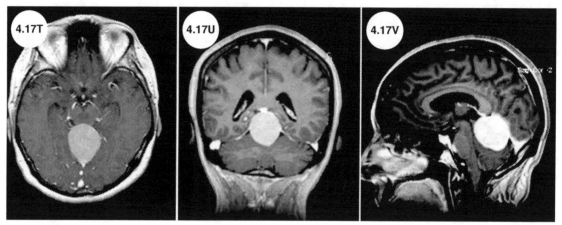

Images 4.17T–4.17V: Postcontrast axial, coronal, and sagittal T1-weighted images demonstrate a meningioma arising from the incisure of the tentorium cerebelli with downward mass effect on the cerebellum.

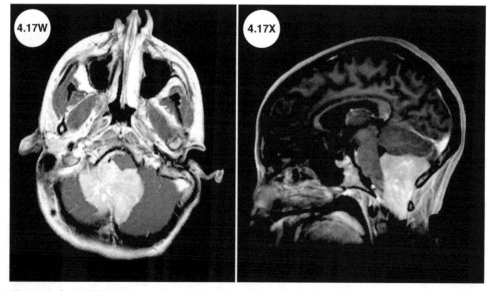

Images 4.17W and 4.17X: Postcontrast axial and sagittal T1-weighted images demonstrate an enhancing mass in the fourth ventricle with significant mass effect on the lower brainstem and cerebellum.

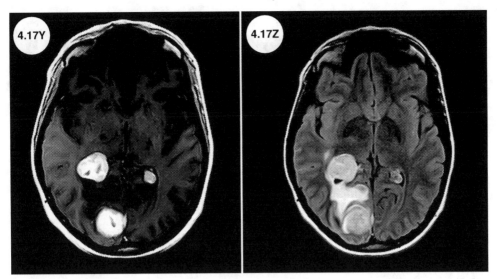

Images 4.17Y and 4.17Z: Postcontrast axial T1-weighted and FLAIR images demonstrate an enhancing mass in the occipital horn of the lateral ventricle and falx cerebri over the occipital lobe. There is mass effect and edema. An additional mass is seen arising from the posteior falx cerebri.

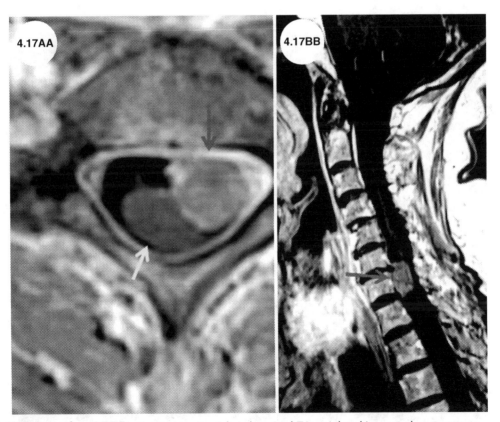

Images 4.17AA and 4.17BB: Postcontrast axial and sagittal T1-weighted images demonstrate a well-circumscribed, extramedullar meningioma (red arrows) with compression of the spinal cord (yellow arrow).

associated with significant amounts of edema, and this is sometimes, though not always, an indicator of a more aggressive tumor. They enhance avidly and homogeneously with the administration of contrast. A characteristic enhancement appearance is the "sunburst" or "spoke wheel" pattern of vasculature created by arterial feeders that radiate into the center of the tumor.

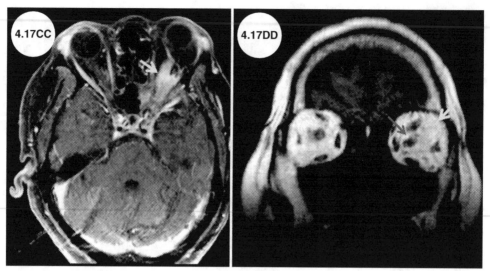

Images 4.17CC and 4.17DD: Postcontrast axial and coronal T1-weighted images demonstrate a well-demarcated enhancing mass superiorly located at the left orbital apex (yellow arrows). The superior rectus muscle is displaced inferiorly and medially as is the optic nerve (red arrow). These tumors may be difficult to differentiate from optic nerve gliomas.

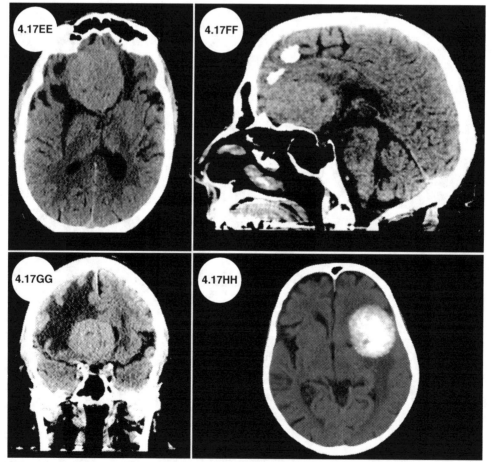

Images 4.17EE–4.17GG: Axial, sagittal, and coronal CT images demonstrate a hyperdense meningioma arising from the planum sphenoidale. **Image 4.17HH:** Axial CT image from a different patient scan shows a heavily calcified meningioma arising from the left sphenoid wing.

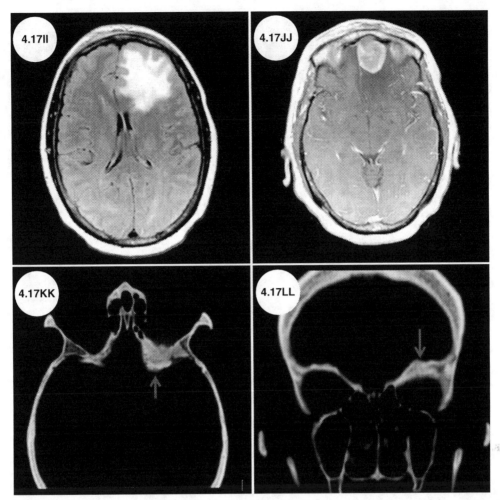

Images 4.17II and 4.17JJ: Axial FLAIR and postcontrast T1-weighted images demonstrate a left subfrontal meningioma with surrounding edema. **Images 4.17KK and 4.17LL:** Axial and coronal CT images demonstrate hyperostosis (red arrows) of the bone in a patient with a meningioma.

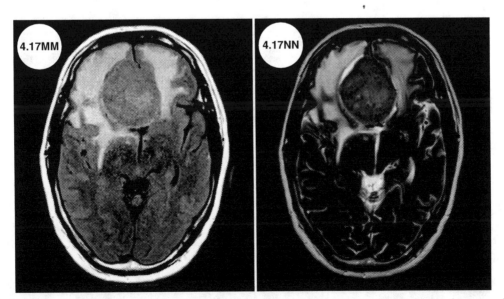

Images 4.17MM–4.17PP: Axial FLAIR, T2-weighted, and pre- and postcontrast T1-weighted images demonstrate the characteristic findings of a meningioma. It is hyperintense on T2-weighted images with edema. It is isointense on T1-weighted images with "sunburst" or "spoke wheel" enhancement on postcontrast images. (*continued*)

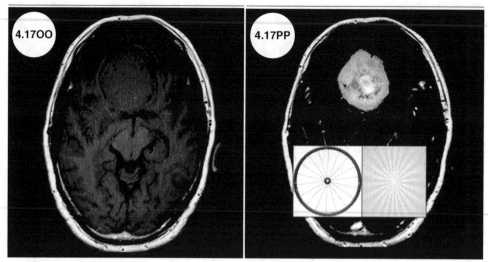

Images 4.17MM–4.17PP: (*continued*)

- A characteristic finding is known as a **dural tail**. This refers to enhancement of the meninges flanking the bulk of the tumor, though this finding is seen in other neoplasms as well.

- In contrast to lower grade meningiomas, more aggressive tumors may display a heterogeneous pattern of enhancement and significant peritumoral edema, though such edema may occur with benign subtypes as well. They may invade the bone and the underlying brain.

- Meningiomas are highly vascular tumors and cerebral angiograms are often performed prior to an operation to better define the vasculature surrounding the meningioma. On angiograms the tumor blush is seen in the arterial phase and remains in the venous phase. Since the finding comes early and stays late, this is called the "mother-in-law" sign.

- Pathologically, meningiomas occur in several types including meningothelial (meningeal cells with indistinct cell borders arranged in whorls), angiomatous, microcystic, and fibrous. These patterns do not correlate with an aggressive phenotype and are generally seen in WHO grade I meningiomas.

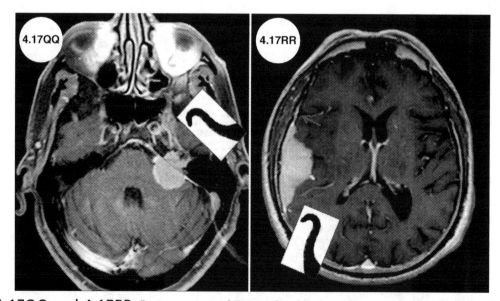

Images 4.17QQ and 4.17RR: Postcontrast axial T1-weighted images demonstrate homogeneously enhancing extraaxial masses in the left cerebellopontine angle and along the right cerebral convexity. In both cases, a characteristic dural tail is seen (red arrows).

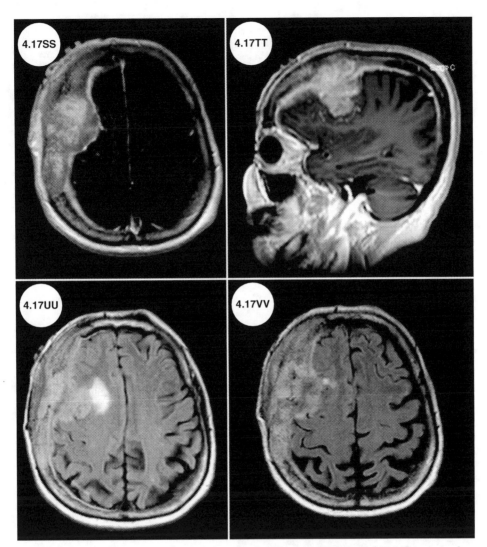

Images 4.17SS–4.17VV: Postcontrast axial and sagittal T1-weighted and axial FLAIR images demonstrate a right frontal convexity meningioma with extensive bony invasion and associated calvarial expansion. The margins of the meningioma with the frontal lobe brain tissue are ill-defined suggesting brain invasion.

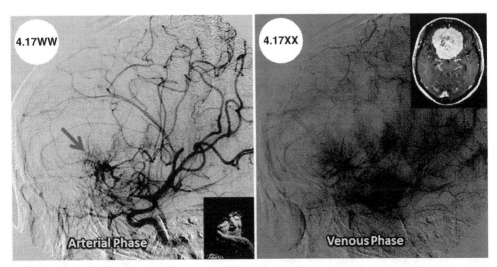

Images 4.17WW and 4.17XX: Catheter angiography reveals tumor blush (red arrows), in both the arterial and venous phases, the "mother-in-law" sign. Inset, an axial postcontrast T1-weighted image shows a large falx meningioma.

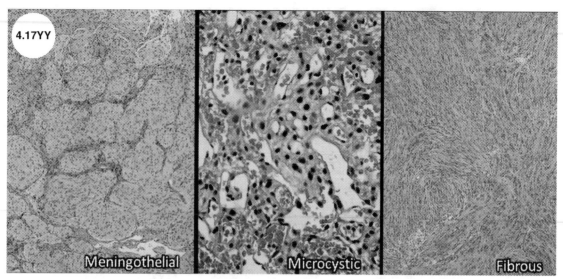

Image 4.17YY: H&E stain showing meningothelial, microcystic, and fibrous meningiomas (image courtesy of Dr. Seema Shroff, Fellow, Neuropathology, NYULMC).

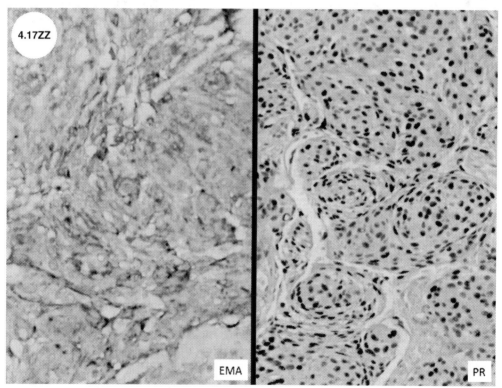

Image 4.17ZZ: Immunostains for epithelial membrane antigen and progesterone receptors (image courtesy of Dr. Seema Shroff, Fellow, Neuropathology, NYULMC).

- Meningioma cells are immunoreactive for epithelial membrane antigen and progesterone receptors.

- Chordoid and clear-cell meningiomas have a higher rate of recurrence and are classified as WHO grade II. Rhabdoid and papillary meningiomas are aggressive neoplasms that warrant WHO grade III.

- Meningiomas with a mitotic count greater than 4/10 high power fields are classified as atypical (WHO grade II) and those with more than 20/10 high power fields are classified as anaplastic (WHO grade III).

- WHO grade I meningiomas have a pushing border against the brain; however, meningiomas with brain invasion have a higher rate of

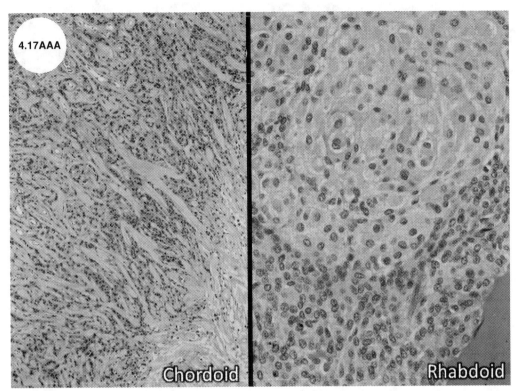

Image 4.17AAA: H&E stain demonstrating chordoid and rhabdoid meningiomas (image courtesy of Dr. Seema Shroff, Fellow, Neuropathology, NYULMC).

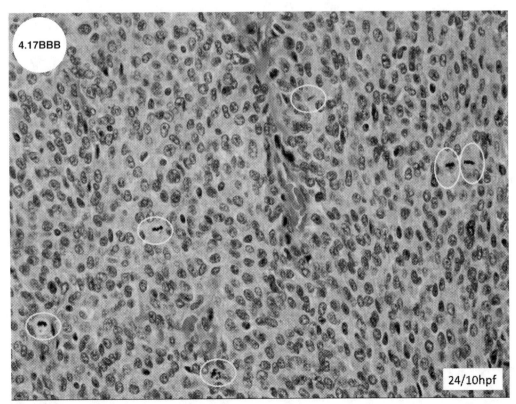

Image 4.17BBB: H&E staining of a meningioma showing multiple mitotic figures (yellow ovals) (image courtesy of Dr. Seema Shroff, Fellow, Neuropathology, NYULMC).

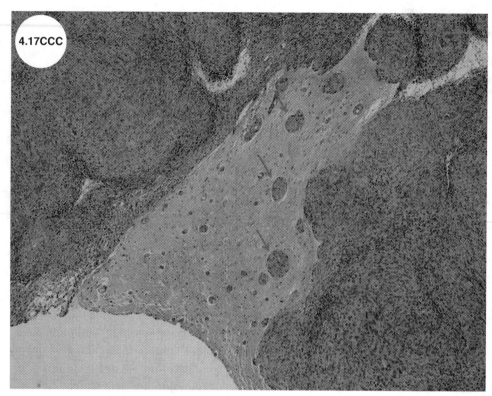

Image 4.17CCC: H&E staining of a meningioma showing brain invasion (red arrows) (image courtesy of Dr. Seema Shroff, Fellow, Neuropathology, NYULMC).

recurrence, warranting classification as WHO grade II.

Treatment

■ Surgical resection is the mainstay of treatment for meningiomas. Larger tumors may require preoperative embolization of the tumor. Up to 25% recur, and the recurrence rate for more malignant tumors is much higher, up to 80%, and radiation may be used for such tumors. SRS is particularly useful for tumors where surgical removal of the tumor is difficult, such as the cavernous sinus. Atypical and malignant meningiomas are associated with an increased risk of local recurrence and decreased overall survival compared with grade I meningiomas. Asymptomatic meningiomas may be followed with repeat imaging. For patients with atypical meningioma, close surveillance serial MRIs are obtained at 3, 6, and 12 months postoperatively, then every 6 to 12 months for 5 years, and then every 1 to 3 years.

References

1. Stessin AM, Schwartz A, Judanin G, et al. Does adjuvant external-beam radiotherapy improve outcomes for nonbenign meningiomas? A Surveillance, Epidemiology, and End Results (SEER)-based analysis. *J Neurosurg.* 2012;117:669.
2. Perry A, Louis DN, Scheithauer BW, et al. Meningiomas. In: Louis DN, Ohgaki H, Wiestler OD, eds. *WHO Classification of Tumours of the Central Nervous System.* Lyon: IARC Press; 2007:164.
3. Longstreth WT, Dennis LK, McGuire VM, et al. Epidemiology of intracranial meningiomas. *Cancer.* 1993;72:639–648.
4. Hsu DW, Efird JT, Hedley-Whyte ET. Progesterone and estrogen receptors in meningiomas: prognostic considerations. *J Neurosurg.* 1997;86:113–120.

4.18 | Vestibular Schwannoma

Case History

A 45-year-old man presented with gradual hearing loss and tinnitus in his left ear. Weber and Rinne tests confirmed the left sensorineural hearing loss.

Diagnosis: Vestibular Schwannoma

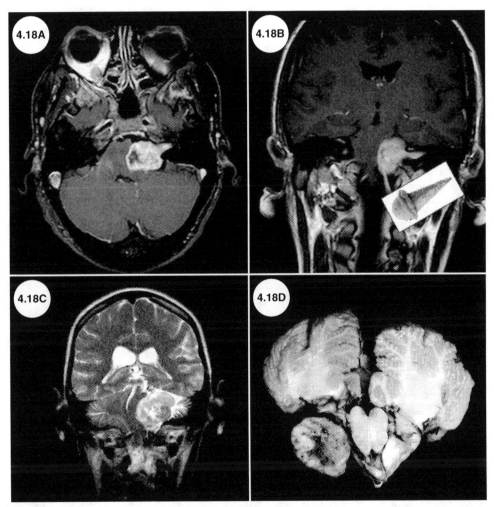

Images 4.18A–4.18C: Postcontrast axial and coronal T1-weighted and coronal T2-weighted images demonstrate an enhancing mass in the left cerebellopontine angle due to a vestibular schwannoma. The lesion arises in the internal auditory meatus and extends into the cerebellopontine angle. The appearance is known as the "ice cream cone" sign. **Image 4.18D:** Gross pathology of a left vestibular schwannoma (image courtesy of Roberta J. Seidman, MD, Associate Professor, Stony Brook School of Medicine, Department of Pathology).

Introduction

■ The most common pathological processes in the CPA masses are schwannomas and meningiomas. Schwannomas arise from Schwann cells, which myelinate axons of the peripheral nervous system. The differential diagnosis of CPA masses can be memorized by the mnemonic SAME (**Table 4.18.1**). Other rare masses, such as lipoma, neurosarcoidosis lesion, cholesterol granuloma, paraganglioma, chordoma, and chondrosarcoma, should also be considered in the differential.

Table 4.18.1 Differential Diagnosis of CPA Masses (Mnemonic SAME)

	Lesion Type	Comments
S	**S**chwannomas: acoustic, vestibular, trigeminal, facial	Low T1, high T2, enhance
A	**A**rachnoid cyst **A**neurysm	Follows CSF, does not enhance High T1 signal from thrombosed berry aneurysm with a calcified rim, and hemosiderin staining
M	**M**eningiomas **M**etastasis	Iso/low T1, iso-high T2, enhance Enhance, usually from breast, lung, malignant melanoma
E	**E**pendymoma **E**pidermoid cyst	Low T1, high T2, enhance Follows CSF signal, does not enhance

CSF, cerebrospinal fluid.

- Schwannomas may arise from any cranial nerve (except the optic and olfactory nerves, which are myelinated by oligodendrocytes) as well as from spinal nerve roots. They most commonly arise from the vestibular portion of the vestibulocochlear nerve and were formerly known as acoustic neuromas. They are almost always benign; however, rare malignant versions have been reported.

- They occur with equal frequency on the superior and inferior branches of the vestibular nerve; only rarely are they derived from the cochlear portion of the VIII nerve.

- They account for about 10% of all intracranial tumors and 80% of CPA tumors. The median age of diagnosis is 50 years. The majority is unilateral. Bilateral schwannomas are limited to patients with neurofibromatosis II.

Clinical Presentation

- Patients present with slowly progressive hearing loss and tinnitus and episodic unsteadiness while walking. True spinning vertigo is uncommon. Patients less commonly develop dizziness or imbalance problems as the lesions grow slowly enough that the brain has time to compensate. Not infrequently, these symptoms go unnoticed and patients present due to mass effect on the brainstem or other cranial neuropathies. Rarely, there may be hemorrhage into the tumor.

- The trigeminal nerve is the second most common nerve from which schwannomas arise. These patients present with facial numbness or trigeminal neuralgia. Facial nerve paresis and ataxia are less common.

- Jugular foramen schwannomas are rare, and presenting symptoms include dizziness, hearing

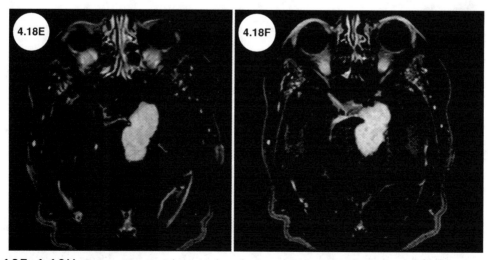

Images 4.18E–4.18H: Postcontrast axial, sagittal, and coronal T1-weighted images demonstrate an enhancing mass entering Meckel's cave with extension into the left CP angle due to schwannoma growing from the trigeminal nerve. (*continued*)

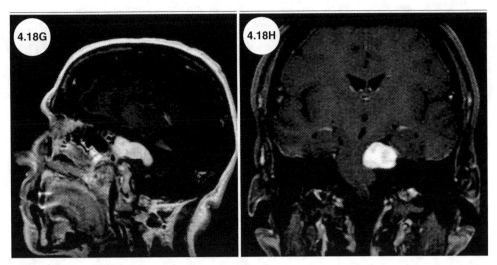

Images 4.18E–4.18H: (*continued*)

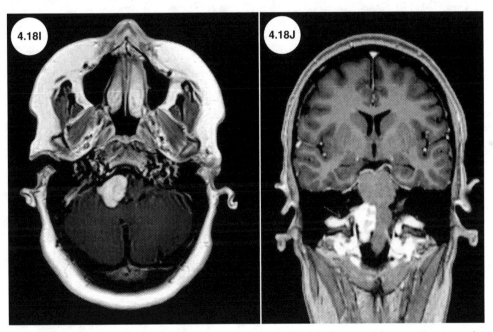

Images 4.18I and 4.18J: Postcontrast axial and coronal T1-weighted images demonstrate an enhancing mass in the right jugular foramen (red arrow) with significant mass effect on the medulla.

loss, ear pain, dysphagia, tongue weakness, and dysphonia.

Radiographic Appearance and Diagnosis

■ They are hypointense on T1-weighted images and hyperintense on T2-weighted images, often with cystic areas. They enhance avidly on postcontrast T1-weighted images. The enhancement is homogeneous with smaller tumors, but often heterogeneous with larger lesions. Other enhancing CPA masses include meningiomas, ependymomas, and other metastasis (**Table 4.18.1**).

■ The tumor originates in the internal auditory meatus and extends into the CPA. This is a characteristic finding for vestibular schwannomas. As shown in **Images 4.18A and 4.18B**, this is known as the "ice cream cone" sign.

■ Widening of internal auditory meatus is best seen on CT and is called a "trumpeted" internal acoustic meatus. This finding is not found with meningiomas, which can also be found in the CPA and have a similar appearance.

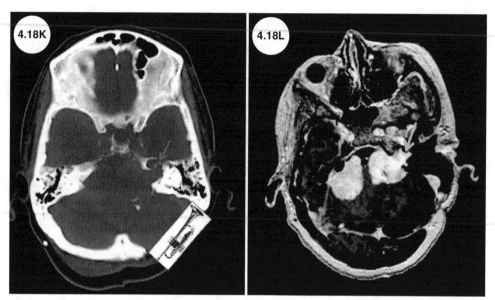

Images 4.18K and 4.18L: Axial CT image demonstrates a "trumpeted internal acoustic meatus" (red arrow). The tumor can be seen within the internal acoustic meatus on postcontrast T1-weighted image as well (blue arrow).

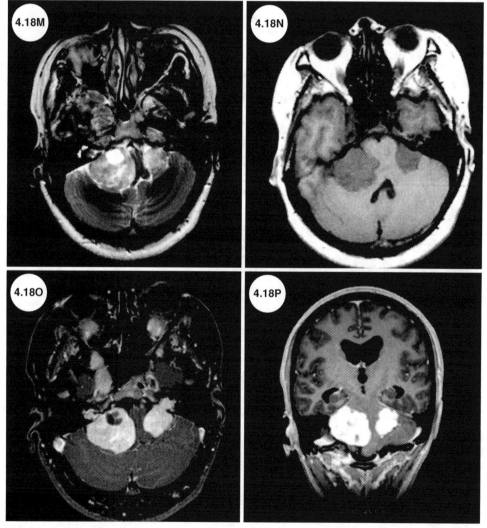

Images 4.18M–4.18P: Axial T2-weighted and noncontrast T1-weighted and postcontrast axial and coronal T1-weighted images demonstrate bilateral vestibular schwannomas in a patient with neurofibromatosis II.

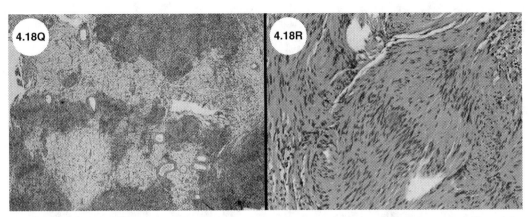

Images 4.18Q and 4.18R: H&E low power view shows alternating Antoni A (cellular and pink) and Antoni B (loose stroma, fewer cells and myxoid changes) areas; image 4.18R shows palisading basophilic nuclei surrounding pink areas referred to as Verocay bodies (images courtesy of Dr. Seema Shroff, Fellow, Neuropathology, NYULMC).

- Bilateral vestibular schwannomas are associated with neurofibromatosis type II.

Treatment

- There are three standard operative approaches for resection of these tumors. These are retromastoid suboccipital (retrosigmoid), translabyrinthine, and middle fossa approaches. The choice of surgical approach depends on the size of the tumor and whether preservation of the cranial nerve function is the goal of the surgery or not. Tumors can be surgically resected to prevent further hearing loss or compression of adjacent brainstem structures. The most common complication is facial nerve damage causing unilateral facial paralysis.

- SRS uses multiple convergent beams to deliver a high single dose of radiation to a radiographically discrete treatment volume. Gamma knife (Elekta), linear accelerator (LINAC), or proton beam machines are used to deliver radiation accurately. Cranial nerve toxicities, cystic degeneration, postradiation tumor expansion, malignant transformation, and local tissue scarring are some of the potential complications of SRS.

- Serial imaging is needed, and therapeutic intervention is indicated if there is evidence of rapid tumor growth (ie, >2.5 mm/year), regardless of tumor size. In other patients with a slower growth, no intervention may be needed and the tumor can be watched on serial imaging.

References

1. Maniakas A, Saliba I. Neurofibromatosis type 2 vestibular schwannoma treatment: a review of the literature, trends, and outcomes. *Otol Neurotol.* January 2014;35(5):889–894.
2. Maniakas A, Saliba I. Conservative management versus stereotactic radiation for vestibular schwannomas: a meta-analysis of patients with more than 5 years' follow-up. *Otol Neurotol.* February 2012;33(2):230–238.
3. Carlson ML, Link MJ, Wanna GB, Driscoll CL. Management of sporadic vestibular schwannoma. *Otolaryngol Clin North Am.* June 2015;48(3):407–422.
4. Vesper, J, Bolke E, Wille C, et al. Current concepts in stereotactic radiosurgery—a neurosurgical and radiooncological point of view. *Eur J Med Res.* 2009;14(3):93–101.
5. Kondziolka D, Lunsford LD, McLaughlin MR, Flickinger JC. Long-term outcomes after radiosurgery for acoustic neuromas. *N Engl J Med.* 1998;339:1426.

4.19 | Glomus Jugulare

Case History

A 70-year-old man presented with dizziness, hoarseness, and hearing loss.

Diagnosis: Glomus Jugulare Tumor

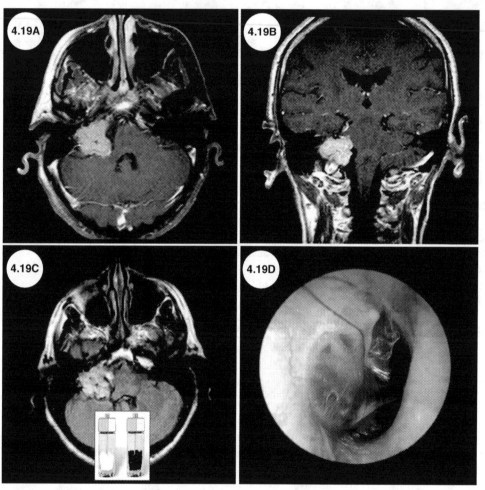

Images 4.19A–4.19C: Postcontrast axial and coronal T1-weighted and axial FLAIR images demonstrate a heterogeneously enhancing mass in the right jugular foramen consistent with a glomus jugulare tumor. This shows the "salt and pepper" appearance of the tumor. **Image 4.19D:** Photograph showing the high vascular nature of glomus jugulare tumors (image credit Dr. Michael Hawke).

Introduction

■ Glomus jugulare tumors are a subtype of paraganglioma, an uncommon neuroendocrine neoplasm. They grow within the jugular foramen, which contains the glossopharyngeal, vagus, and accessory nerves. The jugular foramen also contains nerve fibers known as glomus bodies, which respond to changes in blood pressure and temperature.

Clinical Presentation

■ Glomus jugulare tumors typically occur in patients 60 and older and present with pulsatile tinnitus and hearing loss. Other symptoms occur due to compression of the cranial nerves in the jugular foramen, and may cause dysphagia and dysarthria. Compression of other cranial nerves can lead to tongue and facial weakness. Some patients develop a Horner's syndrome (ptosis, miosis, and anhydrosis).

■ They are benign over 90% of the time.

Radiographic Appearance and Diagnosis

■ They are hyperintense on T2-weighted images and hypointense on unenhanced T1-weighted images. On postcontrast T1-weighted images, they enhance avidly. They are said to have a "salt and pepper" appearance—the "salt" is from hemorrhage, while the "pepper" is from hypervascularity and flow voids.

■ CT scans are important to visualize the surrounding bones, which are frequently eroded by the tumor, which often extends into the middle ear.

Treatment

■ They are treated with surgical resection, though cranial nerve deficits commonly persist after surgery. Radiation therapy is useful in incomplete resection. Recurrence occurs in nearly half of the patients.

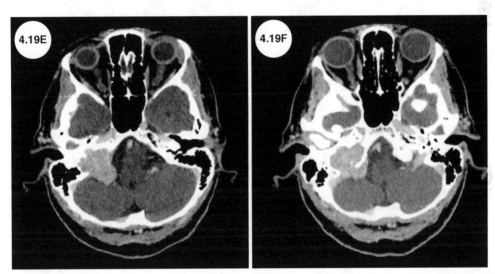

Images 4.19E and 4.19F: Axial CT images with contrast show a hyperdense mass originating from the jugular foramen, which is eroding the temporal bone on the right.

References

1. Jayashankar N, Sankhla S. Current perspectives in the management of glomus jugulare tumors. *Neurol India*. January–February 2015;63(1):83–90.
2. Ivan ME, Sughrue ME, Clark AJ, et al. A meta-analysis of tumor control rates and treatment-related morbidity for patients with glomus jugulare tumors. *J Neurosurg*. May 2011;114(5):1299–1305.
3. Sheehan JP, Tanaka S, Link MJ, et al. Gamma Knife surgery for the management of glomus tumors: a multicenter study. *J Neurosurg*. August 2012;117(2):246–254.
4. Semaan MT, Megerian CA. Current assessment and management of glomus tumors. *Curr Opin Otolaryngol Head Neck Surg*. October 2008;16(5):420–426.

4.20 Esthesioneuroblastoma

Case History

A 53-year-old man presented with frequent nosebleeds and nasal congestion over the course of 6 months. His wife also said that he had become more irritable and had a "shorter fuse" compared to his baseline. On exam, he had a marked decrease in his sense of smell (hyposmia).

Diagnosis: Esthesioneuroblastoma

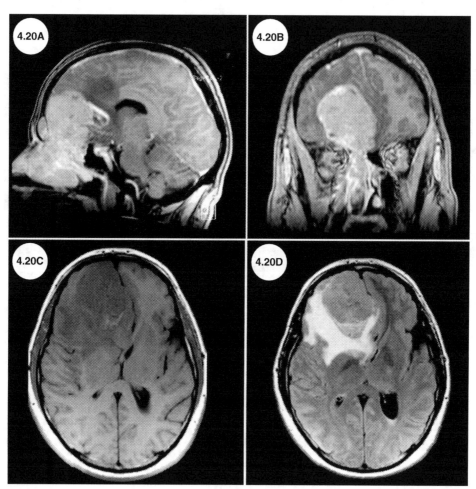

Images 4.20A–4.20D: Postcontrast sagittal and coronal T1-weighted and axial T1-weighted FLAIR images demonstrate a homogeneously enhancing lesion arising from the sinuses, which involves the right medial frontal lobe with significant mass effect, vasogenic edema, and right-to-left midline shift.

Introduction

■ Esthesioneuroblastomas, also known as olfactory neuroblastomas, are rare tumors, believed to originate from olfactory neuroepithelium in the cribriform region of the nasal septum and spread into the nasal and cranial cavities.

Clinical Presentation

■ They usually present with nasal congestion, anosmia, and epistaxis. Approximately 30% extend into the frontal lobes where they can present with seizures, personality changes, or focal neurological deficits.

- Patients usually present between the ages of 50 and 60.

Radiographic Appearance and Diagnosis

- On both T1-weighted and T2-weighted images, they have variable signals and can be hyperintense or hypointense. There is usually avid enhancement on postcontrast T1-weighted images. They are slow-growing tumors and there is often significant tumor burden at the time of presentation. The surrounding bone is often remodeled and destroyed. This is best seen on CT scans.

- A biopsy is required to make a definitive diagnosis, as imaging alone cannot distinguish them from olfactory groove meningiomas or sinonasal carcinomas. They are characterized by small, round, monomorphic cells, which are arranged in sheets or lobules. Immunoreactivity for cytokeratins is exceptional, but these lack immunoreactivity with epithelial membrane antigen.

Treatment

- They are treated with a combination of chemotherapy and radiation. In patients with localized disease, over 60% of patients are alive at 5 years and slightly less than 50% alive at 10 years. Patients with distant metastases have a much worse prognosis.

References

1. Jethanamest D, Morris LG, Sikora AG, Kutler DI. Esthesioneuroblastoma: a population-based analysis of survival and prognostic factors. *Arch Otolaryngol Head Neck Surg.* March 2007;133(3):276–280.
2. Kumar R. Esthesioneuroblastoma: multimodal management and review of literature. *World J Clin Cases.* September 2015;3(9):774–778.
3. Bak M, Wein RO. Esthesioneuroblastoma: a contemporary review of diagnosis and management. *Hematol Oncol Clin North Am.* December 2012;26(6):1185–1207.

4.21 Spinal Epidural Metastases

Case History

A 65-year-old man with a history of prostate cancer presented with lower back pain for the past week. He also said that going up the stairs in his house had been more difficult than usual. On exam, he had severe tenderness to palpation of his thoracic and lumbar spine. He had weakness of his legs and a sensory level at T4. He was diffusely hyperreflexic with upgoing toes bilaterally. His gait was labored and spastic.

Diagnosis: Spinal Epidural Metastases

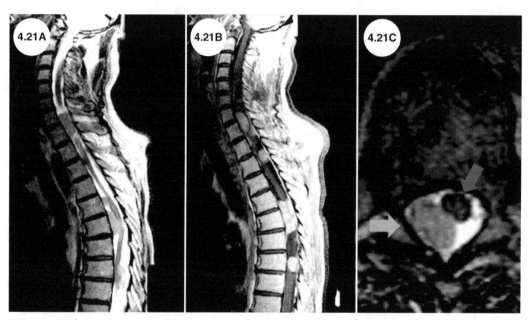

Images 4.21A and 4.21B: Sagittal T2-weighted and postcontrast sagittal T1-weighted images demonstrate multiple spinal epidural metastases with significant cord compression. **Image 4.21C:** Axial T2-weighted image demonstrates the spinal cord (blue arrow) being compressed and displaced to the right by a tumor (red arrow).

Introduction

■ The vertebral column is a highly vascular structure and as such it is a common location for metastases to the epidural location. Epidural metastases to the spinal canal arise most commonly from breast, lung, or prostate cancers. Other frequent primary cancers include: thyroid, renal, melanoma, and blood dyscrasias such as lymphoma and multiple myeloma. Spinal cord compression occurs most frequently at the thoracic level.

Clinical Presentation

■ Patients present with pain, weakness, sensory loss, and bowel/bladder incontinence.

■ Neurological exam will reveal a varying degree of myelopathic signs below the level of lesion. These include spastic paraparesis or quadriparesis, sensory loss, hyperreflexia and pathological reflexes, and loss of rectal sphincter tone.

Radiographic Appearance and Diagnosis

■ MRI with contrast is the imaging modality of choice. The lesions typically enhance with the administration of contrast. They compress the spinal cord, distorting its normal architecture. Hyperintensity within the cord is common on T2-weighted images.

- CSF analysis may show a marked elevated protein if there is blockage of CSF flow within the spinal canal.

- In patients with an unknown primary, biopsy of the lesion should be undertaken.

Treatment

- Spinal cord compression is a neurological emergency. Once myelopathic symptoms develop, they may progress rapidly leading to permanent injury. Patients who have motor deficits that persist beyond 24 hours usually do not recover. The immediate administration of high-dose intravenous (IV) corticosteroids is required in all patients with spinal cord compression from metastases.

- Radiotherapy is useful even in patients whose tumors are classically resistant to this treatment. Decompressive surgery should be used in patients with rapidly progressive neurological deficits or in patients whose symptoms progress despite the use of radiotherapy.

Reference

1. Shah LM, Salzman KL. Imaging of spinal metastatic disease. *Int J Surg Oncol.* 2011;2011:769753.

4.22 | Cerebral Metastases

Case History

A 67-year-old man presented with a partial seizure with secondary generalization. His daughter said that he had been increasingly confused over the past few weeks.

Diagnosis: Cerebral Metastases

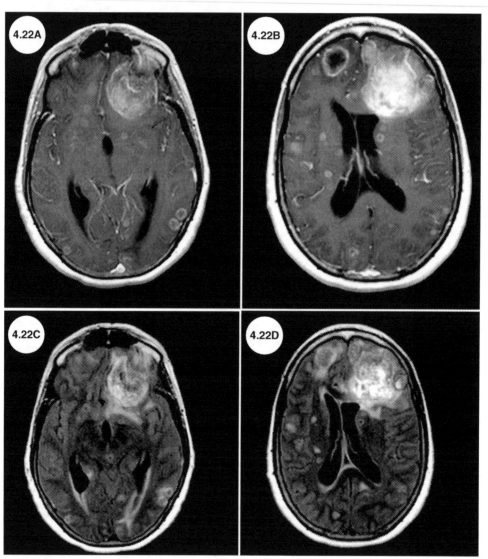

Images 4.22A–4.22D: Postcontrast axial T1-weighted and FLAIR images demonstrate extensive metastases, both intraparenchymal and leptomeningeal with mass effect and edema.

Introduction

■ Up to 20% of patients with cancer will develop a metastatic lesion to the brain, making brain metastases much more common than primary

brain tumors. There are nearly 100,000 such cases annually in the United States.

■ Lung cancers account for 50% of all brain metastases followed by breast cancer, melanoma, renal cell carcinomas, and gastrointestinal malignancies.

- The tumors with the highest propensity to hemorrhage are melanoma, renal cell carcinoma, choriocarcinoma, and papillary thyroid cancer. At times, breast/lung or hepatocellular carcinoma can present with hemorrhagic intracranial metastases.

Clinical Presentation

- Patients present with headaches, seizures, cognitive slowing, personality change, or focal neurological deficits depending on the number, size, and location of the tumors.

Radiographic Appearance and Diagnosis

- There is a variable appearance on both CT and MRI. On CT, the tumor may be hypodense, isodense, or hyperdense to the brain. On T1-weighted images, metastases are hypointense unless there is hemorrhage. On T2-weighted images, they may be hyperintense or hypointense. There is often peritumoral edema and mass effect. With the addition of contrast, there is avid enhancement, which may be solid, ring-shaped, or punctate.

- Hemorrhage is the presenting symptom in about half of these tumors.

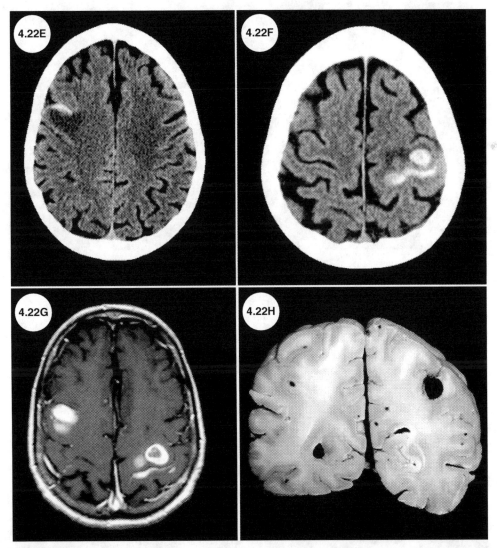

Images 4.22E–4.22G: Axial CT images and postcontrast T1-weighted images demonstrate hemorrhagic metastatic lesions in a patient with melanoma. There is both solid and ring-enhancing with the addition of contrast.
Image 4.22H: Gross pathology of hemorrhagic metastatic melanoma (image courtesy Roberta J. Seidman, MD, Associate Professor, Stony Brook School of Medicine, Department of Pathology).

■ Metastases to the brain occur when tumor cells spread via the bloodstream, and they are most commonly found at the gray–white junction, where there is relatively slow blood flow. In cases with an unknown primary, a biopsy is needed to confirm the diagnosis.

■ Immunohistochemistry for breast cancer can be estrogen receptor, progesterone receptor, and HER2/neu positive. The BRST-2 immunohistochemistry labeling for GCDFP is a relatively specific marker of tumors of breast origin (refer to **Image 4.22O**). Immunohistochemistry (IHC) markers are used for metastatic brain tumors

without unknown primary. The immunoreactivity for cytokeratin (CK)-7 and thyroid transcription factor-1 (TTF-1) favor a lung primary whereas immunoreactivity for CK20 and CDX-2 favors lower gastrointestinal malignancies (**Image 4.22P**). Carcinomas immunoreactive for CK7 and CDX-2 are compatible with metastases from an upper gastrointestinal primary, most commonly the stomach.

■ Tumors in the cerebellum are very likely to be metastatic disease in adults.

■ Nearly half of metastases are single lesions, and these may be indistinguishable from primary

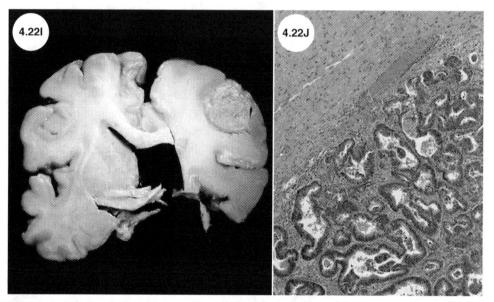

Image 4.22I: Gross pathology of a metastatic carcinoma at the gray–white junction (image courtesy Roberta J. Seidman, MD, Associate Professor, Stony Brook School of Medicine, Department of Pathology). **Image 4.22J:** H&E stain demonstrates an adenocarcinoma infiltrating the brain (image credit Jensflorian).

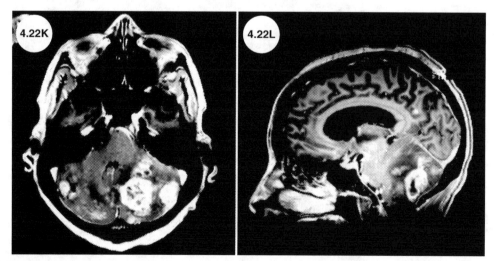

Images 4.22K–4.22N: Axial, sagittal, and coronal postcontrast T1-weighted images and sagittal FLAIR MRI demonstrate multiple enhancing masses in the cerebellum with edema and significant mass effect on the fourth ventricle. Metastatic lesions are also visible in the brain. (*continued*)

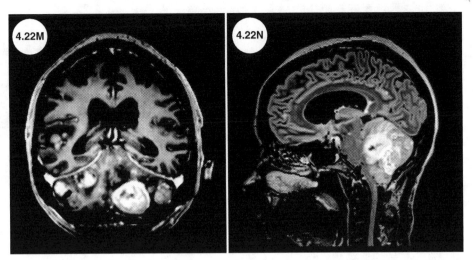

Images 4.22K–4.22N: *(continued)*

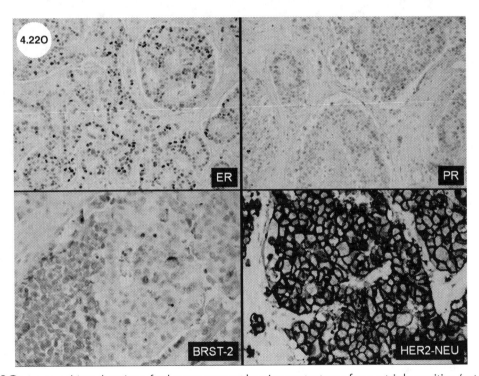

Image 4.22O: Immunohistochemistry for breast cancer showing metastases from a triple positive (estrogen receptor, progesterone receptor, and Her2-Neu) with breast carcinoma as primary. The BRST-2 immunohistochemistry labeling for GCDFP is a relatively specific marker of tumors of breast origin (image courtesy of Dr. Seema Shroff, Fellow, Neuropathology, NYULMC).

brain tumors. About 33% of patients with a metastatic brain lesion do not have a known primary, and a search for the primary tumor is mandatory. In about 30% to 40% of cases, these studies do not reveal the primary tumor.

Treatment

■ As with primary brain tumors, glucocorticoids are used to reduce edema and improve

symptoms, often dramatically over the course of a day or two. The treatment strategies for brain metastases are listed in **Table 4.22.1** and range from IV/oral steroids, chemotherapy, surgery, whole brain radiation therapy (WBRT), or more localized radiation, or a combination of these.

■ Single brain lesions can be surgically excised, though this does not improve the overall survival. There is some evidence that resection of up

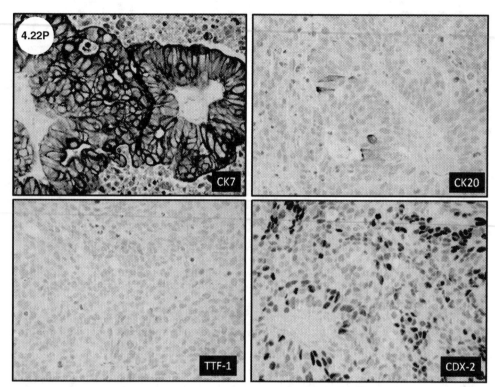

Image 4.22P: Most commonly used initial IHCs for metastatic brain tumors include CK7 and TTF-1, which favor a lung primary, whereas carcinomas immunoreactive for CK7 and CDX-2, as shown are compatible with metastases from an upper gastrointestinal primary, most commonly the stomach (image courtesy of Dr. Seema Shroff, Fellow, Neuropathology, NYULMC).

Table 4.22.1 Treatment Approaches for Intracranial Metastases

Corticosteroids
WBRT
Surgery +/- WBRT
Surgery +/- localized radiation
WBRT + radiation sensitizers
WBRT + chemotherapy
SRS +/-WBRT
Chemotherapy

WBRT, whole brain radiation therapy, SRS, stereotactic radiosurgery.

to three lesions can be beneficial. When numerous lesions are present, treatment with whole brain radiation is indicated.

■ SRS can be considered when metastatic lesion is radiographically distinct on neuroimaging, pseudospherical in shape, and displacing the normal brain tissue with minimal invasion of normal brain. The ideal size of metastatic lesion at presentation should be 3 cm or less for SRS.

■ Chemotherapy is indicated if the primary tumor is sensitive.

■ The use of prophylactic anticonvulsant therapy is not recommended, though seizures occur in about 30% of patients with cerebral metastases.

References

1. Posner JB. Management of brain metastases. *Rev Neurol (Paris)*. 1992;148(6–7):477–487.
2. Wen PY, Loeffler JS. Management of brain metastases. *Oncology (Huntingt)*. July 1999;13(7):941–954, 957–961; discussion 961–962, 9.
3. Sze G, Milano E, Johnson C. Detection of brain metastases: comparison of contrast-enhanced MR with unenhanced MR and enhanced CT. *AJNR Am J Neuroradiol*. July–August 1990;11(4):785–791.
4. Barajas RF Jr, Cha S. Imaging diagnosis of brain metastasis. *Prog Neurol Surg*. 2012;25:55–73.
5. Ozawa Y, Omae M, Fujii M, et al. Management of brain metastasis with magnetic resonance imaging and stereotactic irradiation attenuated benefits of prophylactic cranial irradiation in patients with limited-stage small cell lung cancer. *BMC Cancer*. August 2015;15:589.
6. Fink KR, Fink JR. Imaging of brain metastases. *Surg Neurol Int*. 2013;4(Suppl. 4):S209–S219.

CHAPTER 5

PITUITARY DISORDERS

5.1 | Pituitary Adenoma

Case History

A 37-year-old woman presented with headaches and blurry vision. She was found to have a bitemporal hemianopsia on examination.

Diagnosis: Pituitary Adenoma

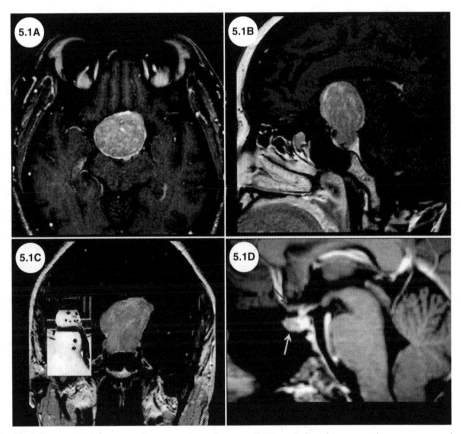

Images 5.1A–5.1C: Postcontrast axial, sagittal, and coronal T1-weighted images demonstrate a large complex multilobulated mass in the sellar/suprasellar area. The sella turcica is massively expanded. The tumor shows the characteristic "snowman" appearance. **Image 5.1D**: Postcontrast sagittal T1-weighted image of a normal MRI. The pituitary gland (yellow arrow) and stalk normally enhance and are seen below the optic chiasm (red arrow).

Introduction

- Pituitary adenomas are slow-growing, benign tumors that arise from one of the cell types in the anterior lobe of the pituitary gland. They are the most common tumor in the sellar region, and comprise about 10% of primary intracranial tumors.

- Macroadenomas are larger than 10 mm, while microadenomas are smaller than this. They are often incidental findings.

Clinical Presentation

- Though the majority of pituitary tumors do not secrete hormones, most patients nonetheless present due to endocrine dysfunction. There is no relationship between the size of a tumor and the probability of it being hormonally active. The three most common hormonally active tumors are presented in **Table 5.1.1**.

- In addition to causing endocrine dysfunction via the oversecretion of pituitary hormones,

Table 5.1.1 Characteristics of Hormonally Active Tumors

Tumor Type	Clinical Features	Diagnosis	Comments
Prolactinoma	Amenorrhea in women; galactorrhea, sexual dysfunction, alopecia, and weight gain in either sex	Elevated prolactin level	Dopamine agonists, such as bromocriptine, inhibit the release of prolactin. Dopamine-blocking agents, such as typical antipsychotics and antiemetics, can cause elevated prolactin levels and the same symptoms as a prolactinoma.
Growth-Hormone Secreting Tumors	Gigantism, if they present before puberty, or acromegaly, if they present after puberty	Serum IGF; GH levels after oral glucose loading	Patients with acromegaly present with enlargement of the hands, feet, and jaw as well as thickening of the cranial vault and frontal bossing. The symptoms progress slowly, such that patients are often not aware of the changes in their physical appearances.
ACTH-Secreting Tumors	A puffy round face (termed "moon facies"), abdominal obesity, hypertension, diabetes, edema, a compromised immune system, lethargy, poor wound healing, avascular necrosis of the femoral head, osteoporosis, sexual dysfunction, edema, and a panoply of psychiatric symptoms	24-hour urinary-free cortisol; dexamethasone suppression test (normal subjects will have a low serum cortisol in the morning after being given dexamethasone the previous night); ACTH assay	Tumors that secrete adrenocorticotrophic hormone (ACTH) cause *Cushing's disease*, while glucocorticoid excess from any cause is known as *Cushing's syndrome*. The ACTH level is high or normal in Cushing's disease, but suppressed in Cushing's syndrome from other causes, such as prolonged administration of steroids.
Thyrotropinoma	Palpitations, weight loss, insomnia, nervousness, anxiety, goiter	T3, T4, thyroid stimulating hormone (TSH), free T3 and free T4, anti-thyroid peroxidase, thyroid stimulating immunoglobulin	Beta-blockers, methimazole, propylthiouracil, radioactive iodine.

any sellar or suprasellar mass may present with panhypopituitarism if there is compression of the pituitary gland or stalk. Symptoms of panhypopituitarism include lethargy, growth failure, diabetes insipidus, hypogonadism, and hypoadrenalism.

- Tumors that are not hormonally active present due to mass effect on adjacent brain structures. Such tumors present with headaches, cranial neuropathies if there is involvement of the cavernous sinus, or a bitemporal hemianopsia if there is compression of the optic chiasm. Less commonly, there may be monocular visual loss if there is involvement of the optic nerve or a homonymous hemianopsia if the optic tract is affected distal to the optic chiasm. Very large tumors may cause personality changes if there is involvement of the frontal lobe, or seizures if there is involvement of the medial temporal lobe. In rare cases, patients may suffer

pituitary apoplexy with potentially devastating consequences.

Radiographic Appearance and Diagnosis

- The evaluation of a patient with a suspected pituitary disorder should include:

  - **Neuroimaging:** On CT, adenomas appear as hyperdense masses emerging from the sella turcica with upward deviation of the optic chiasm. Computed tomography angiography is extremely useful in preoperative planning for macroadenomas. The relationship of the tumor to the anterior cerebral arteries and optic nerve is critical to the surgeon. MRI brain sagittal, coronal, and axial images with and without contrast with attention to sella turcica can help differentiate a sellar mass (**Table 5.1.2**).

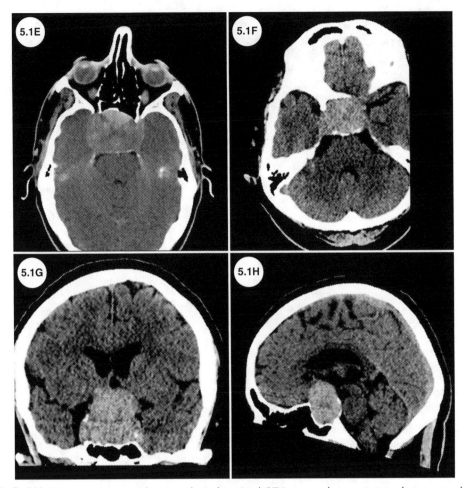

Images 5.1E–5.1H: Non-contrast axial, coronal, and sagittal CT images demonstrate a large complex multilobulated mass in the sellar/suprasellar area. The sella turcica is massively expanded.

Adenomas are typically isodense to gray matter on both T1-weighted images and T2-weighted images, though larger lesions may have a more heterogeneous appearance due to hemorrhage, cystic changes, or necrosis. They enhance homogenously with the addition of contrast. The sella turcica is expanded, and large tumors expand after

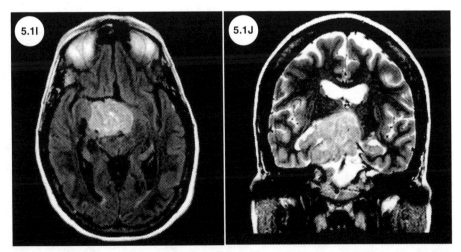

Images 5.1I–5.1L: Axial fluid-attenuated inversion recovery, coronal T2-weighted, and postcontrast axial and coronal T1-weighted images demonstrate a large pituitary adenoma. It is hyperintense on T2-weighted imaging and can be seen encasing the carotid arteries (red arrows). (*continued*)

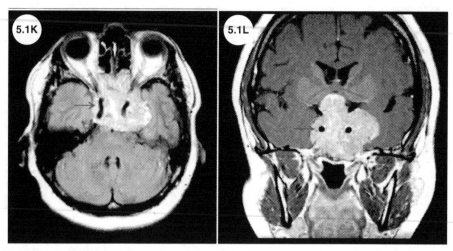

Images 5.1I–5.1L: *(continued)*

emerging from its confines, creating the "snowman sign." There is often invasion of the cavernous sinus, and the tumor encases the internal carotid artery.

- **Visual field testing:** Formal visual testing is important even on patients with grossly intact visual fields.

- **Endocrinological evaluation:** Patients should be screened carefully for endocrine dysfunction and electrolyte disturbances. Specific tests include prolactin level, thyroid function tests, 24-hour urine cortisol, follicle-stimulating hormone (FSH), and lymphocytic hypophysitis (LH) levels, growth hormone (GH) assays, and insulin-like growth factor (IGF) to screen for GH irregularities.

- Ultimately, pathological examination is needed to confirm the diagnosis.

Table 5.1.2 Differential Diagnosis of a Sellar Mass

Pituitary adenoma
Rathke's cleft cyst
Craniopharyngioma
Meningioma
Germinoma
Chordoma
Carcinoma
Epidermoid, dermoid cyst, and teratomas
Pituitary sarcoid
Aneurysm
Abscess
Hypothalamic hamartoma, glioma, and gangliocytoma
Metastases
Histiocytosis X
Infiltrative lesions (hereditary hemochromatosis)
Lymphocytic hypophysitis

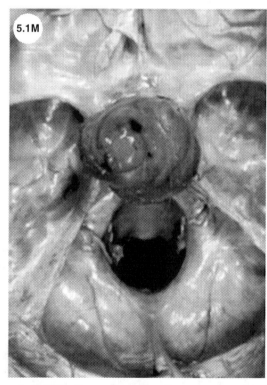

Image 5.1M: Gross specimen demonstrates a pituitary adenoma (image credit WikiDocs, www.wikidoc.org/index.php/File:Gross_pituitary_adenoma_A..jpg).

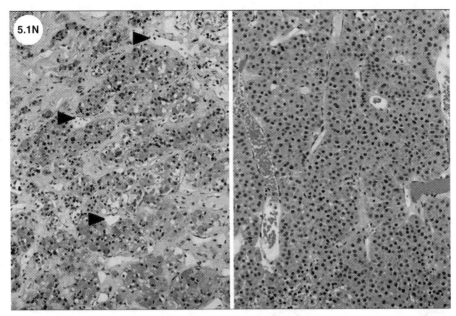

Image 5.1N: Hematoxylin and eosin stain: Left image shows normal pituitary gland. Note the heterogeneity of the cells, arranged in acinar clusters interspersed with sinusoids (black arrowheads). There is a mixture of acidophils, basophils, and chromophobe cells. The right image shows pituitary adenoma with sheets of monomorphous cells and loss of acinar pattern (image credit Dr. Seema Shroff, Fellow, Neuropathology, NYULMC).

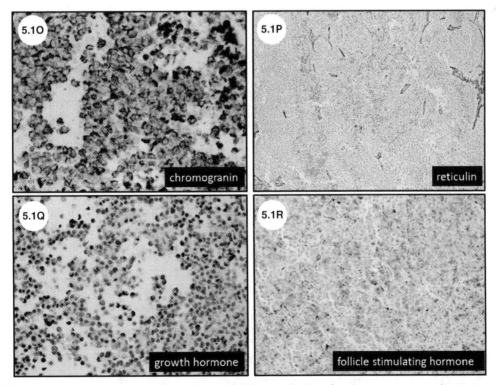

Image 5.1O: Pituitary glandular as well as adenoma cells are positive for chromogranin and synaptophysin (neuronal markers). **Image 5.1P:** Normal pituitary acini are outlined by reticulin; however, the acinar pattern is lost in adenomas, and they show sheet like growth. **Images 5.1Q and 5.1R:** Pituitary adenomas may be silent or secrete hormones. Markers for growth hormone and follicle stimulating hormone are shown in two separate patients.

Treatment

■ Symptomatic tumors are treated primarily with surgery, which is curative in most cases. The transsphenoidal approach using endoscopic techniques is preferred, though larger and more invasive adenomas may require a transfrontal resection. Risks of transsphenoidal surgery include postoperative infarction and hemorrhage, diabetes insipidus, fluid and electrolyte disturbances, cerebrospinal fluid (CSF) rhinorrhea, meningitis, and cranial nerves III, IV, VI palsies.

■ Medically, therapy is an option in hormonally active tumors. Dopamine agonists such as bromocriptine are used in tumors that secrete prolactin. In tumors that secrete GH or TSH, somatostatin analogues are used.

■ Small tumors can be effectively targeted by a focused beam of radiation therapy (RT) referred to as "stereotactic radiosurgery." There should be at least 5 mm separation between the tumor and chiasma/optic nerve before considering radiosurgery as an option. In certain cases, adjunctive, stereotactic radiotherapy is used, especially in the case of nonfunctioning tumors that are unable to be completely resected.

■ Patients with panhypopituitarism are treated with hormone replacement therapy.

References

1. Syro LV, Rotondo F, Ramirez A, et al. Progress in the diagnosis and classification of pituitary adenomas. *Front Endocrinol (Lausanne)*. June 2015;6:97.
2. Oldfield EH, Merrill MJ. Apoplexy of pituitary adenomas: the perfect storm. *J Neurosurg*. June 2015;122(6):1444–1449.
3. Melmed S. Pituitary tumors. *Endocrinol Metab Clin North Am*. March 2015;44(1):1–9.
4. Melmed S. Pathogenesis of pituitary tumors. *Nat Rev Endocrinol*. May 2011;7(5):257–266.

5.2 | Craniopharyngioma

Case History

A 20-year-old man developed gradual, but severe visual loss and also failed to develop secondary sexual characteristics.

Diagnosis: Craniopharyngioma

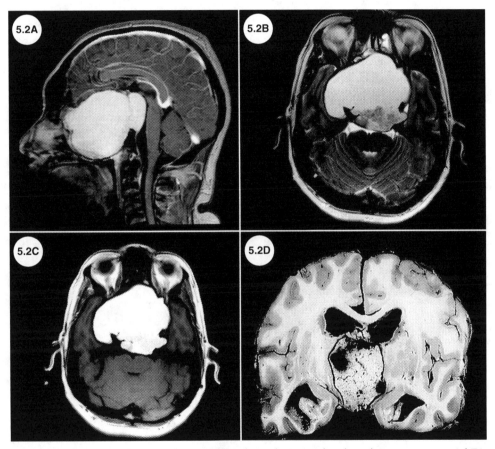

Images 5.2A–5.2C: Postcontrast sagittal T1-weighted, axial T2-weighted, and non-contrast axial T1-weighted images demonstrate an enormous, hyperintense cystic pituitary mass, which has expanded the sella turcica, with mass effect on the brainstem and both medial temporal lobes. **Image 5.2D:** Gross pathology of a craniopharyngioma (image credit The Armed Forces Institute of Pathology).

Introduction

■ Craniopharyngiomas are slow-growing, WHO grade I tumors, which account for 2% of all intracranial neoplasms and 5% to 10% of childhood intracranial neoplasms. They arise from the cells along the pituitary stalk that are derived from remnants of Rathke's pouch and the craniopharyngeal duct.

■ The peak incidence is in children aged 5 to 15 years. A second peak occurs later in life, between ages 50 and 60 years. There is no sexual predilection, but these tumors are more common in Africa, the Far East, and Japan.

Clinical Presentation

■ The common presenting symptoms of these tumors are:

- **Visual disturbances** due to compression of the optic chiasm; more common in adults than children
- **Endocrine dysfunction** due to compression of the pituitary or hypothalamus; these presentations include short stature, delayed puberty in children, amenorrhea, sleep disturbances, changes in appetite and weight, and diabetes insipidus
- **Cranial nerve dysfunction**
- **Symptoms of increased intracranial pressure**
- **Cognitive and personality changes** due to extension in the frontal or temporal lobes
- **Chemical meningitis** if there is rupture of the cyst

Radiographic Appearance and Diagnosis

■ The appearance of craniopharyngiomas varies on MRI; these are typically multilobular, multicystic lesions in the suprasellar/intrasellar region, which are hypointense on T1-weighted images and hyperintense on T2-weighted images. The appearance depends on the exact components of the fluid in the cyst. The cyst is typically hyperintense on T2-weighted images but has a highly variable signal on T1-weighted images. With the administration of contrast, there is often enhancement around the edge of the cyst as well as enhancement of any solid components.

■ Calcifications are common in the cyst wall and/or solid component. They are best seen on CT scans. Fine flaky calcification suggests fast-growing tumors, whereas dense calcification is seen in slowly growing craniopharyngiomas.

■ It is rare to find craniopharyngiomas completely confined to the intrasellar compartment. About 70% are combined suprasellar and intrasellar. They can extend anteriorly to the prechiasmatic cistern and subfrontal spaces, posteriorly into the prepontine and interpeduncular cisterns, cerebellopontine angle, third ventricle, posterior fossa, and foramen magnum, and laterally toward the subtemporal spaces.

- **Classification:** These tumors have been classified based on their location, vertical extension, or subtypes. Hoffman et al classified these tumors as **intrasellar, prechiasmatic, and retrochiasmatic.** Samii and Samii et al divided these tumors into five grades based on their vertical projection as follows:
- **Grade I:** intrasellar or infradiaphragmatic
- **Grade II:** localized to the cistern with or without an intrasellar component
- **Grade III:** reaches the lower half of the third ventricle
- **Grade IV:** reaches the upper half of the third ventricle
- **Grade V:** tumor dome reaches the septum pellucidum or lateral ventricles

■ Craniopharyngioma comprises three clinically, histologically, and genetically distinct subtypes as follows (**Table 5.2.1**):

- **Adamantinomatous** (most common)

Table 5.2.1 Characteristics of Common Subtypes of Craniopharyngiomas

	Adamantinomatous	Papillary
Frequency	More common	Less common
Age of onset	Occurs at a younger age but also seen in adults	Occurs typically in adults
MRI brain	Complex multilobular, and commonly calcified and cystic	Calcification is less common. Commonly solid, well circumscribed
Genetic	Mutation in β-catenin present in 70% of cases of this subtype	Lack of β-catenin mutation
Histology	Complex epithelial pattern with peripherally palisading cells and wet keratin, calcification, foreign body giant cells, and cholesterol clefts, keratinized "ghost cells"	Composed of simple squamous epithelium and fibrovascular islands of connective tissue; keratin nodules are not seen
Prognosis	High rates of recurrence are seen within the first five years and usually after subtotal or partial resection	Readily resected surgically and recurs less often

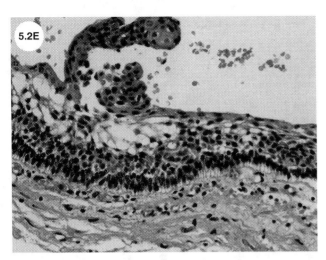

Image 5.2E: Adamantinomatous craniopharyngioma showing sheets of keratinized cells of stratified squamous epithelium with a palisading basal layer with "piano key" appearance. The epithelium may be more flattened in cystic cavities with loose matrix (stellate reticulum) (image credit Dr. Seema Shroff, Fellow, Neuropathology, NYULMC).

- Papillary
- Mixed (15%)

■ Complete endocrinological evaluation is necessary to uncover hypopituitarism, particularly GH, cortisol, and thyroid hormone.

Treatment

■ **Radical surgery** is the treatment of choice in most cases, as craniopharyngiomas are benign tumors and many affected patients are young. The surgical approach is influenced by the tumor location with respect to sella, chiasm, and third ventricle. Anterior midline (transsphenoidal, subfrontal), anterolateral (pterional, orbitozygomatic), transpetrosal, subtemporal, intraventricular (transcallosal–transventricular, transcortical–transventricular translamina terminalis), or a combination of these approaches is used to tackle such tumors. There have been anecdotal case reports of craniopharyngioma seeding along the surgical access route and through the CSF pathways. Cystic lesion aspiration with implantation of an Ommaya reservoir or intracavitary instillation of a radioisotope (brachytherapy) may be employed in treating cystic craniopharyngiomas.

■ **Radiation therapy (RT)** can be used to treat patients with residual disease who have undergone a partial surgical resection or to treat disease that has recurred following what was initially thought to be a gross total resection. Fractionated stereotactic radiosurgery (FSRT), stereotactic radiation therapy (SRT), proton beam RT, and intensity modulated RT (IMRT) are various currently employed RT techniques. In a retrospective series, the recurrence rate was significantly higher in patients receiving ≤54 Gy compared with higher doses (50% versus 15%). The rates of radiation-induced endocrine, neurological, and vascular sequelae are low with doses less than 61 Gy.

■ **Hormonal replacement therapy** is needed for patients with endocrinological dysfunction; thyroid supplements for hypothyroidism, intranasal and intravenous supplementation with desmopressin in patients with diabetes insipidus. High doses of hydrocortisone may be required to treat symptoms of hypoadrenalism postoperatively.

■ Tumor recurrence is a very common phenomenon even after complete resection and postoperative radiotherapy. To avoid adhesions from the previous surgery, a different surgical approach can be selected.

References

1. Fernandez-Miranda JC, Gardner PA, Snyderman CH, et al. Craniopharyngioma: a pathologic, clinical, and surgical review. *Head Neck.* July 2012;34(7):1036–1044.
2. Kuratsu J, Usio Y. Epidemiological study of primary intracranial tumor in childhood. A population based survey in Kumamoto Prefecture, Japan. *Pediatr Neurosurg.* 1996;25:946–50.
3. Izuora GI, Ikerionwu S, Saddeqi N, Iloeje SO. Childhood intracranial neoplasms Enugu, Nigeria. *West Africa Journal of Med.* 1989;8:171–174.
4. Zada G, Lin N, Ojerholm E, Ramkissoon S, Laws ER. Craniopharyngioma and other cystic epithelial lesions of the sellar region: a review of clinical, imaging, and histopathological relationships. *Neurosurg Focus.* April 2010;28(4):E4.
5. Hoffman HJ, De Silva M, Humphreys RP, et al. Aggressive surgical management of craniopharyngiomas in children. *J Neurosurg.* 1992;76:47–52.
6. Samii M, Tatagiba M. Surgical management of craniopharyngiomas: a review. *Neurol Med Chir.* (Tokyo). 1997;37:141–149.
7. Samii M, Samii A. Surgical management of craniopharyngiomas. In: Schmidek HH, ed. *Schmidek and Sweet Operative Neurological Techniques: Indications, Methods, and Results.* 4th ed. Philadelphia, PA: WB Saunders; 2000:489–502.
8. Lin A, Bluml S, Mamelak AN. Efficacy of proton magnetic resonance spectroscopy in clinical decision making for patients with suspected malignant brain tumors. *J Neurooncol.* 1999;45:69.
9. Thiel A, Pietrzyk U, Sturm V, et al. Enhanced accuracy in differential diagnosis of radiation necrosis by positron emission tomography-magnetic resonance imaging coregistration: technical case report. *Neurosurgery.* 2000;46:232.

5.3 | Rathke's Cleft Cyst

Case History

A 34-year-old woman developed headaches and "blurry vision." She was found to have bitemporal hemianopsia on exam.

Diagnosis: Rathke's Cleft Cyst

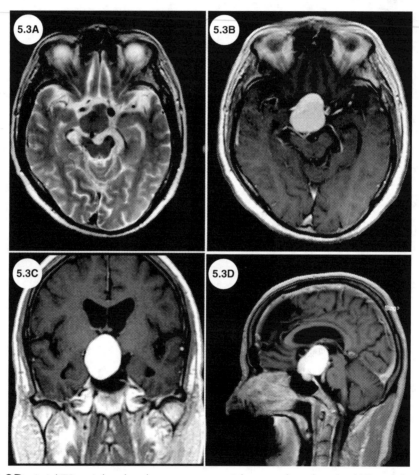

Images 5.3A–5.3D: Axial T2-weighted and postcontrast axial, coronal, and sagittal T1-weighted images demonstrate a large well-defined sellar/suprasellar T1-bright mass. The bulk of the lesion demonstrates T2-hypointense signal and T1-hyperintense suprasellar mass consistent with a giant Rathke's cleft cyst.

Introduction

■ A Rathke's cleft cyst (also known as a **pars intermedia cyst)** is a benign, fluid-filled cyst typically located in the center of the pituitary gland. They are congenital malformations due to incomplete development of Rathke's pouch.

■ Unlike craniopharyngiomas, which are more common in men, Rathke's cleft cysts are twice as common in women.

Clinical Presentation

■ Most often, they are incidental findings. Large cysts may extend into the suprasellar cistern where they can present with visual disturbances, endocrine dysfunction, and headaches. The most common endocrine disturbances are diabetes insipidus and increased prolactin levels due to compression of the pituitary stalk.

Radiographic Appearance and Diagnosis

- The cyst arises in the sella turcica with slightly more than half extending into the suprasellar region. The MRI signal depends on the protein contents of the cyst. On T1-weighted images, half are hyperintense and half are hypointense. On T2-weighted images, most are hyperintense, but about 25% are hypointense. They do not enhance with the administration of contrast, other than a thin rim on the periphery.

- An intracystic nodule that is hyperintense on T1-weighted images and hypointense on T2-weighted images is highly specific and can be found in up to 80% of cases.

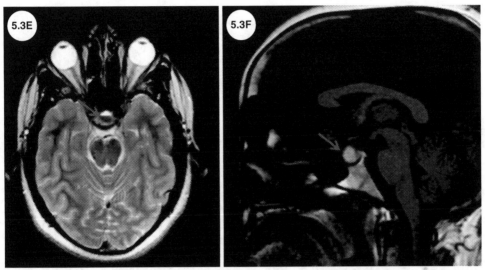

Images 5.3E and 5.3F: Axial T2-weighted and postcontrast sagittal T1-weighted images demonstrate a sellar mass with a nodule that is hyperintense on T1-weighted images and hypointense on T2-weighted images (red arrows).

Treatment

- Symptomatic cysts can be drained surgically.

References

1. Larkin S, Karavitaki N, Ansorge O. Rathke's cleft cyst. *Handb Clin Neurol*. 2014;124:255–269.
2. Trifanescu R, Ansorge O, Wass JA, Grossman AB, Karavitaki N. Rathke's cleft cysts. *Clin Endocrinol (Oxf)*. February 2012;76(2):151–160.
3. Han SJ, Rolston JD, Jahangiri A, Aghi MK. Rathke's cleft cysts: review of natural history and surgical outcomes. *J Neurooncol*. April 2014;117(2):197–203.

5.4 | Lymphocytic Hypophysitis

Case History

A 19-year-old woman developed a severe headache and vision loss postpartum.

Diagnosis: Lymphocytic Hypophysitis

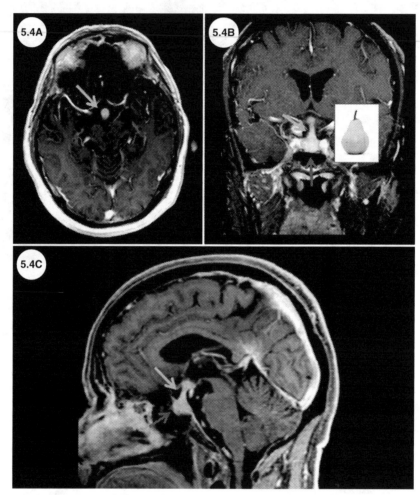

Images 5.4A–5.4C: Postcontrast axial, coronal, and sagittal T1-weighted images demonstrate enlargement and enhancement of the pituitary gland (red arrows) and stalk (blue arrows). This creates a "pear-shaped" lesion.

Introduction

■ Lymphocytic hypophysitis (LH) is an autoimmune disease that is characterized by lymphocytic infiltration of the hypophysis or infundibulum. It is pathologically related to orbital pseudotumor and Tolosa–Hunt syndrome. It is a rare cause of pituitary hypofunction.

■ It classically affects pregnant young women in third trimester or the postpartum period, but can be seen in both men and women at any age.

Clinical Presentation

■ Patients present with headache, the most common symptom, and hypopituitarism (fatigue, decreased libido, amenorrhea). Large lesions may cause visual disturbances due to mass effect on the optic chiasm or cranial neuropathies due to involvement of the cavernous sinus.

■ Involvement of the posterior pituitary presents with diabetes insipidus.

Radiographic Appearance and Diagnosis

- MRI is the imaging modality of choice to evaluate pituitary lesions. The lesion is isointense on T1-weighted images, and there is enhancement of the pituitary gland and stalk. The pituitary gland and stalk are "pear-shaped." The pituitary stalk enhances normally, but is markedly enlarged in LH.

- Most commonly, the anterior pituitary gland is affected, termed lymphocytic adenohypophysitis.

- When the entire pituitary gland is affected, the condition is termed lymphocytic infundibulo-panhypophysitis. In rare cases, the posterior pituitary alone is affected. This is called lymphocytic infundibular neurohypophysitis.

- All patients with suspected LH should have a thorough endocrine evaluation and visual field testing.

- A variety of other lesions can have a similar appearance, including adenomas, germinomas, tuberculosis, IgG4-related hypophysitis, CTL4-blockade-related hypophysitis, sarcoidosis, metastatic disease, lymphomas, or hypothalamic gliomas. In children, the most common etiology is eosinophilic granulomatous disease of the pituitary stalk (also known as Langerhans cell histiocytosis). The most common presentation is diabetes insipidus.

Treatment

- LH is treated with glucocorticoids and hormone replacement if needed. Recognition is important

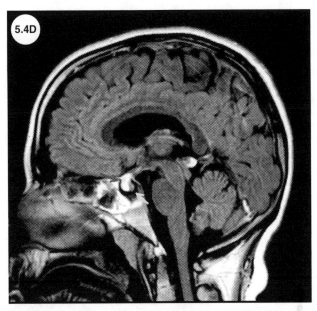

Image 5.4D: Postcontrast sagittal T1-weighted image demonstrates enlargement and enhancement of the anterior pituitary gland and stalk (red arrow) with sparing of the posterior pituitary (yellow arrow).

as it is usually self-limited, and patients can be spared surgery if the lesion is not confused with a pituitary adenoma. Chronic immunosuppression might be needed in refractory patients and surgery is indicated for patients with refractory headaches or potential visual loss.

References

1. Molitch ME, Gillam MP. Lymphocytic hypophysitis. *Horm Res.* 2007;68(Suppl. 5):145–150.
2. Rivera JA. Lymphocytic hypophysitis: disease spectrum and approach to diagnosis and therapy. *Pituitary.* 2006;9(1):35–45.

5.5 | Pituitary Apoplexy

Case History

A 63-year-old woman presented with the sudden onset of a severe headache along with confusion and blurry vision. On exam she was lethargic but able to answer simple questions. She had bilateral abducens nerve palsies.

Diagnosis: Pituitary Apoplexy

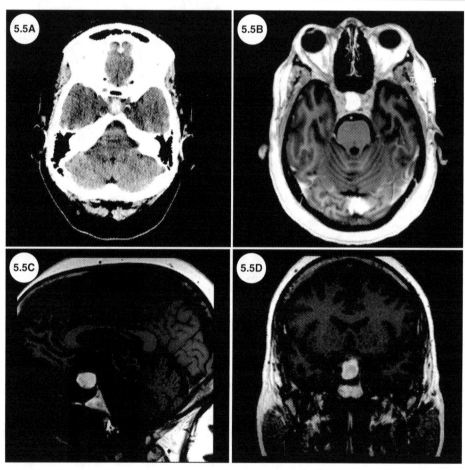

Images 5.5A–5.5D: Axial CT image and axial, sagittal, and coronal T1-weighted images demonstrate acute blood products (red arrow) in the pituitary gland in a patient with pituitary apoplexy.

Introduction

- Pituitary apoplexy occurs when there is an acute hemorrhage within or a necrotic infarction of the pituitary gland. It most often occurs in a preexisting adenoma and can be the presenting feature of the tumor. It may also occur in patients with a variety of systemic diseases such as hypertension, diabetes, or sickle cell disease. It is known as Sheehan's syndrome when it occurs in postpartum women, as normal enlargement of the pituitary gland during pregnancy is a predisposing factor to hemorrhage.

Clinical Presentation

- Patients present with the sudden onset of a severe headache, visual loss, ophthalmoplegia, and altered mental status. Other common symptoms include nausea/vomiting and photophobia.

Radiographic Appearance and Diagnosis

- CT scans will reveal the hemorrhage only if there is gross intracranial blood.
- MRI will show a pituitary lesion with variable signal on both T1-weighted and T2-weighted images depending on the age of the blood products and whether there is an underlying adenoma. A fluid level is often seen. Enhancement on postcontrast images may occur.

Treatment

- For most patients, pituitary apoplexy is a neurosurgical emergency as a subarachnoid hemorrhage can be fatal. Any patient with visual changes or loss of consciousness should undergo emergent surgical decompression. Patients with no visual disturbances or mental status changes can be monitored with serial imaging and treated with glucocorticoids. Hypopituitarism is common even in treated patients.

References

1. Briet C, Salenave S, Bonneville JF, Laws ER, Chanson P. Pituitary apoplexy. *Endocr Rev.* September 2015;36(6):622–645. doi:10.1210/er.2015-1042.
2. Briet C, Salenave S, Chanson P. Pituitary apoplexy. *Endocrinol Metab Clin North Am.* March 2015;44(1):199–209.
3. Piantanida E, Gallo D, Lombardi V, et al. Pituitary apoplexy during pregnancy: a rare, but dangerous headache. *J Endocrinol Invest.* September 2014;37(9):789–797.

CHAPTER 6
CYSTIC LESIONS

6.1 Arachnoid Cyst

Case History

A 56-year-old man presented with a headache, which was thought to be chronic tension headache with normal neurological examination. An incidental finding was noted on the brain MRI.

Diagnosis: Arachnoid Cyst

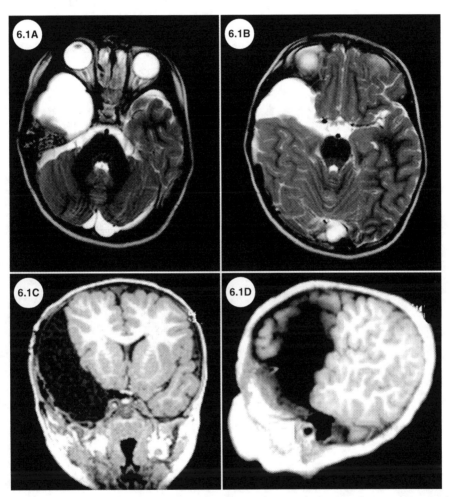

Images 6.1A–6.1D: Axial T2-weighted images (6.1A, 6.1B) and coronal (6.1C) and sagittal T1-weighted image (6.1D) demonstrate a large cystic, extraaxial lesion in the middle cranial fossa; it follows the CSF signal on all pulse sequences.

Introduction

- Arachnoid cysts (ACs) are benign sacs filled with cerebrospinal fluid (CSF) that are formed between the inner and outer layers of the arachnoid. They are usually congenital abnormalities caused by a failure of the arachnoid membrane to fuse and dysgenesis of the embryonic development of subarachnoid space, allowing for the flow of CSF into a cleft beneath the arachnoid.

- These are typically congenital but can develop after trauma, subarachnoid hemorrhage, meningitis, or mastoiditis.

Clinical Presentation

- Most cysts are incidental findings, but can cause symptoms due to compression of the brainstem, hypothalamus, or optic chiasm. Large cysts may cause hypoplasia of the adjacent brain structures.

- ACs are more common in males than females.

Radiographic Appearance and Diagnosis

- On CT and all MRI sequences, they follow the signal intensity of CSF. They are most commonly confused with epidermoid cysts, but ACs have smooth margins, in contrast to epidermoid cysts, which have uneven borders.

- These can cause bone remodeling and macro-crania.

- They are most commonly found in the middle cranial fossa outside of the temporal lobe.

- The Galassi classification system is used to describe middle cranial fossa ACs:

    - **Type I:** small size, located in the anterior temporal lobe and exerts no mass effect

    - **Type II:** medium-size cysts located in the anterior and middle temporal fossa can cause displacement of the temporal lobe.

    - **Type III:** constitutes a large oval or round cyst that fills the entire temporal fossa and exerts large mass effect

- About 10% to 15% of ACs are found in the suprasellar region. The can also be found in the cerebral convexity, cisternal spaces (quadrigeminal or suprasellar cistern), cerebellopontine angle, posterior fossa, the interhemispheric fissure, within the ventricle and the spinal canal.

Treatment

- Symptomatic ACs can be surgically drained by either craniotomy (fenestration or excision) or placement of a cystoperitoneal shunt.

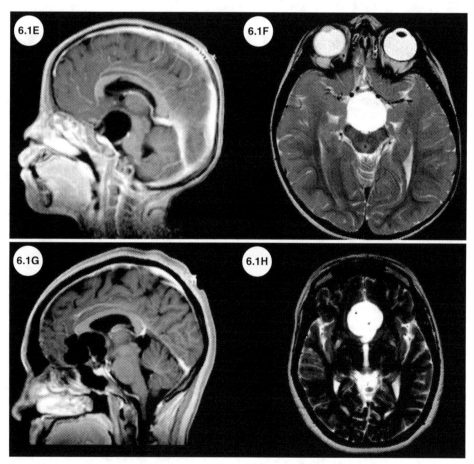

Images 6.1E and 6.1F: Sagittal T1-weighted image and axial T2-weighted image demonstrate a suprasellar cyst. **Images 6.1G and 6.1H:** Sagittal T1-weighted image and axial T2-weighted image demonstrate an interhemispheric cyst.

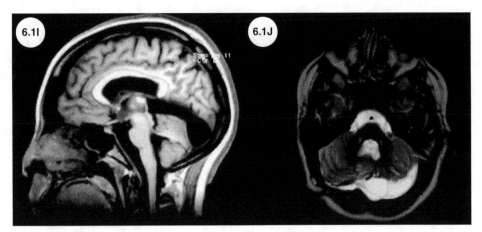

Images 6.1I and 6.1J: Sagittal T1-weighted image and axial T2-weighted image demonstrate a posterior fossa cyst. All cysts follow the isointense CSF signal on all pulse sequences.

References

1. Pradilla G, Jallo G. Arachnoid cysts: case series and review of the literature. *Neurosurg Focus*. February 2007;22(2):E7.
2. Westermaier T, Schweitzer T, Ernestus RI. Arachnoid cysts. *Adv Exp Med Biol*. 2012;724:37–50.
3. von Wild K. Arachnoid cysts of the middle cranial fossa. *Neurochirurgia (Stuttg)*. November 1992;35(6):177–182.
4. Osborn AG, Preece MT. Intracranial cysts: radiologic-pathologic correlation and imaging approach. *Radiology*. 2006;239(3):650–664.

6.2 | Colloid Cyst of Third Ventricle

Case History

A 34-year-old man developed severe headaches and transient visual blurring whenever he stood up after lying down. On several occasions, he lost consciousness after a particularly severe headache.

Diagnosis: Colloid Cyst of Third Ventricle

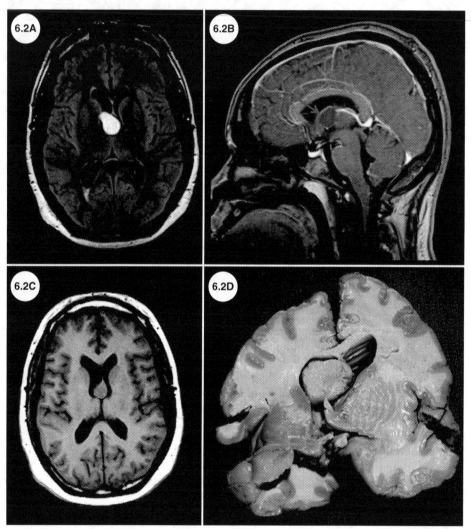

Images 6.2A–6.2C: Axial fluid-attenuated inversion recovery, postcontrast sagittal T1-weighted, and noncontrast axial T1-weighted images demonstrate a hyperintense cyst in the foramen of Monro. There is subtle enhancement around the rim of the cyst (red arrow). **Image 6.2D:** Gross pathology of a colloid cyst.

Introduction

■ Colloid cysts of the third ventricle are a type of neuroepithelial cyst. They are benign growths typically found in the anterior part of the third ventricle, adjacent to the fornix. Other benign cysts are encountered around several sites in and around the central nervous system (CNS; see **Table 6.2.1**).

Unless otherwise stated, all pathology images in this chapter are from the website http://medicine.stonybrookmedicine.edu/pathology/neuropathology and are reproduced with permission of the author, Roberta J. Seidman, MD, Associate Professor.

▓ They are uncommon, accounting for 1% to 2% of intracranial tumors; these are considered to be congenital and typically present in patients between the ages of 20 and 50 years.

Table 6.2.1 Cysts Around the Midline of the Brain and Spinal Cord

Colloid cyst of third ventricle
Epidermoid cyst in parasellar region
Rathke's cleft cyst
Epidermoid cyst in cerebellopontine angle
Dermoid cyst in cerebellar vermis
Ependymal cyst of cervical region
Epidermoid cyst in thoracic canal
Neurenteric cyst in lumbar region
Dermoid cyst in conus

Clinical Presentation

▓ In the vast majority of cases, these cysts are found incidentally and are asymptomatic.

▓ These may produce headache, papilledema, and vision changes or present with hydrocephalus and symptoms of increased intracranial pressure (ICP). It can cause transient obstruction of CSF flow through the foramen of Monro through a ball-valve mechanism. Occasionally, sudden dramatic increases in ICP can lead to a loss of consciousness or even death if the obstruction does not resolve spontaneously.

Radiographic Appearance and Diagnosis

▓ They are filled with a variety of components including CSF, mucoid content, cholesterol, proteins, and water content. This leads to a highly variable appearance. Depending on the exact contents of the cyst it can be isointense or hyperintense to CSF on MRI.

▓ With contrast administration, there is sometimes a rim of enhancement, perhaps representing stretched venous structures, but not solid enhancement. Neuroepithelial cysts may occur in any section of the ventricular system, and in such instances they are usually incidental findings.

▓ Nearly all colloid cysts are found in the anterior part of the third ventricle but rarely these can be seen in the posterior part of the third ventricle, lateral ventricles, or even fourth ventricles. Colloid cysts of the third ventricle can cause enlarged lateral ventricles and even hydrocephalus.

▓ **Table 6.2.2** lists other masses near the foramen of Monro, which should be considered in the differential diagnosis of colloid cysts of third ventricle.

Table 6.2.2 Differential Diagnosis of Other Masses Arising From the Foramen of Monro

Pediatric	Adult
Subependymal giant cell astrocytomas	Aneurysm
Subependymal nodules in tuberous sclerosis	Cysticercus cyst
Central neurocytoma	Meningioma
Pilocytic astrocytoma	Lymphoma
Choroid plexus papilloma	Intraventricular metastasis
Glioma	Glioma
Germinoma	Ependymal cyst
Craniopharyngioma	Pituitary adenoma

▓ On immunohistochemical profile, the cysts show endodermal differentiation and their walls are lined by a columnar or cuboidal epithelium; mucin producing goblet cells in the epithelium of the colloid cyst can be stained with periodic acid-Schiff–diastase.

Treatment

▓ Colloid cyst, although a benign tumor, is surgically challenging because of its deep midline location. Early detection and total excision of the colloid cyst carry an excellent prognosis.

▓ Endoscopic removal of colloid cysts in the third ventricle is a safe and effective approach compared with transcallosal craniotomy. The endoscopic approach is associated with a shorter operative time, shorter hospital stay, and lower infection rate than the transcallosal approach. However, more patients treated endoscopically needed a reoperation for residual cyst.

▓ A small number of these patients may need a transcallosal craniotomy to remove residual cysts, and this usually ensures gratifying and lasting results.

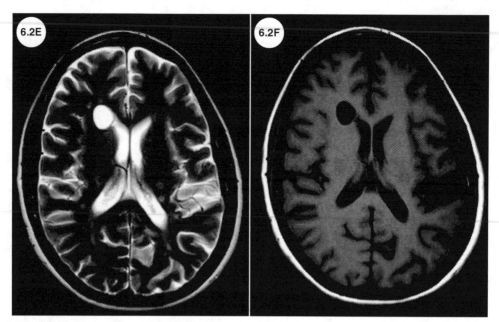

Images 6.2E and 6.2F: Axial T2-weighted and T1-weighted images demonstrate a neuroepithelial cyst in association with the frontal horn of the right lateral ventricle.

References

1. Ravnik J, Bunc G, Grcar A, Zunic M, Velnar T. Colloid cysts of the third ventricle exhibit various clinical presentation: a review of three cases. *Bosn J Basic Med Sci.* August 2014;14(3):132–135.
2. Desai KI, Nadkarni TD, Muzumdar DP, Goel AH. Surgical management of colloid cyst of the third ventricle—a study of 105 cases. *Surg Neurol.* May 2002;57(5):295–302.
3. Kumar V, Behari S, Kumar Singh R, Jain M, Jaiswal AK, Jain VK. Pediatric colloid cysts of the third ventricle: management considerations. *Acta Neurochir (Wien).* March 2010;152(3):451–461.
4. Abdou MS, Cohen AR. Endoscopic treatment of colloid cysts of the third ventricle. Technical note and review of the literature. *J Neurosurg.* 1998;89(6):1062–1068.

6.3 Epidermoid Cyst

Case History

A 40-year-old woman presented with right facial pain. The patient was diagnosed with right trigeminal neuralgia.

Diagnosis: Epidermoid Cyst

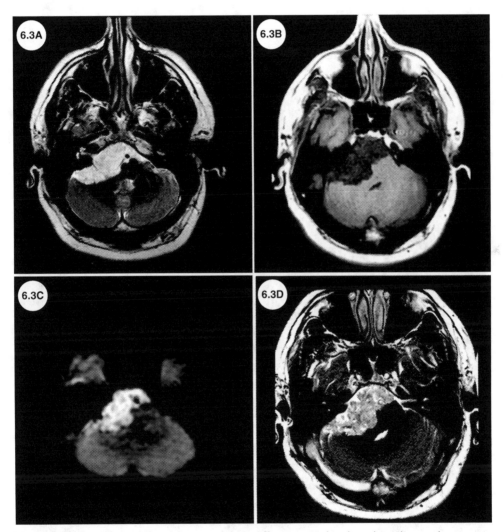

Images 6.3A–6.3D: Axial T2-weighted, T1-weighted, diffusion-weighted, and gradient echo sequence images demonstrate a cystic lesion in the right cerebellopontine angle. The diffusion-weighted image demonstrates restricted diffusion.

Introduction

■ Epidermoid cysts are congenital, and mainly intracranial cysts, most commonly found near the cerebellopontine angle, parasellar regions

and cranial diploë spaces, pineal region, or near foramen magnum.

■ They are composed of epidermal cells, which are believed to arise from embryonic epidermal rests. Mature epidermal cells are found in the center of the cyst, which frequently desquamate into the cyst center, which is also composed of keratin and cholesterol crystals. Proliferative epidermal cells line the periphery of the cyst.

- They are rare, accounting for less than 1% of all intracranial tumors.

Clinical Presentation

- They are often incidental findings, but may become symptomatic in patients in their 20s or 30s and cause headaches, seizures, or mass effect on surrounding structures.

Radiographic Appearance and Diagnosis

- They are isointense to CSF on all MRI sequences and demonstrate restricted diffusion. There may be a thin rim of enhancement with the addition of contrast.

- On gross pathology they have a smooth gray surface and friable waxy material inside. These are called "pearly tumors" due to their appearance (Image 6.3H). Microscopically, these cysts are lined by stratified squamous epithelium.

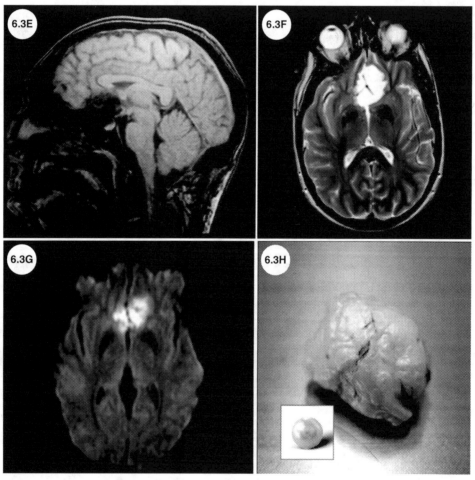

Images 6.3E–6.3G: Sagittal T1-weighted and axial T2-weighted images demonstrate a cystic lesion isointense to CSF in the suprasellar region. The diffusion-weighted image demonstrates restricted diffusion. Image 6.3H: Gross pathology of an epidermoid cyst; these cysts are known as "pearly tumors" (image credit Jensflorian).

- They are similar in appearance to arachnoid cysts; however, epidermoid cysts tend to have a jagged border, unlike arachnoid cysts, which have smooth borders. Additionally, arachnoid cysts do not demonstrate restricted diffusion.

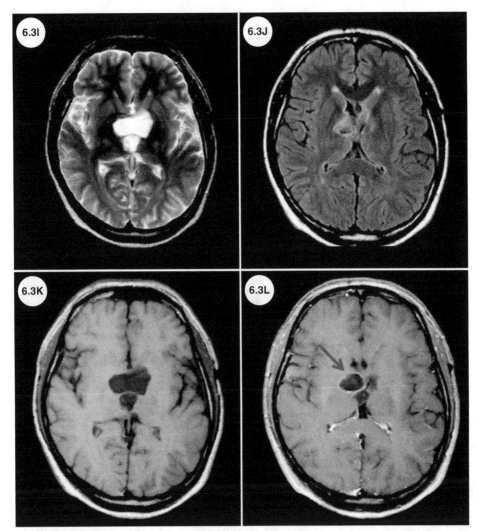

Images 6.3I–6.3L: Axial T2-weighted, fluid-attenuated inversion recovery, and pre- and postcontrast T1-weighted images demonstrate a cystic, midline lesion isointense to CSF. There is enhancement around the periphery with the addition of contrast (red arrow).

Treatment

▓ Symptomatic cysts can be surgically excised.

References

1. Hu XY, Hu CH, Fang XM, Cui L, Zhang QH. Intraparenchymal epidermoid cysts in the brain: diagnostic value of MR diffusion-weighted imaging. *Clin Radiol*. July 2008;63(7): 813–818.

2. Krass J, Hahn Y, Karami K, Babu S, Pieper DR. Endoscopic assisted resection of prepontine epidermoid cysts. *J Neurol Surg A Cent Eur Neurosurg*. March 2014;75(2):120–125.

6.4 Ruptured Dermoid Cyst

Case History

A 30-year-old woman presented with the sudden onset of a severe headache.

Diagnosis: Ruptured Dermoid Cyst

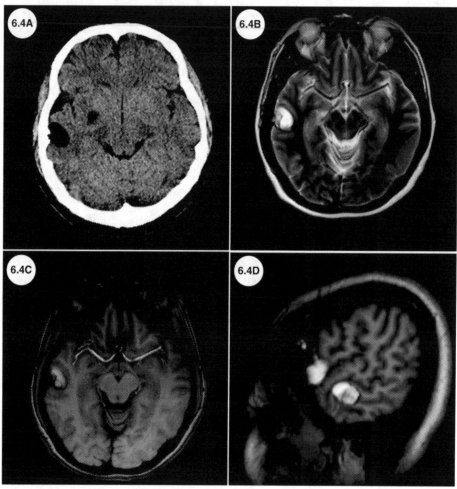

Image 6.4A–6.4D: Axial CT, T2-weighted, and postcontrast axial and sagittal T1-weighted images demonstrate two hypodense and hyperintense, extraaxial, globular masses over the right temporal lobe. On all sequences, the lesion has the signal characteristics of fat, and is consistent with a ruptured dermoid cyst.

Introduction

■ Dermoid cysts are congenital lesions believed to arise from embryonic skin tissue that remains trapped in the CNS during closure of the neural tube. Both dermoid cysts and epidermoid cysts are lined by stratified squamous epithelium. Dermoids are composed of elements of the dermis, which includes hair follicles, sweat and sebaceous glands, and epidermis, while epidermoid cysts are composed only of desquamated squamous epithelium.

■ They are rare, accounting for less than 0.5% of intracranial tumors.

■ They are often incidental findings, but when symptomatic tend to present before the age of 30.

Clinical Presentation

- They occur most frequently in the cerebellopontine angle or in the midline areas of the brain, including the fourth ventricle. They are also found in the lumbosacral spinal cord where they present with a myelopathy or cauda equina syndrome.

- They can gradually enlarge and cause symptoms due to mass effect on adjacent structures. Importantly, they may rupture into the subarachnoid space or ventricles, leading to a severe headache and symptoms of meningeal irritation due to chemical meningitis. This can lead to significant morbidity due to vasospasm and ischemia.

Radiographic Appearance and Diagnosis

- On CT, dermoids are isodense to CSF. Calcification is common as well. On unenhanced T1-weighted images, they are hyperintense and there is no enhancement with the administration of contrast. There may be pial enhancement if there is chemical meningitis due to cyst rupture. There is a variable appearance on T2-weighted images.

Treatment

- Symptomatic cysts can be surgically excised with excellent outcomes.

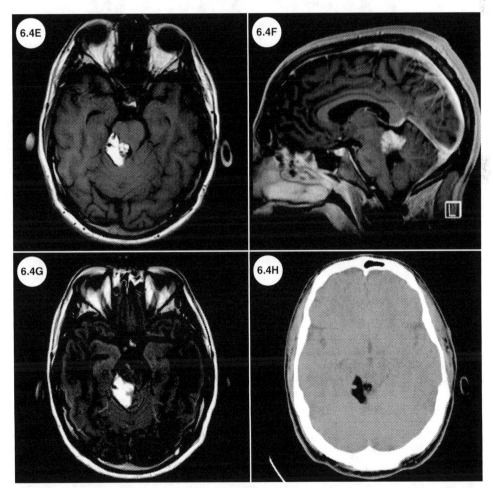

Images 6.4E–6.4H: Noncontrast axial T1-weighted, postcontrast sagittal T1-weighted, axial fluid-attenuated inversion recovery, and axial CT images demonstrate a hyperintense, hypodense lesion in the right posterior lateral mesencephalic cistern.

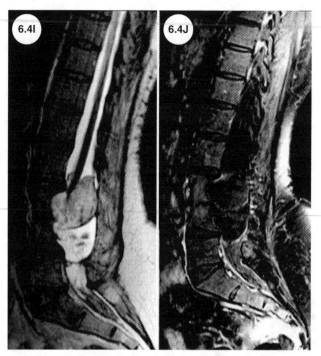

Images 6.4I and 6.4J: Sagittal T2-weighted and postcontrast fat-suppressed T1-weighted images demonstrate an intradural, extramedullary heterogeneous mass insinuating around the conus medullaris and extending throughout the lumbar spine. The inferior component of the mass has signal characteristics similar to the CSF.

References

1. Esquenazi Y, Kerr K, Bhattacharjee MB, Tandon N. Traumatic rupture of an intracranial dermoid cyst: Case report and literature review. *Surg Neurol Int*. June 2013;4:80.

2. Zhang Y, Cheng JL, Zhang L, et al. Magnetic resonance imaging of ruptured spinal dermoid tumors with spread of fatty droplets in the central spinal canal and/or spinal subarachnoidal space. *J Neuroimaging*. January 2013;23(1):71–74.

CHAPTER 7

DEMYELINATING DISEASES

7.1 Multiple Sclerosis

Case History

A 30-year-old female presented with double vision and ataxia. Three years earlier she had an episode where she lost vision in her left eye for two weeks. On exam, she was mildly ataxic, with brisk reflexes, and both horizontal and vertical nystagmus.

Diagnosis: Multiple Sclerosis

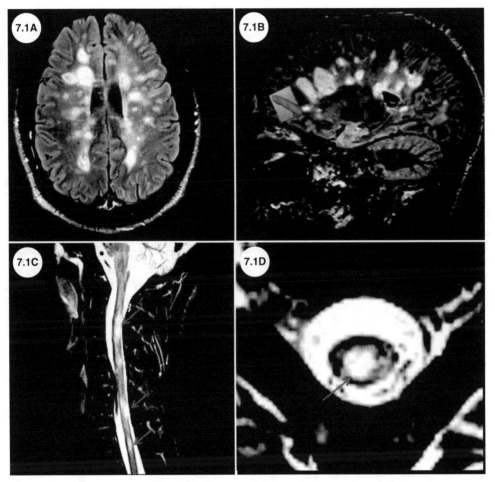

Images 7.1A and 7.1B: Axial and sagittal fluid-attenuated inversion recovery (FLAIR) images demonstrate Dawson's fingers, the oval-shaped periventricular lesions of multiple sclerosis. **Images 7.1C and 7.1D:** Sagittal short tau inversion recovery (STIR) and axial T2-weighted images demonstrate innumerable demyelinating plaques (red arrows) in the cervical spine and brainstem.

Introduction

■ Multiple sclerosis (MS) is an immune-mediated demyelinating disorder of the central nervous system (CNS) that affects about 1:750 people, or nearly 400,000 people in the United States. Aside from trauma, it is the leading cause of neurological disability in young people.

Unless otherwise stated, all pathology images in this chapter are from the website http://medicine.stonybrookmedicine.edu/pathology/neuropathology and are reproduced with permission of the author, Roberta J. Seidman, MD, Associate Professor. Unauthorized reproduction is prohibited.

■ MS is primarily considered a demyelinating disease as the myelin sheath is targeted by the immune system. Nonetheless, demyelination only reflects a portion of the pathology in MS. Axonal loss following demyelination is thought to be a major cause of permanent disability in MS.

■ Its cause is unknown, but has been associated with certain viral infections, growing up far away from the equator, low vitamin D levels, and genetics. The gene most strongly implicated in MS is the *HLA-DR2* gene, though over 100 genetic variants, mostly related to immune function, have been identified in MS. Cigarette smoking is the only behavior that poses a risk for MS.

■ It typically affects patients 20 to 40 years of age, and rarely presents after age 60 or before 10. Women are affected more than twice as often as men. It is more common in persons of Caucasian ancestry. Though the disease is less common in African Americans, it tends to have a more severe course in this population.

Clinical Presentation

■ Sensory disturbances are the most common presentation followed by motor disturbances and optic neuritis. Diplopia, vertigo, ataxia, and bowel/bladder dysfunction are less common initial symptoms. Psychiatric disturbances and aphasias are rare as initial presentations.

■ MS presents as a relapsing–remitting disease (relapsing–remitting MS [RRMS]) 85% of the time, meaning patients suffer a neurological symptom that then abates. Discrete episodes of neurological dysfunction develop over hours to days and are called relapses, flares, attacks, or exacerbations. Attacks may be quite devastating, though most patients recover well. Occasionally, however, attacks can be debilitating if left untreated, especially if the brainstem or spinal cord is involved. During a severe exacerbation, inflammatory damage to myelin can also damage the underlying axon, which can lead to poor recovery and permanent disability. Though the patient may be left with residual disability from attacks, there is no or little progression of disability independent of attacks.

■ Over time patients with RRMS evolve into a secondary progressive phase (secondary progressive MS [SPMS]) where disability accumulates gradually without overt relapses.

■ About 10% of patients present with a progressive form of the disease at onset without clear relapses, known as primary progressive MS (PPMS). Unlike RRMS, PPMS presents equally in men and women, and tends to occur at an older age. Certain presentations, such as optic neuritis, that are common in RRMS, are rare in PPMS, and enhancing MRI lesions indicative of active inflammation are less common in PPMS compared to RRMS. Generally, PPMS patients have a more rapid accumulation of disability compared to patients with RRMS, though there are exceptions.

■ There is a large degree of variation in the disability caused by MS. About 33% of patients develop no life-altering disability, 33% of patients develop enough disability to impair vigorous activities but not routine activities, and 33% of patients develop significant disability such that they cannot live independently. MS is only very rarely a fatal disease, but severely affected patients may have a slightly shortened life expectancy.

Radiographic Appearance and Diagnosis

■ The typical brain lesions are ovoid foci of T2/fluid-attenuated inversion recovery (FLAIR) hyperintensity that radiate away from the ventricles. These periventricular lesions are called **Dawson's fingers** and are best appreciated on sagittal FLAIR images. For every clinical relapse the patient experiences, the MRI shows 5 to 10 times as many lesions.

■ **Juxtacortical** lesions about the cortex.

■ **Infratentorial** lesions are in the brainstem and cerebellum and are best seen on T2-weighted images.

■ Lesions in the corpus callosum are very typical for MS, although they are not part of the diagnostic criteria for MS. These lesions are best seen on sagittal FLAIR images.

■ Significant brain atrophy is typically a feature of advanced disease; however, some degree of atrophy is often present even in early MS.

■ Damage to the spinal cord causes significant weakness, sensory symptoms, and bowel/bladder dysfunction. While brain lesions are often clinically silent, this is less commonly the case for spinal cord lesions. As in the brain, spinal cord lesions are discrete plaques within the white

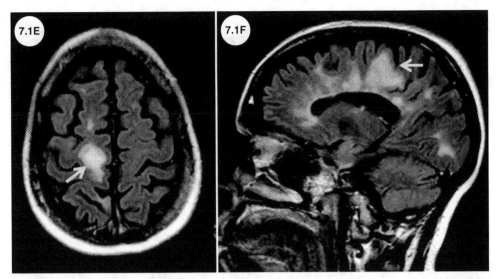

Images 7.1E and 7.1F: Axial and sagittal FLAIR images demonstrate a large juxtacortical lesion (yellow arrows).

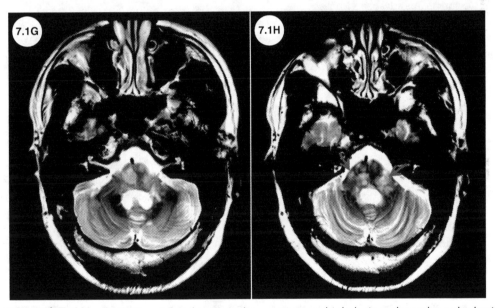

Images 7.1G and 7.1H: Axial T2-weighted images demonstrate multiple lesions throughout the brainstem and cerebellum (red arrows) in a patient with multiple sclerosis (MS).

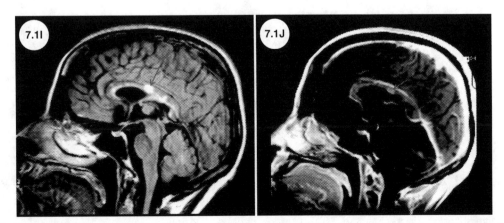

Images 7.1I and 7.1J: Sagittal FLAIR and postcontrast sagittal T1-weighted images demonstrate lesions throughout the corpus callosum, the largest of which is enhancing (red arrows).

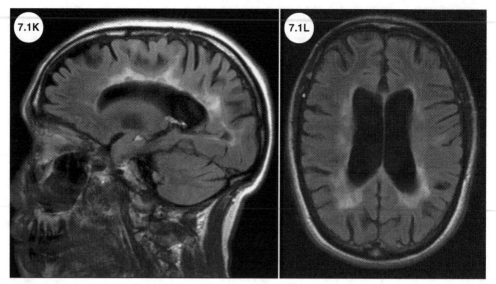

Images 7.1K and 7.1L: Sagittal and axial FLAIR images demonstrate cerebral atrophy and ventricular enlargement in a patient with advanced MS.

matter, though over time they become more confluent. On axial imaging, these lesions are typically on the periphery of the spinal cord.

- Actively inflamed lesions demonstrate enhancement after the administration of gadolinium. Enhancement patterns include solid enhancement, "ring-enhancing" lesions, and "horseshoe" enhancement, often with the opening of the horseshoe pointing to the cortex. There may be edema around active lesions, best visualized on T2-weighted images.

- Actively inflamed lesions in the spinal cord also enhance.

- In addition to enhancement, active lesions in MS may demonstrate restricted diffusion.

- Older lesions reflect irreversible demyelination and axonal loss. They appear hypointense on T1-weighted images and are referred to as "black holes."

- Some patients present with a large area of demyelination referred to as a tumefactive lesion. Patients may present with aphasia, visual field deficits, cognitive and personality changes, neglect syndromes, weakness, and sensory deficits. Both the clinical presentation and the radiographic appearance of the lesions can mimic a neoplasm or an

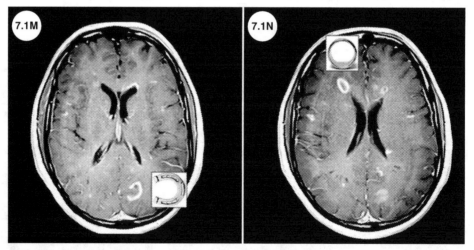

Images 7.1M and 7.1N: Postcontrast axial T1-weighted images demonstrate numerous enhancing lesions, including solidly enhancing, ring-enhancing, and horseshoe-enhancing lesions.

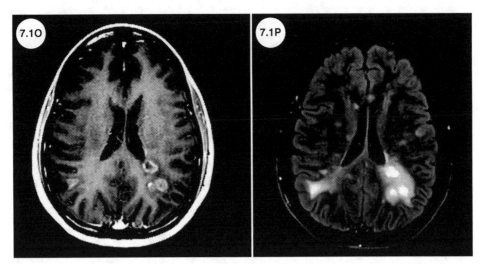

Images 7.1O and 7.1P: Axial FLAIR image demonstrates edema around the lesions.

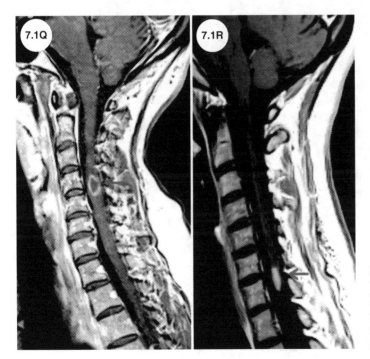

Images 7.1Q and 7.1R: Sagittal postcontrast T1-weighted images demonstrate enhancing lesions (red arrows) in the spinal cord in patients with MS. Like brain lesions, the lesions can have a ring-like appearance or a solid pattern of enhancement.

abscess, and a biopsy may need to be undertaken before the correct diagnosis is made.

- CT scans may be helpful in distinguishing tumefactive demyelinating lesions from neoplastic disease. Demyelinating lesions are typically hypodense, whereas neoplasms are typically hyperdense due to increased cellularity.

- Occasionally, tumefactive lesions in MS may take on a target, or **"onion-like,"** appearance,

where circles of demyelination alternate with rings of relatively preserved myelin. This pattern is known as Balo's concentric sclerosis. Characteristically, this radiographic pattern is associated with a more fulminant onset and atypical clinical presentation for MS (behavioral changes, aphasia, headaches, and seizures), as well as a more rapid course.

- The diagnosis of MS requires patients have two discrete episodes of neurological dysfunction, at

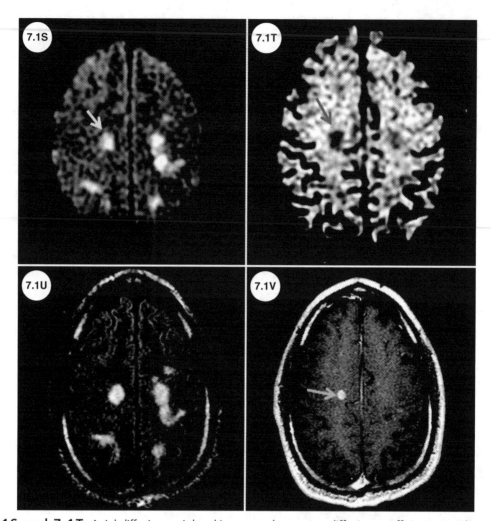

Images 7.1S and 7.1T: Axial-diffusion-weighted image and apparent diffusion coefficient map demonstrate an area of restricted diffusion (yellow and red arrows) in an active MS plaque. **Images 7.1U and 7.1V:** Axial FLAIR and postcontrast T1-weighted images demonstrate other lesions typical for MS and enhancement of the active lesion (blue arrow).

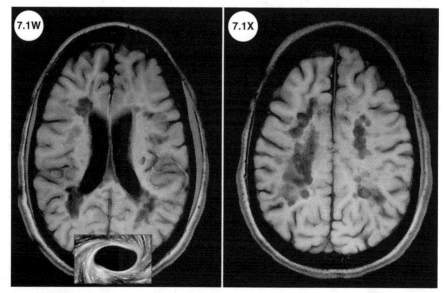

Images 7.1W and 7.1X: Axial T1-weighted images demonstrate multiple "black holes" in a patient with advanced MS.

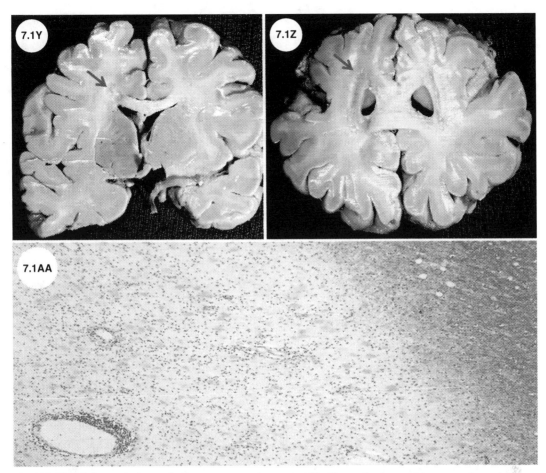

Images 7.1Y–7.1AA: Pathological specimens are shown in MS. The red arrows point to periventricular demyelination in the gross specimens (image credit Roberta J. Seidman, MD). Klüver–Barrera stain demonstrates a classic sharply demarcated demyelinating plaque in the spinal cord in a patient with MS (image credit Marvin101).

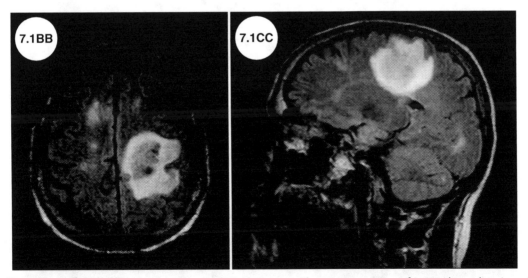

Images 7.1BB and 7.1CC: Axial and sagittal FLAIR images demonstrate a tumefactive demyelinating plaque in the left frontal lobe. The lesion is in the white matter and there is minimal mass effect. Other lesions characteristic for MS are seen in the right frontal lobe.

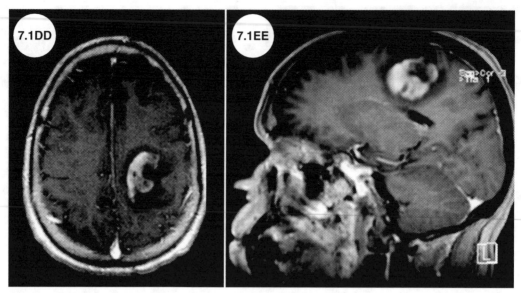

Images 7.1DD and 7.1EE: Axial and sagittal postcontrast T1-weighted images demonstrate a tumefactive demyelinating plaque in the posterior left frontal lobe with heterogeneous enhancement.

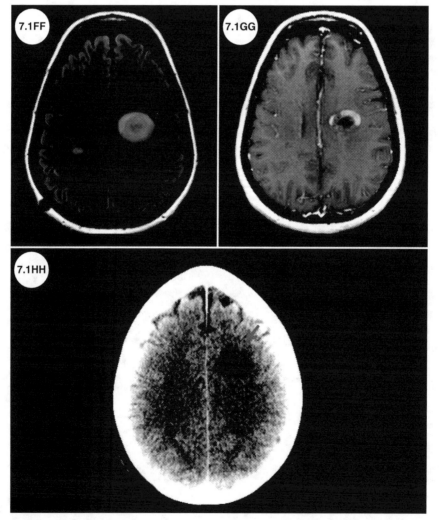

Images 7.1FF and 7.1GG: Axial FLAIR and postcontrast T1-weighted images demonstrate a large demyelinating plaque in the left frontal lobe with incomplete, peripheral enhancement. **Image 7.1HH:** Axial CT image demonstrates that the lesion is hypodense (red arrow).

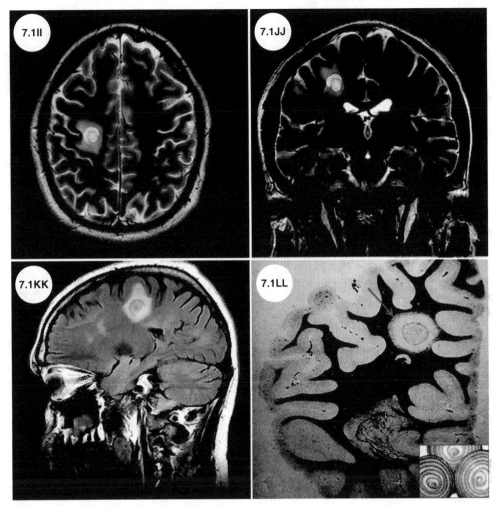

Images 7.1II–7.1LL: Axial and coronal T2-weighted and sagittal FLAIR images demonstrate a lesion characteristic of Balo's concentric sclerosis in the left frontal lobe, as well as a histological specimen showing the characteristic "onion" rings of demyelination.

Source: Khonsari RH, Calvez V. The origins of concentric demyelination: self-organization in the human brain. *PLoS One.* 2007;2(1):e150.

least 30 days apart, in different locations of the CNS. Alternatively, the diagnosis can be made in patients who have had one relapse but show evidence of dissemination in time and space based on MRI. Patients who have had a single attack but do not meet formal criteria for MS are said to have clinically isolated syndrome (CIS), while patients who have imaging consistent with MS discovered incidentally are said to have radiographically isolated syndrome (RIS). The criteria for diagnosing MS are as follows.

- *Dissemination in space (DIS) is:*
  - One or more T2 lesions in at least two out of four areas of the CNS: periventricular, juxtacortical, infratentorial, or spinal cord
  - Gadolinium enhancement of lesions is not required for DIS

- *Dissemination in time is:*
  - A new T2 and/or gadolinium-enhancing lesion(s) on follow-up MRI, with reference to a baseline scan, irrespective of the timing of the baseline MRI or
  - Simultaneous presence of asymptomatic gadolinium-enhancing and nonenhancing lesions at any time

Treatment

Treatment of Relapses

- Attacks are treated with intravenous steroids. The usual course is 5 days of intravenous methylprednisolone at 1 g/day. Adrenocorticotropic hormone (ACTH) can be used as an alternative to steroids. Severe attacks can be treated with plasmapheresis.

■ Treating relapses speeds up the rate at which patients recover from attacks, and in patients suffering their first attacks it delays the likelihood of developing MS over the next 2 years. However, the use of steroids does not have a clear long-term impact on the course of disease.

Disease-Modifying Therapies

■ Disease-modifying medications in RRMS are the injectable medications, interferon beta and glatiramer acetate, the oral medications, fingolimod, teriflunomide, and dimethyl fumarate, and monoclonal antibodies, natalizumab and alemtuzumab, and the chemotherapeutic agent mitoxantrone. These are all indicated for patients still having relapses, but other than mitoxantrone, they do not have a role in the progressive phase of the illness.

■ Traditionally, the first-line treatment was with either interferon beta or with glatiramer acetate. They reduce relapses by about 30% compared to placebo, reduce new MRI lesions, and slow the accumulation of disability. These are very safe medicines with years of experience; however, they are all injections, which are intolerable to many patients. The interferons can cause flu-like symptoms, and glatiramer acetate can be associated with local injection-site reactions, including lipoatrophy with prolonged use. Many patients experience "needle fatigue" with prolonged use.

■ Oral agents include fingolimod, teriflunomide, and dimethyl fumarate.

■ **Fingolimod** is a once daily pill that blocks lymphocyte egress from lymph nodes by acting as a sphingosine-1-phosphate receptor modulator. It was found superior to intramuscular interferon beta in a head-to-head trial in reducing relapses. It has been associated with reversible macular edema and transient bradycardia during the administration of the first dose. There have been three cases thus far of progressive multifocal leukoencephalopathy (PML) in patients treated with fingolimod as well as several deaths due to complications of varicella zoster virus infection. Considering the medication has been taken by about 135,000 patients thus far, the overall risk of infection does not seem high. Birth defects have been reported in women who became pregnant while taking fingolimod. Therefore, all women of childbearing potential should be advised to use effective birth control while on the medication

■ **Teriflunomide** blocks proliferation and functioning of activated T and B lymphocytes, which are thought to be especially damaging in MS, by selectively and reversibly inhibiting dihydroorotate dehydrogenase, a mitochondrial enzyme involved in the de novo pyrimidine synthesis pathway. In clinical trials, it reduced relapses by 30% to 40% compared to placebo. No serious side effects have emerged, though it is category X in pregnancy.

■ **Dimethyl fumarate** is a pill taken twice daily. It has been used in Europe for decades for psoriasis and was approved for MS in the United States in 2013. There were several cases of PML in patients treated for psoriasis and there have been four cases of PML in MS patients thus far, though over 170,000 patients have taken the medication. Significant and sustained leukopenia seems to be a risk factor for PML. It frequently causes stomach upset and flushing. Though these diminish over time, many patients are unable to tolerate the medication.

■ **Natalizumab** is a monoclonal antibody that prevents lymphocytes from crossing the blood–brain barrier. It is a monthly infusion, and is more effective than the intramuscular interferon beta, reducing relapses by 66%. It can cause PML, which has been fatal in approximately 100 MS patients to date. An antibody test to detect infection with the JC virus is available. Patients without antibodies to the JC virus can take natalizumab with a very low risk of PML (less than 1:10,000). Patients with an elevated antibody level can have a risk of PML that is over 1% after two years of treatment. Prior treatment with immunosuppressant agents doubles the risk. In patients who are JC virus antibody positive, the benefits have to be carefully weighed against the risks.

■ **Alemtuzumab** is a monoclonal antibody directed at CD52 (a protein on the surface of immune cells) that is currently approved for the treatment of B-cell chronic lymphocytic leukemia. It is approved for patients who failed other therapies. It is given by intravenous infusion for 5 days initially and for 3 days one year later. The most common side effects of alemtuzumab are other autoimmune disorders, the most serious of which is immune thrombocytopenic purpura (ITP), which led to a fatal intracranial hemorrhage in one study patient. Patients must therefore have monthly laboratory monitoring for 48 months after their last dose.

Treatment of Symptoms

■ Management of MS also means treating the physical, cognitive, psychiatric, and social disabilities that accompany the illness.

References

1. Oreja-Guevara C. Overview of magnetic resonance imaging for management of relapsing-remitting multiple sclerosis in everyday practice. *Eur J Neurol*. October 2015;22(Suppl. 2):22–27.

2. Milo R, Miller A. Revised diagnostic criteria of multiple sclerosis. *Autoimmun Rev*. April–May 2014;13(4–5):518–524.

3. Wingerchuk DM, Carter JL. Multiple sclerosis: current and emerging disease-modifying therapies and treatment strategies. *Mayo Clin Proc*. February 2014;89(2):225–240.

4. Cross AH, Naismith RT. Established and novel disease-modifying treatments in multiple sclerosis. *J Intern Med*. April 2014;275(4):350–363.

5. Feinstein A, Freeman J, Lo AC. Treatment of progressive multiple sclerosis: what works, what does not, and what is needed. *Lancet Neurol*. February 2015;14(2):194–207.

6. Ben-Zacharia AB. Therapeutics for multiple sclerosis symptoms. *Mt Sinai J Med*. March–April 2011;78(2):176–191.

7. Khonsari RH, Calvez V. The origins of concentric demyelination: self-organization in the human brain. *PLoS One*. 2007;2(1):e150.

7.2 Optic Neuritis

Case History

A 29-year-old woman presented with blurry vision and pain in her left eye for 3 days.

Diagnosis: Optic Neuritis

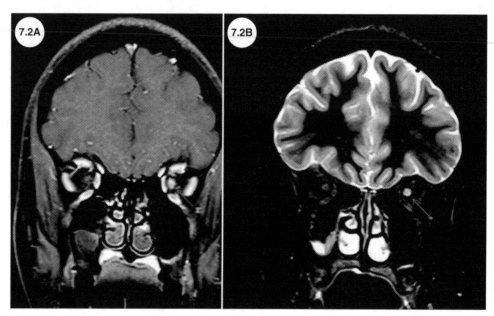

Images 7.2A and 7.2B: Postcontrast fat-suppressed coronal T1-weighted and T2-weighted images demonstrate enhancement and hyperintensity of the left optic nerve (red arrows).

Introduction

■ Optic neuritis (ON) is an inflammatory demyelinating disorder of the optic nerve that typically affects young adults, most often in patients with multiple sclerosis (MS).

■ Besides MS, a number of inflammatory and autoimmune conditions can lead to optic neuropathies. These include rheumatologic conditions (systemic lupus erythematosus, Sjogren's syndrome, Behçet disease), sarcoidosis, uveitis-associated optic neuropathy, chronic recurrent inflammatory ON, acute disseminated encephalomyelitis (ADEM), and optic perineuritis. Bilateral inflammation of the optic nerves, chiasm, and longitudinally extensive myelitis are characteristics of neuromyelitis optica (NMO). Infectious causes include Lyme disease, HIV, and other viral infections. Some cases are isolated in nature.

Clinical Presentation

■ Patients complain of blurry vision, as if they are looking through wax paper or a dirty window. The most subtle symptom is decreased perception of the color red. The vast majority have pain with eye movement. Symptoms progress over hours to days. Complete visual loss is uncommon, as is visual loss that progresses over weeks to months.

Radiographic Appearance and Diagnosis

■ All patients with suspected ON should have a contrast-enhanced MRI of the brain and orbits. This will typically reveal hyperintensity, swelling, and enhancement of the affected nerve, best seen on coronal T2-weighted and fat-suppressed postcontrast T1-weighted images. With chronic ON, the nerve may be atrophied.

- Examination of the pupils using the "swinging flashlight test" will reveal a relative afferent pupillary defect. Fundoscopic exam is typically normal in the acute phase leading to the adage, "the patient sees nothing and the doctor sees nothing." Over time, optic pallor may be observed.

- Bilateral ON is highly suggestive of NMO. Inflammation of the optic nerve in NMO is typically more posterior, often involving the optic chiasm, and is longitudinally extensive compared to ON in MS.

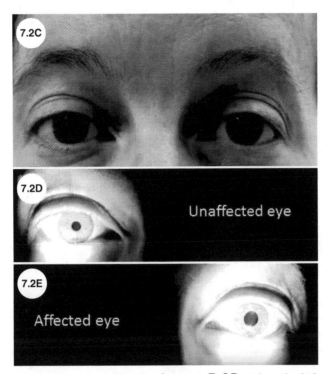

Image 7.2C: In bright light the pupils are equal in size. **Image 7.2D**: When the light is shone in the unaffected eye, both eyes constrict normally. **Image 7.2E**: When the light is shone in the affected eye, it perceives little or no light and the pupils dilate.

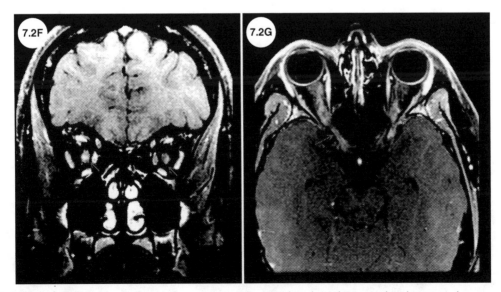

Images 7.2F and 7.2G: Postcontrast fat-suppressed coronal and axial T1-weighted images demonstrate enhancement of both optic nerves (red arrows) in a patient with NMO.

Treatment

■ ON is treated with a 3-day course of intravenous (IV) methylprednisolone (1 g) followed by an oral prednisone taper. This hastens clinical recovery but does not have a clear, long-term impact on overall visual acuity. Most patients recover, though often incompletely. Many have residual color deficits, usually of the color red, and difficulty seeing in a low-contrast environment.

■ The probability of a patient developing clinically definite MS (CDMS) is directly related to the presence of T2 hyperintensities on the initial MRI, which are found in up to 70% of patients with isolated ON. After 15 years of follow-up, only 25% of patients with a normal MRI developed MS, while 72% of patients with even one lesion went on to develop MS. Treatment with IV steroids may delay the progression to CDMS at 2 years, but not beyond that.

■ Most clinicians would suggest starting disease-modifying treatments for MS in a patient with an abnormal brain MRI. This has been shown to delay progression to CDMS in patients with a single clinical episode. However, this comes with the risk of treating patients who might never develop MS or have only a very mild disease course.

References

1. Optic Neuritis Study Group. Multiple sclerosis risk after optic neuritis: final optic neuritis treatment trial follow-up. *Arch Neurol.* June 2008;65(6):727–732.
2. Dooley MC, Foroozan R. Optic neuritis. *J Ophthalmic Vis Res.* July 2010;5(3):182–187.
3. Kale N. Management of optic neuritis as a clinically first event of multiple sclerosis. *Curr Opin Ophthalmol.* November 2012;23(6):472–476.

7.3 Neuromyelitis Optica

Case History

A 24-year-old Hispanic woman presented with severe, bilateral visual loss over the course of 3 days.

Diagnosis: Neuromyelitis Optica

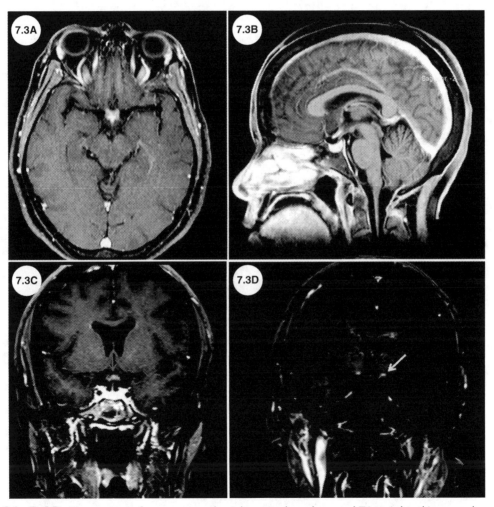

Images 7.3A–7.3D: Postcontrast fat-suppressed axial, sagittal, and coronal T1-weighted images demonstrate enhancement of the optic chiasm (red arrows) and optic tracts bilaterally (the yellow arrow points to the left optic tract).

Introduction

■ Neuromyelitis optica (NMO) is an inflammatory disease that presents with pathology of the optic nerves/chiasm, spinal cord, brainstem, or, less commonly, the brain.

■ It is an uncommon disease that affects 0.5 to 5 per 100,000 persons. It is more than 10 times more common in women than in men, whereas MS is only 2 to 3 times more common in women. Unlike MS, it is more common in African Americans, Asians, and Hispanics than Caucasians. It typically presents between the ages of 30 and 40, though it may present at any age.

Clinical Presentation

- Patients present with acute relapses, typically ON, which may be bilateral, transverse myelitis, or brainstem syndromes that present with nausea, vomiting, and intractable hiccups. Patients with brain lesions present with narcolepsy, excessive sleepiness, obesity, and autonomic dysfunction due to lesions in the hypothalamus.

- In patients with bilateral ON, there will be an afferent pupillary defect in each eye. As such, each pupil will be poorly reactive to light. In patients with significant visual loss, fundoscopic exam will reveal optic nerve pallor.

- Attacks in NMO often leave permanent disability and are generally more devastating than typical attacks of MS. With repeated attacks, there is significant atrophy of the spinal cord and optic nerves with resultant disability, which is crippling and permanent. Without treatment, the 5-year mortality reaches 30%. Unlike MS, there is no progression of disability independent of relapses.

- Patients with NMO have a high incidence of other autoimmune disorders.

Radiographic Appearance and Diagnosis

- The formal criteria for NMO are divided into two categories: those with NMO-IgG seropositivity and those without this antibody. The NMO antibody is directed against the aquaporin-4 water channel on astrocyte foot processes of the blood–brain barrier. It is positive in about 75% of patients with a clinical symptom consistent with NMO, and its presence is nearly 100% specific for NMO.

- Patients with NMO-IgG seropositivity have to have one core clinical characteristic and no better clinical explanation for their symptoms. Core clinical characteristics include:

  - **Optic neuritis:** Inflammation of the optic nerves is often bilateral and frequently involves the posterior part of the optic nerves and the optic chiasm, even at times extending into the optic tracts. In contrast, optic neuritis due to MS typically involves the more anterior part of the optic nerve and the lesion is much shorter.

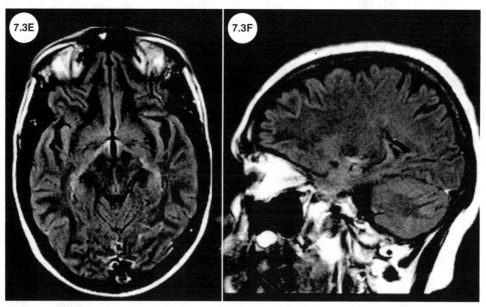

Images 7.3E and 7.3F: Axial and sagittal fluid-attenuated inversion recovery (FLAIR) images demonstrate hyperintensity of the optic tracts (red arrows) in a patient with NMO.

- **Acute myelitis:** A hallmark of NMO is longitudinally extensive transverse myelitis, meaning that the lesion is greater than

three spinal cord segments in length. There is often significant edema and enhancement during periods of active inflammation to such a degree that NMO lesions have been mistaken for neoplastic disease. Unlike in MS, where the lesion tends to be on the periphery of the cord, spinal lesions in NMO tend to be located centrally in the gray matter. Though any section of the spine can be affected, the cervical cord is most commonly affected, and the lesion often extends into the medulla. In some cases, the inflammation and swelling have been severe enough to mimic a tumor, leading to a cord biopsy.

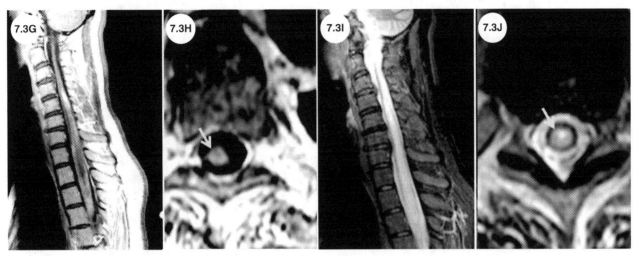

Images 7.3G–7.3J: Sagittal and axial postcontrast T1-weighted and T2-weighted images demonstrate enhancement and hyperintensity throughout the entire cervical spinal cord in a patient with NMO. On axial images the lesion is the center of the spinal cord (yellow arrows).

- Some NMO lesions present with hyperintensities of the anterior horn cells, the "owl's eye" sign, and this may mimic acute spinal infarcts.

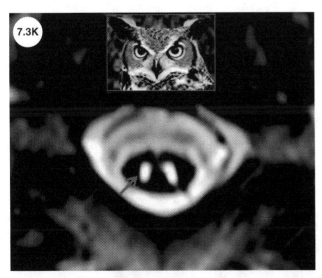

Image 7.3K: Axial T2-weighted image demonstrates hyperintensity of the anterior horn cells (red arrow), the "owl's eye" sign, in a patient with NMO.

- **Area postrema or other brainstem syndromes:** Lesions in the brainstem, often near the area postrema, are also common in NMO and present with hiccups, nausea, and vomiting.

- **Narcolepsy with a diencephalic lesion.** Brain lesions are seen in almost 90% of patients over time. The lesions correspond to regions of high AQP4 expression. In addition to the area postrema, the thalamus and hypothalamus are frequent targets.

- **Symptomatic brain lesion:** Periventricular brain lesions may be seen in NMO; however, the lesions typically line the ventricles and do not appear like Dawson's fingers as seen in MS. Some patients may develop large cerebral lesions mimicking tumefactive MS.

- Corticospinal tract lesions have been described as well, and were in fact, the most common brain abnormality in a cohort of Korean patients with NMO. They typically involve the posterior limb of the internal capsule and cerebral peduncle in the midbrain.

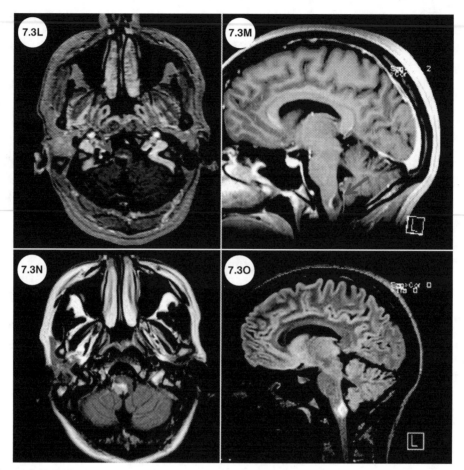

Images 7.3L and 7.3M: Postcontrast axial and sagittal T1-weighted images demonstrate a peripherally enhancing lesion in the medulla on the left (red arrows). **Images 7.3N and 7.3O:** Axial and sagittal FLAIR images demonstrate hyperintense lesion in the medulla.

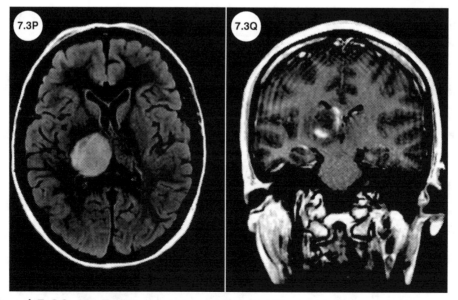

Images 7.3P and 7.3Q: Axial FLAIR and postcontrast coronal T1-weighted images demonstrate a large right thalamic lesion with ring enhancement in a patient with NMO.

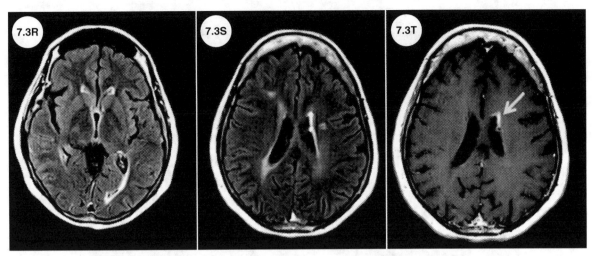

Images 7.3R–7.3T: Axial FLAIR images and postcontrast axial T1-weighted images demonstrate hyperintensity of the ventricular walls, including an enhancing lesion abutting the left lateral ventricle in the frontal lobe (yellow arrow).

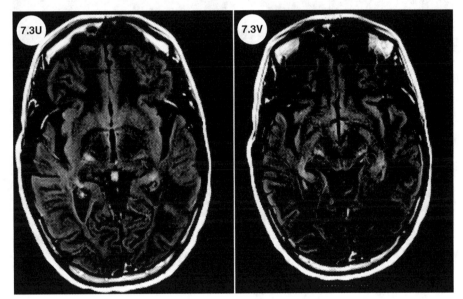

Images 7.3U and 7.3V: Axial FLAIR images demonstrate hyperintensity of the corticospinal tract bilaterally (red arrows) in a patient with *systemic lupus erythematosus* who was later diagnosed with NMO.

- Occasionally, large areas of demyelination may occur in the lobes of the brain.

- Patients who are negative for the NMO-IgG antibody must have two core clinical syndromes. These include ON involving more than half of the optic nerve or chiasm, longitudinally extensive transverse myelitis, or a dorsal medullary syndrome. This syndrome occurs equally in men and women and is more common in Caucasians. Simultaneous ON and transverse myelitis are common as the initial presentation.

- Cerebrospinal fluid (CSF) analysis in NMO typically shows up to several hundred mononuclear cells and increased protein. In contrast to MS, oligoclonal bands are present in only about 25% of cases.

Treatment

- Like MS, relapses in NMO are treated with IV and plasmapheresis for severe relapses.

- There are no completed, randomized, clinical trials of disease-modifying treatments in NMO, but small series support the use of immunosuppressive agents such as mycophenolate mofetil and azathioprine. The monoclonal antibody

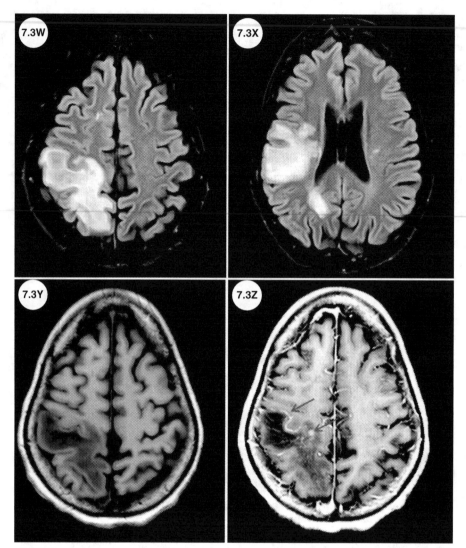

Images 7.3W–7.3Z: Axial FLAIR images and pre- and postcontrast axial T1-weighted images demonstrate a large, tumefactive demyelinating lesion in the right frontal, parietal, and occipital lobes, with peripheral enhancement (red arrows) in a patient with NMO.

rituximab, which eliminates circulating B-cells, has shown the greatest efficacy. The anti-interleukin-6 receptor antibody, tocilizumab, has shown promise in a small series of patients. Patients are often maintained on oral glucocorticoids as well. The disease-modifying agents in MS do not play a role in NMO, and they may worsen the disease.

References

1. Wingerchuk DM, Banwell B, Bennett JL, et al. International consensus diagnostic criteria for neuromyelitis optica spectrum disorders. *Neurology*. July 2015;85(2):177–189.

2. Vodopivec I, Matiello M, Prasad S. Treatment of neuromyelitis optica. *Curr Opin Ophthalmol*. September 2015;26(6):476–483.

3. Trebst C, Jarius S, Berthele A, et al. Update on the diagnosis and treatment of neuromyelitis optica: recommendations of the Neuromyelitis Optica Study Group (NEMOS). *J Neurol*. January 2014;261(1):1–16.

4. Drori T, Chapman J. Diagnosis and classification of neuromyelitis optica (Devic's syndrome). *Autoimmun Rev*. April–May 2014;13(4–5):531–533.

5. Kim W, Kim S-H, Huh S-Y, Kim HJ. Brain abnormalities in neuromyelitis optica spectrum disorder. *Mult Scler Int*. 2012;2012:1–10.

7.4 Acute Disseminated Encephalomyelitis

Case History

An 8-year-old child presented with encephalopathy and seizures.

Diagnosis: Acute Disseminated Encephalomyelitis

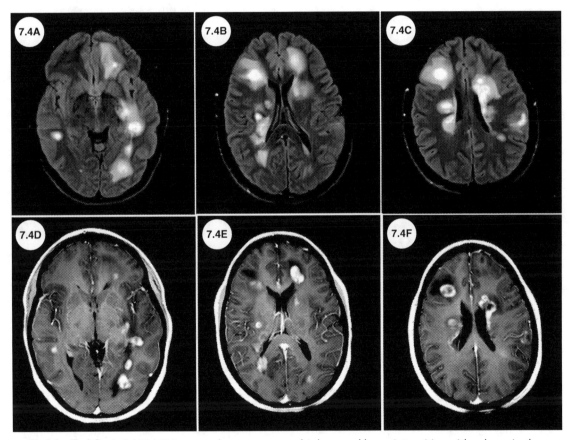

Images 7.4A–7.4C: Axial FLAIR images demonstrate multiple round hyperintensities with edema in the subcortical and periventricular white matter. **Images 7.4D–7.4F:** Postcontrast T1-weighted images demonstrate enhancement of every lesion.

Introduction

■ Acute disseminated encephalomyelitis (ADEM) is an immune-mediated, inflammatory demyelinating disorder that occurs during or after a systemic illness. It is an uncommon disease, with an estimated incidence of 0.4 cases per 100,000 people per year.

■ It is typically a childhood disease, though it has been reported at every age. The mean age is approximately 5 years, with a slight male predominance. This is likely the result of increased exposure to infections and vaccinations in children, though the incidence of ADEM with vaccines is much lower than the diseases they prevent.

- Measles infection carries the highest risk of ADEM. Influenza A and B, parainfluenza, mumps, rubella, varicella, herpes simplex virus 1, human herpesvirus-6, Epstein–Barr virus, cytomegalovirus, hepatitis A and B, and Coxsackie virus are all commonly associated with ADEM. Immunizations against measles, mumps, rubella, DPT, varicella, mumps, rubeola, influenza, Japanese encephalitis type B, and poliomyelitis are also less commonly associated with ADEM. There is generally a 30-day latency period between illness and onset of neurological dysfunction.

Clinical Presentation

- Patients present with a prodrome of headache, lethargy, myalgia, malaise, fever, and nausea/vomiting. This is followed days to weeks later by a combination of encephalopathy, seizures, cranial neuropathies, weakness, sensory deficits, ataxia, meningismus, headaches, and involuntary movements. Transverse myelitis and ON can precede ADEM.

- ADEM is usually monophasic, but relapses occur in 10% of patients. A relapse is defined as new neurological dysfunction following a month of resolution of previous symptoms.

Radiographic Appearance and Diagnosis

- The diagnosis is based on characteristic MRI findings and clinical presentation. T2-weighted images demonstrate multifocal white matter hyperintensities in the cerebral hemispheres, brainstem, cerebellum, spinal cord, or optic nerves. Most of the lesions enhance with the administration of contrast in a solid, ring, or horseshoe appearance. A lack of enhancement does not rule out the diagnosis. Restricted diffusion is common on the periphery of the lesion.

- Serum is typically normal, though there can be a leukocytosis. CSF may show mild lymphocytic pleocytosis and elevated protein. Oligoclonal bands or an elevated IgG index in the CSF are present much less frequently than in MS.

- Electroencephalogram (EEG) during the acute phase can show generalized or focal slowing with high-amplitude theta or delta waves.

Treatment

- There is empirical evidence of improved outcomes using high-dose IV steroids, which may be followed by oral steroids and intravenous immunoglobulin (IVIG). For more aggressive cases, plasmapheresis can be used.

- Mortality is highest in the first week, but most survivors do well, with the majority having made a complete recovery by 1 month. Neurocognitive deficits and seizures are the most common sequelae. The risk of developing MS has ranged from 10% to 57% in different studies. Older patients had a higher risk, and those with mental status changes had a lower risk.

References

1. Steiner I, Kennedy PG. Acute disseminated encephalomyelitis: current knowledge and open questions. *J Neurovirol.* June 2015;21(5):473–479.
2. Alper G. Acute disseminated encephalomyelitis. *J Child Neurol.* November 2012;27(11):1408–1425.
3. Marin SE, Callen DJ. The magnetic resonance imaging appearance of monophasic acute disseminated encephalomyelitis: an update post application of the 2007 consensus criteria. *Neuroimaging Clin N Am.* May 2013;23(2):245–266.
4. Scolding N. Acute disseminated encephalomyelitis and other inflammatory demyelinating variants. *Handb Clin Neurol.* 2014;122:601–611.
5. Dale RC, Branson JA. Acute disseminated encephalomyelitis or multiple sclerosis: can the initial presentation help in establishing a correct diagnosis? *Arch Dis Child.* June 2005;90(6):636–639.
6. Mikaeloff Y, Suissa S, Vallée L, et al. First episode of acute CNS inflammatory demyelination in childhood: prognostic factors for multiple sclerosis and disability. *J Pediatr.* February 2004;144(2):246–252.

7.5   Susac's Syndrome

Case History

A 28-year-old woman presented with encephalopathy and hearing loss.

Diagnosis: Susac's Syndrome

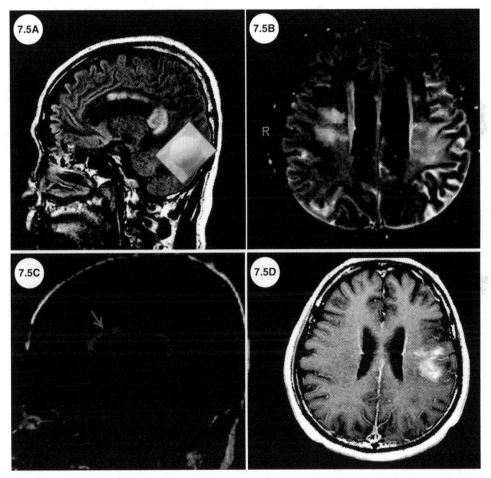

Images 7.5A and 7.5B: Sagittal and axial FLAIR images demonstrate "snowball" lesions in the corpus callosum, numerous white matter hyperintensities, the largest in the left frontal lobe. There is also significant hyperintensity of the leptomeninges. **Images 7.5C and 7.5D:** Sagittal T1-weighted and postcontrast axial T1-weighted images demonstrate hypointensities (red arrow) in the center of the corpus callosum and enhancement of the lesion in the left frontal lobe.

Introduction

- Susac's syndrome (also known as retinocochleo-cerebral vasculopathy) is a rare microangiopathy that affects the brain, eyes, and ears. It is thought to be an autoimmune reaction against endothelial cells in blood vessels.

- It can occur at any age, but most characteristically affects females between the ages of 20 and 40.

Clinical Presentation and Diagnosis

▨ It is characterized by the triad of encephalopathy, branch retinal artery occlusion (BRAO), and hearing loss, though not all three features are present in every patient.

1. **Encephalopathy:** The features of encephalopathy can be quite varied, including headaches, psychiatric disturbances, cognitive changes, seizures, ataxia, aphasia, and frank dementia.

2. **Branch retinal artery occlusion:** BRAO causes visual loss and is best evaluated using fluorescein angiography.

3. **Hearing loss:** The hearing loss is due to cochlear end arteriole occlusion. It may be unilateral or bilateral and may be severe and acute or mild and insidious. Audiometry reveals bilateral sensorineural hearing loss, with low to moderate range frequencies preferentially affected. Vertigo and tinnitus are common.

Radiographic Appearance and Diagnosis

▨ Imaging findings include hyperintensities in the white matter and corpus callosum on T2-weighted images. The lesions in the corpus callosum are round, having a "snowball" appearance. Hypointensities in the corpus callosum on T1-weighted images are also typical. Abnormalities are found in the gray matter in up to 70% of patients and the leptomeninges in 30%. Acute lesions typically enhance with the administration of contrast. The appearance may be very similar to MS, though hearing loss and acute encephalopathy are not common features of MS.

Treatment

▨ High-dose steroids combined with IVIG is the preferred treatment. Oral immunosuppressants (mycophenolate mofetil, azathioprine) or rituximab may be used in refractory cases. Many cases, especially the encephalopathic form, resolve spontaneously.

References

1. Rennebohm RM, Susac JO. Treatment of Susac's syndrome. *J Neurol Sci.* June 2007;257(1–2):215–220.
2. Rennebohm R, Susac JO, Egan RA, Daroff RB. Susac's syndrome—update. *J Neurol Sci.* December 2010;299(1–2):86–91.
3. Rennebohm RM, Egan RA, Susac JO. Treatment of Susac's syndrome. *Curr Treat Options Neurol.* January 2008;10(1):67–74.

7.6 Adrenoleukodystrophy

Case History

An 8-year-old boy presented with progressive dementia, blindness, and seizures.

Diagnosis: Adrenoleukodystrophy

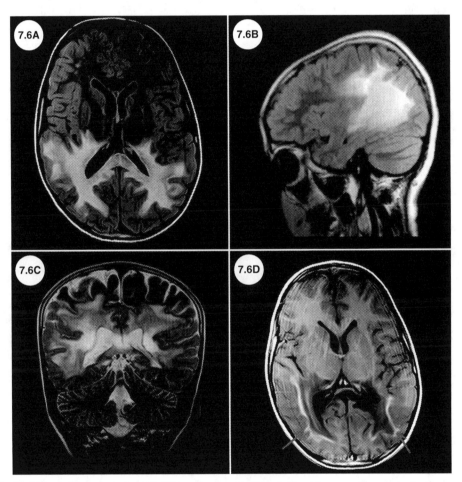

Images 7.6A–7.6C: Axial and sagittal FLAIR and coronal T2-weighted images demonstrate the confluent white matter hyperintensity in the parietal and occipital lobes, extending across the splenium of the corpus callosum.
Image 7.6D: Axial postcontrast T1-weighted image demonstrates enhancement along the margins (red arrows).

Introduction

■ Adrenoleukodystrophy is an X-linked recessive genetic disorder due to a deficiency of acyl coenzyme A synthetase (ABCD1), a peroxisomal protein needed to break down very long chain fatty acids (VLCFAs). These VLCFAs, particularly cerotic acid, accumulate in central nervous system (CNS) myelin and the adrenal gland. The abnormal gene is located on the X chromosome.

■ It is rare, affecting 1 in 20,000 to 50,000 people.

Clinical Presentation

■ There is a wide phenotypic variation, even in the same family and genotype.

■ They are classified as follows:

1. **Childhood cerebral:** The most severe form affects males between the ages of 3 and 10

years. Patients present with either symptoms of adrenal insufficiency or neurological symptoms, which include dementia, deafness, blindness, or seizures. In patients with neurological disease, life expectancy is only several years. This affects about 35% of patients.

2. **Adolescent cerebral:** similar to childhood cerebral, but symptoms develop between the ages of 10 and 20.

3. **Adult cerebral:** presents in adulthood with dementia and psychiatric symptoms.

4. **Adrenomyeloneuropathy (AMN):** a combination of progressive neuropathy and paraparesis. About 50% of patients present with AMN.

5. **Addison's disease:** isolated adrenal insufficiency.

■ About 50% of women develop symptoms. They most frequently present later in life with features of AMN. Most have a mild myelopathy, but some have a more severe myeloneuropathy. Cerebral involvement occurs in less than 2% of affected women.

Radiographic Appearance and Diagnosis

■ There are symmetric T2-weighted abnormalities of the white matter in the posterior parts of the brain and splenium of the corpus callosum. The white matter is divided into three zones:

1. The **central zone** is an area of irreversible scarring axonal destruction, gliosis, and cavitation, which is markedly hyperintense on T2-weighted images.

2. The **intermediate zone** is an area of active demyelination, perivascular lymphocytic infiltrates, and breakdown of the blood–brain barrier. This is isointense or mildly hypointense on T2-weighted images.

3. The **outer zone** is the leading edge, with active demyelination and preservation of axons. This is moderately hypointense on T2-weighted images, and about 50% of cases demonstrate enhancement on the margins with the addition of contrast.

■ The diagnosis is confirmed by finding elevated levels of VLCFAs and a mutation in the *ABCD1* gene.

Treatment

■ A mixture of unsaturated fatty acids glycerol trioleate and glyceryl trierucate in a 4:1 ratio (Lorenzo's oil) inhibits fatty acid elongation, but does not stop neurological progression. Dietary restriction of VLCFAs is of limited value as they are produced endogenously. Adrenal insufficiency is treated with hormone replacement.

■ Stem cell transplants can stop the demyelination, but are ineffective and may even worsen disease once neurological disease has begun.

References

1. Engelen M, Kemp S, Poll-The BT. X-linked adrenoleukodystrophy: pathogenesis and treatment. *Curr Neurol Neurosci Rep.* October 2014;14(10):486.
2. Cappa M, Bizzarri C, Vollono C, Petroni A, Banni S. Adrenoleukodystrophy. *Endocr Dev.* 2011;20:149–160.
3. Siddiqui S, Pawar G, Hogg JP. MRI in X-linked adrenoleukodystrophy. *Neurology.* January 2015;84(2):211.

7.7 Adult Polyglucosan Body Disease

Case History

A 56-year-old man presented with progressive leg weakness and urinary incontinence.

Diagnosis: Adult polyglucosan body disease

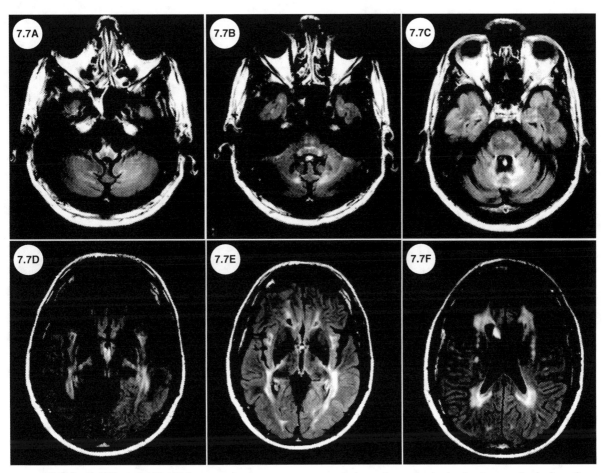

Images 7.7A–7.7F: Axial FLAIR images demonstrate symmetric hyperintensity in the brainstem (including the corticospinal tract and medial lemniscus), deep cerebellar nuclei, external capsule, and periventricular white matter. The medulla is atrophied.

Introduction

- Adult polyglucosan body disease (APBD) is a rare, autosomal-recessive glycogen storage disorder. It is a disorder of the *GBE1* gene, which produces glycogen branching enzyme. Abnormal glycogen molecules, called polyglucosan bodies,

accumulate within multiple cells, though neurons are particularly vulnerable. Axons of the peripheral nervous system (PNS) are affected as well.

- It typically presents in the sixth decade and is more common in people of Ashkenazi Jewish heritage.

Clinical Presentation

■ Neurogenic bladder is a universal symptom, and over 90% of patients experience progressive paraparesis, gait disturbances, and sensory loss in the legs. Mild executive dysfunction occurs in about 50% of patients.

Radiographic Appearance and Diagnosis

■ T2-weighted images show symmetric white matter hyperintensities in the periventricular regions, posterior limb of the internal capsule, insula, external capsule, corticospinal tracts and medial lemniscus in the brainstem, and the cerebellum around the fourth ventricle. All patients have atrophy of the medulla and spine. General atrophy of the brain and cerebellum is common as well.

■ A peripheral nerve biopsy will show characteristic polyglucosan bodies within nerve tubes.

■ The diagnosis can be confirmed by molecular genetic testing of the glycogen branching enzyme gene.

Treatment

■ There is no specific treatment other than symptomatic relief. Patients become wheelchair-bound in their 60s and death occurs in their 70s.

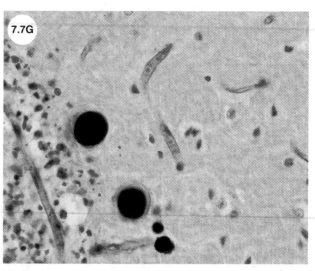

Image 7.7G: Polyglucosan bodies (photo credit Marvin101).

References

1. Mochel F, Schiffmann R, Steenweg ME, et al. Adult polyglucosan body disease: Natural history and key magnetic resonance imaging findings. *Ann Neurol.* September 2012;72(3):433–441.
2. Klein CJ. Adult polyglucosan body disease. *Gene Reviews.*

7.8 Krabbe's Disease

Case History

An 18-month-old child developed seizures and started losing weight. On examination the child had nystagmus and hearing loss.

Diagnosis: Krabbe's Disease

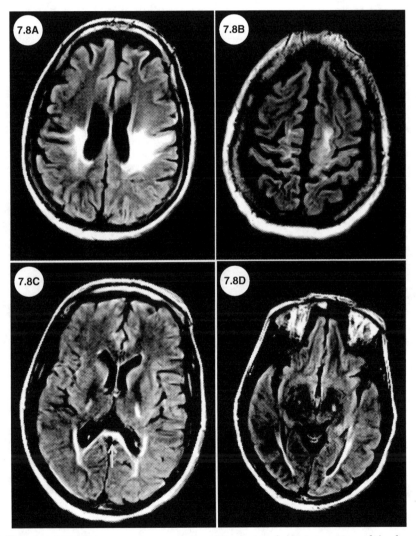

Images 7.8A–7.8D: Axial FLAIR images demonstrate white matter hyperintensities of the frontal lobes bilaterally, descending down into the corticospinal tract (red arrows), and splenium of the corpus callosum (yellow arrow).

Introduction

■ Krabbe's disease, also known as globoid cell leukodystrophy, is an autosomal-recessive lysosomal storage disease caused by accumulation of galactocerebroside and psychosine. There is

apoptosis and gliosis of oligodendrocytes with resultant demyelination. The underlying defect is the deficiency of the b-galactocerebrosidase enzyme, which localizes to chromosome 14q31.

■ It is rare, affecting approximately 1 in 100,000 individuals.

Clinical Presentation

■ It typically presents in infants less than 2 years old with irritability, weakness, poor feeding, fevers, sensorineural deafness, spasticity, nystagmus, and failure to reach cognitive milestones. Eventually, muscle weakness prevents chewing, swallowing, and respiration. Visual loss and seizures are common.

■ Late-onset forms can affect children or teenagers. Rarely, it can manifest in patients older than 40. It presents with progressive visual loss and gait difficulties. As the disease progresses, patients develop spastic paraparesis or quadriparesis. Slowly progressive dementia and cortical visual loss are common, as are seizures.

Radiographic Appearance and Diagnosis

■ On T2-weighted images multiple white matter tracts of the cerebellum and brain are affected.

These include the corticospinal tract, splenium of corpus callosum, and optic radiations. The corticospinal tract may be hyperintense throughout its course in the brain and brainstem.

■ Galactocerebrosidase enzyme activity is 0% to 5% of normal activity in leukocytes.

Treatment

■ Bone marrow transplantation and transplantation of umbilical-cord blood have demonstrated mild benefit when given early in the disease course.

References

1. Leite CC, Lucato LT, Santos GT, Kok F, Brandão AR, Castillo M. Imaging of adult leukodystrophies. *Arq Neuropsiquiatr.* August 2014;72(8):625–632.
2. Escolar ML, Poe MD, Provenzale JM, Richards KC, et al. Transplantation of umbilical-cord blood in babies with infantile Krabbe's disease. *N Engl J Med.* May 2005;352(20): 2069–2081.

7.9 Metachromatic Leukodystrophy

Case History

A 14-month-old girl lost the ability to walk as well as the several words she had learned.

Diagnosis: Metachromatic Leukodystrophy

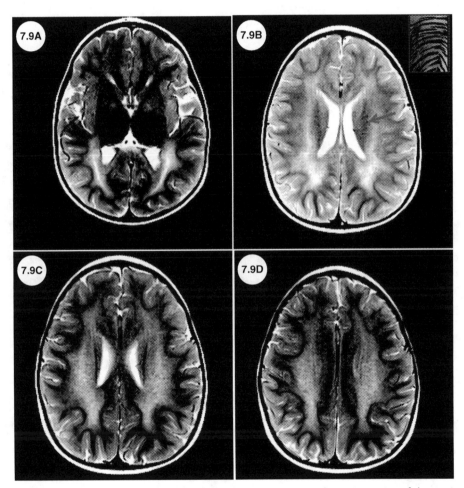

Images 7.9A–7.9D: Axial T2-weighted images demonstrate symmetric hyperintensity of the periventricular white matter. Areas of striped hyperintensity (red arrow) within the white matter create the characteristic "tigroid" appearance.

Introduction

■ Metachromatic leukodystrophy (MLD) is a lysosomal storage disorder that is inherited in an autosomal-recessive fashion. Mutation occurs in the *ARSA* gene, which codes for the enzyme arylsulfatase A. This enzyme breaks down sulfatides in lysosomes. Sulfatides accumulate in oligodendrocytes, leading to widespread demyelination.

■ It occurs in approximately 1 in 40,000 to 160,000 newborns, making it the most common hereditary leukodystrophy.

Clinical Presentation

- MLD has three forms: late infantile, juvenile, and adult. The severity of symptoms depends on the age of onset. In the most common form, children develop symptoms between 12 and 18 months. Affected children lose developmental milestones, and both motor and language skills regress. Involvement of the PNS leads to sensory loss. Patients develop progressive visual and hearing loss and dysphagia. Most patients develop seizures. Patients become progressively demented, weak, and rigid leading to death by age 5.

- Approximately 25% of patients have a juvenile form where symptoms present after 4 years, primarily with cognitive and behavioral disturbances. Progression is slower, and patients may live into early adulthood.

- The adult form affects about 20% of individuals. Symptoms first appear in teenagers and young adults, primarily with behavioral disturbances or frank psychosis. Patients may live up to 30 years after disease onset.

Radiographic Appearance and Diagnosis

- The findings are best appreciated on T2-weighted images. There is symmetrical hyperintensity of the periventricular white matter, which is said to show a "tigroid pattern" due to dark stripes that appear within the hyperintense area. Enhancement of cranial nerves may be seen with the addition of contrast.

- Diagnostic tests include arylsulfatase A enzyme activity in leukocytes, which will be less than

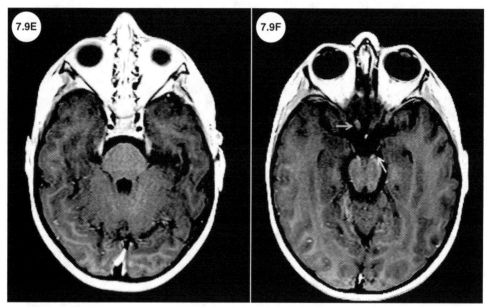

Images 7.9E and 7.9F: Postcontrast axial T1-weighted images demonstrate enhancement of the trigeminal nerve (red arrow), optic nerves (blue arrow), and oculomotor nerve (yellow arrow).

10% of normal, urinary excretion of sulfatides, and genetic testing of the *ARSA* gene.

Treatment

- At present, there is no direct treatment, though trials involving bone marrow and stem cell transplantation are ongoing. Seizure control is with standard antiseizure medications, combined with physical and occupational therapy.

References

1. van Rappard DF, Boelens JJ, Wolf NI. Metachromatic leukodystrophy: disease spectrum and approaches for treatment. *Best Pract Res Clin Endocrinol Metab*. March 2015;29(2):261–273.
2. Fluharty AL. Arylsulfatase a deficiency. *Gene Reviews*.
3. Gieselmann V, Krägeloh-Mann I. Metachromatic leukodystrophy—an update. *Neuropediatrics*. February 2010;41(1):1–6.
4. Kohlschütter A. Lysosomal leukodystrophies: Krabbe disease and metachromatic leukodystrophy. *Handb Clin Neurol*. 2013;113:1611–1618.

CHAPTER 8

EPILEPSY

8.1 Temporal Lobe Epilepsy

Case History

A 25-year-old woman had repeated episodes of the sudden onset of fear on unpleasant odor. These were followed by her losing consciousness for several minutes and making bizarre lip-smacking movements.

Diagnosis: Temporal Lobe Epilepsy

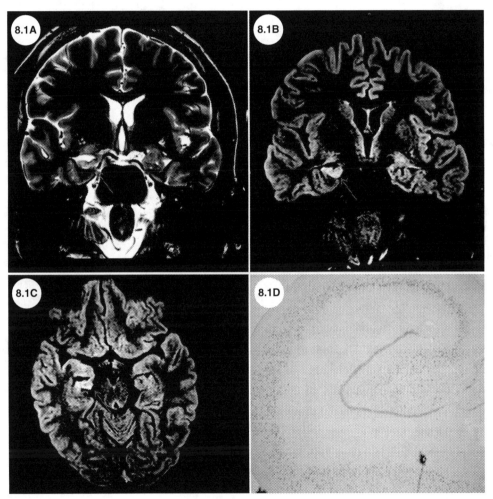

Images 8.1A–8.1C: Coronal T2-weighted and coronal and axial FLAIR images demonstrate hyperintensity and atrophy of the right hippocampus (red arrow). Mild enlargement of the temporal horn is noted. **Image 8.1D:** Pathological demonstration of hippocampal sclerosis (image courtesy of Dr. Seema Shroff, Fellow, Neuropathology, NYULMC).

Introduction

■ A seizure is defined by the International League Against Epilepsy (ILAE) as "abnormal excessive or synchronous neuronal activity in the brain." Epilepsy is defined as recurrent, unprovoked seizures due to inherent neuronal hyperexcitability. Seizures can be provoked or unprovoked. Examples of provoked seizures include metabolic derangements, such as hyponatremia, drug withdrawal (alcohol and benzodiazepines being the most common), or drug intoxication.

■ The lifetime risk of epilepsy is about 3% and about 10% of adults will have a seizure at some point in their lives. The rate of epilepsy is high in early childhood (ages 0–14.) In children, genetic factors, congenital malformations, trauma, and neoplasms are the cause of most seizures. The risk of epilepsy declines significantly until the age of 60, at which vascular disease, neoplasms, trauma, infections, and neurodegenerative disorders are responsible for most seizures. In this age group, vascular disease is the leading cause of seizures, accounting for over 50%.

■ There are two broad classifications of epilepsy: focal and generalized seizures.

Focal Seizures

■ Focal seizures are those that have their onset at a specific brain location due to some localized pathology of the cerebral cortex. These may be related to some focal brain lesion such as an infection, tumor, or injury, though in most cases the cause is unknown. Partial seizures are further divided into simple and complex seizures, depending on whether or not a patient's consciousness is impaired. A **simple partial seizure** does not affect consciousness. Partial seizures may manifest with motor, sensory, autonomic, or psychiatric symptoms, often a sense of overwhelming fear or depersonalization. **Complex partial seizures** affect consciousness and are most commonly associated with abnormalities of the medial temporal lobe. Simple partial seizures may spread and evolve into complex partial seizures. They may further spread throughout the entire brain, in which case they are called **secondarily generalized** seizures. An aura (warning) is an abnormal sensation that may precede a partial seizure.

Generalized Seizures

■ Primary generalized seizures involve both cerebral hemispheres at once without a localized area of onset. The etiology of these seizures is often hereditary. Auras do not occur in primarily generalized seizures. Generalized seizures, whether primary or secondary, always involve the impairment of consciousness, even if only for a few seconds. Types of primary generalized seizures include:

■ **Absence seizures:** Absence seizures are divided into typical and atypical forms. Typical absence seizures are characterized by brief (less than 10 seconds) episodes of unresponsiveness after which patients rapidly return to baseline, often unaware that they had a seizure. There may be subtle eye-blinking or facial movements. These seizures can be provoked by hyperventilation or photic stimulation. Atypical absence seizures are longer (up to 30 seconds) with more pronounced motor movements, and postictal confusion.

■ **Myoclonic seizures:** Myoclonic seizures are characterized by rapid, "shock-like" jerks of individual muscles or the entire body.

■ **Tonic–clonic seizures:** In the tonic phase of the seizure, the patient abruptly loses consciousness followed by a loud vocalization (the epileptic cry) as air is expelled from the lungs against a close glottis. The skeletal muscles tense and the patient falls to the ground if standing. After 10 to 30 seconds, the clonic phase begins. It is characterized by dramatic muscle contraction and relaxation of progressively increasing duration. Patients may bite their tongues due to contracture of the jaw muscles, and the eyes are open in almost all cases. There are increases in heart rate, blood pressure, pupillary dilation, and salivation. The entire seizure lasts 1 to 3 minutes. Patients are often confused after the seizure, and in some cases may become frankly psychotic, a state termed postictal psychosis. Bowel and bladder incontinence are common in the postictal phase. Todd's paralysis refers to motor weakness that persists after a seizure, sometimes as long as 24 hours. Patients may exhibit persistent symptoms other than weakness, such as aphasia, though this is less common. This is the most common type of seizure, experienced by about 10% of patients with epilepsy.

■ **Clonic seizures:** Clonic seizures are similar to tonic seizures, but without the tonic component. They usually start before the age of 3.

■ **Tonic seizures:** Tonic seizures are characterized by tonic spasms of the facial and truncal muscles, with flexion or extension of the extremities. The patient often falls to the ground, and serious injury may result. These seizures usually being in early childhood.

■ **Atonic seizures:** Atonic seizures, also known as drop attacks, are characterized by the sudden weakness of postural muscles. They can be mild and result in a mere head drop, or severe and result in a complete loss of postural tone and severe injuries.

■ The localized and generalized categories are divided into three further categories: idiopathic (unknown or inherited cause), symptomatic (identifiable cause), and cryptogenic (brain lesion is suspected, but cannot be identified).

■ Another method of classifying seizures is by dividing them into epilepsy syndromes as defined by the ILAE. Epilepsy syndromes are defined by a cluster of features including the type of seizure, its localization, frequency, precipitating factors, age at onset, additional features of neurological or systemic disease, genetic factors, prognosis, and suggested treatments.

▨ **West syndrome:** West syndrome occurs in children aged 3 months to 2 years, most commonly in infants aged 8 to 9 months. It is defined by the triad of mental retardation, seizures known as infantile spasms (IS), and a pathognomonic EEG pattern (high-amplitude waves and a background of irregular spikes) called hypsarrhythmia. The most common cause is tuberous sclerosis, though it may be idiopathic. The prognosis is related to the underlying cause, though most children have significant cognitive disability and other seizures, including Lennox–Gastaut syndrome (LGS). It is treated with adrenocorticotropic hormone (ACTH) and conventional antiepileptic drugs (AEDs).

▨ **Lennox–Gastaut syndrome:** LGS develops in children aged 2 to 18 years old. It is characterized by a variety of generalized seizures (astatic seizures [drop attacks], tonic seizures, tonic–clonic seizures, atypical absence seizures, and less frequently, complex partial seizures) and developmental delay. The characteristic EEG shows slow spike-wave complexes of 2 Hz. AEDs are rarely effective in stopping the seizures.

▨ **Juvenile myoclonic epilepsy:** Juvenile myoclonic epilepsy (JME) is a primarily generalized epilepsy that develops in teenagers and young adults who are otherwise healthy and without neurological deficits. As the name implies, patients most often experience myoclonic jerks, though other seizure types occur as well. The jerks are most common early in the morning, and patients are often thought to "be clumsy." The EEG has a characteristic pattern, showing generalized 4 to 6 Hz spike-wave discharges or multiple spike discharges. They are triggered by sleep deprivation, and a classic presentation is that of a teenager who has a generalized seizure after staying up all night. Patients will need life-long treatment with AEDs, and avoidance of triggers, namely sleep deprivation.

▨ **Benign centrotemporal epilepsy of childhood:** Benign centrotemporal epilepsy of childhood (also known as benign Rolandic epilepsy) occurs in otherwise healthy children 3 to 13 years old. The seizures almost always occur at night and the most common type of seizure is a partial seizure involving the facial muscles. Speech arrest and drooling are common. For such seizures, no treatment is required, and the seizures always remit during puberty. In some circumstances, the seizures may generalize and AEDs may be required in such children. The characteristic EEG shows epileptic spike discharges originating from the centrotemporal scalp over the central sulcus (the Rolandic sulcus), which most commonly occur during the early stages of sleep.

▨ **Benign occipital epilepsy of childhood:** Benign occipital epilepsy of childhood (BOEC) occurs in children younger than 10 and is characterized by seizures on one half of the body and a variety of visual distortions including loss of vision or positive visual phenomena typically described in migraines, such as scintillating scotomas or brightly colored patterns or shapes (fortification spectra). As in migraines, headaches and nausea are common. The EEG reveals spikes originating from the occipital lobes.

▨ **Landau–Kleffner syndrome:** Landau–Kleffner syndrome (also known as acquired epileptic aphasia) is characterized by seizures and a progressive aphasia. It usually starts as a receptive aphasia, but may eventually develop into a global aphasia or even a complete auditory agnosia. It occurs in children between the ages of 5 and 7 who were previously healthy. Spontaneous remission may occur.

▨ **Progressive myoclonic epilepsies:** The progressive myoclonic epilepsies (PMEs) are a collection of disorders characterized by progressive cognitive decline and seizures. Myoclonic seizures are the most common, though tonic–clonic seizures may occur. Specific examples of PMEs include Unverricht–Lundborg disease (Baltic myoclonus); myoclonus epilepsy and ragged red fibers (MERRF); Lafora disease; neuronal ceroid lipofuscinosis; and type I Sialidosis. The most common of these is Unverricht–Lundborg disease, which occurs in children between ages 6 and 15. It is an autosomal-recessive inherited disorder that begins in children aged 6 to 18 with seizures and cognitive decline over the course of several decades. MERRF is a mitochondrial disorder characterized by both myoclonic and generalized tonic–clonic seizures (GTCs). Other features include developmental delay, deafness, and exercise intolerance.

- **Febrile seizures:** Febrile seizures occur in children aged 6 months to 6 years when there is a rapid rise in temperature. Boys are affected at twice the rate of girls. A simple febrile seizure is a generalized seizure that lasts less than 15 minutes (usually much less) and does not recur in a 24-hour period. In contrast, any seizure that is partial in onset, lasts for more than 15 minutes, or recurs in a 24-hour period is termed a complex febrile seizure. Risk factors for developing seizures later in life include complex partial seizures, an abnormal neurological exam, or nonfebrile seizures in a first degree relative. For most children, no treatment is required. Technically, febrile seizures are classified as a seizure condition that does not require the diagnosis of epilepsy.

- **Reflex seizures:** Reflex seizures are those which are triggered in response to a sensory stimulus. The stimuli are most commonly visual and include television and video games. Other stimuli known to cause seizures include reading and the startle response. Most seizures are generalized tonic–clonic.

- **Symptomatic localization-related epilepsies:** Symptomatic localization-related epilepsies are defined by the lobe of the brain in which the seizure originates. Epilepsies arising from lobes of the brain, other than the medial temporal lobes, are often due to tumors, infarcts, vascular malformations, traumatic injuries, or infectious processes such as neurocysticercosis. It is important to note that any lesion must affect the cerebral cortex in order to cause a seizure, and lesions of the white matter, basal ganglia, thalamus, and brainstem are not associated with seizures. Patients with seizures arising from the frontal lobes often have bizarre, seemingly purposeful motor behaviors that are often mistaken for nonepileptic seizures.

Clinical Presentation

- Temporal lobe epilepsy (TLE) is a specific type of complex partial seizure, which as the name implies, arises from the medial temporal lobes. Though this is the most common origin of the focal epilepsies, other lobes of the brain can serve as seizure foci as well. The medial temporal lobe contains several important structures, namely the hippocampus, the amygdala, and the olfactory cortex. These structures are an integral part of the limbic system.

- The clinical features of the aura in patients with TLE reflect the anatomy of the medial temporal lobe. Déjà vu is a feeling of increased familiarity reflecting seizure activity in the hippocampus. Some patients experience the opposite, jamais vu, where familiar situations suddenly seem unrecognizable. Patients may also experience a strong feeling of fear due to activation of the amygdala, and patients may experience unpleasant odors, often described as if something is burning.

- Patients with TLE typically have a preceding aura, which can be:

  - **Somatosensory and special sensory:** epigastric sensations or rising surge, metallic taste in mouth, strange smell, vertigo, visual, hearing
  - **Psychic:** déjà vu (recalled emotions or memories), jamais vu (feelings of unfamiliarity), sudden intense emotions, depersonalization and derealization, extreme fear, anxiety
  - **Autonomic:** abdominal pain, dilated eyes, sweating, piloerection, flushed face, nausea, palpitations, profuse salivation (slobbering), changes in heart rate

- Automatisms are also common in temporal lobe seizures. There can be oro-masticatory manual/pedalor reactive automatisms.

- Motionless stare, behavioral arrest, speech arrest, unilateral dystonic posturing, periods of confusion, disorientation, and decreased responsiveness are common clinical features seen during dyscognitive seizures.

Radiographic Appearance and Diagnosis

- The MRI with epilepsy protocol includes T1-inversion prepared, gradient echo, echoplanar, true inversion recovery image, T2-fast spin echo, fluid-attenuated inversion recovery (FLAIR), and 3D volume acquisition of thin temporal cuts. The most common identifiable lesion on the brain MRI is mesial temporal sclerosis (MTS). In patients with TLE, subtle anatomic features of the medial temporal lobes and pathologies like MTS or incomplete hippocampal inversion are best appreciated in an oblique coronal plane. This orientation is orthogonal to the long axis of the temporal lobe and reduces volume averaging problems for the thin laminar appearance of the hippocampus. Oblique coronal temporal high-resolution T2-weighted and FLAIR are the best sequences to diagnose MTS.

■ MTS is characterized by hippocampal atrophy, increased T2 signal, and abnormal morphology or loss of internal architecture of hippocampus. In 10% of the cases, MTS can be bilateral.

■ Secondary findings may include dilatation of the temporal horn of the lateral ventricle, loss of gray–white matter differentiation in the temporal lobe, or decreased white matter in the adjacent temporal lobe (eg, collateral eminence and temporal stem). There can be atrophy of the ipsilateral fornix and mammillary body. High-resolution 3D T1-weighted images are also useful when performing hippocampal volumetric analyses.

■ The presurgical evaluation is done to determine if the patient has a single epileptogenic focus that is not in "eloquent" cortex and can therefore be resected without causing an unacceptable neurological deficit. Corroborative evidence from various forms of noninvasive advanced imaging summarized in **Table 8.1.1**, the neuropsychological testing, and neuropsychiatric evaluation help determine whether a patient is a good surgical candidate or not. Seizures originating from medial temporal structures such as hippocampi are most amenable to surgical cure.

■ Video EEG monitoring of patients' typical seizures with scalp EEG is the cornerstone of the epilepsy surgery evaluation. Supervised medication withdrawal and provocation procedures (eg, sleep deprivation, hyperventilation, photic stimulation) are often necessary to facilitate seizures.

Treatment

■ In a patient presenting with a seizure, the first goal is to attend to a patient's respiratory and cardiovascular status, and to terminate seizures if they are ongoing. In patients without a known history of epilepsy, investigations should be immediately undertaken to rule out potentially devastating and treatable conditions such as tumors, hemorrhages, metabolic derangements,

Table 8.1.1 Presurgical Evaluation of Patients With Focal Seizures

MRI	To look for any structural lesion such as MTS, cortical dysplasia, low-grade tumors (ganglioglioma, DNET etc.), malrotated hippocampus, encephalitis, cavernoma, AVM, or rare causes such as encephalocele of the sphenoid wing
VEEG	Differentiates epileptic from nonepileptic events; determines if seizures originate from a single focus or multiple foci
Wada	Language memory test; tells which side is controlling the language in the brain and gives individual scores of memory on each side of the brain
PET	Directly measures neurometabolic activity and receptor binding; regional reduction in glucose uptake (hypometabolism) during the interictal state in FDG-PET
SPECT *ictal interictal* SISCOM	Hyperperfusion of the seizure focus Hypoperfusion of the seizure focus Subtraction ictal SPECT co-registered to MRI
MEG, MSI	Localizes source of epileptiform discharges; when it is combined with structural imaging, it is called magnetic source imaging mainly used for co-registration with MRI to give MSI in three-dimensional space
fMRI	Identifies eloquent cortices such as language, motor, somatosensory, visual, auditory
DWI	Sensitive to the translational motion of water molecules in a lesion and helps identify strokes, neoplastic lesions, or abscesses
DTI	Helps precise delineation of white matter tracts in the brain; identifies eloquent white matter tracts, such as the arcuate fasciculus or the anterior extent of Meyer's loop
MRS	Differentiates between dysplastic versus neoplastic masses, recurrent brain neoplasm versus radiation injury, or between an abscess versus a tumor; decreased NAA and decreased NAA/Cho and NAA/Cr ratios and decreased myoinositol in ipsilateral temporal lobe and increased lipid and lactate soon after a seizure

AVM, arteriovenous malformation; DTI, diffusion tensor imaging; DWI, diffusion-weighted image; FDG-PET, fludeoxyglucose-PET; fMRI, functional magnetic resonance imaging; MEG, magnetoencephalogram; MRS, magnetic resonance spectroscopy; MSI, magnetic source imaging; NAA, N-acetyl aspartate; NAA/Cho, NAA/Choline; NAA/Cr, NAA/Creatine; SISCOM, subtraction ictal SPECT co-registered to MRI; SPECT, single photon emission computed tomography; VEEG, video EEG.

or central nervous system (CNS) infections that can present with seizures.

▪ Status epilepticus (SE) is a life-threatening condition defined as a seizure lasting longer than 30 minutes, or recurrent seizures without regaining consciousness between seizures for greater than 30 minutes. Benzodiazepines are the preferred initial management due to their rapid onset of action. Note that intravenous (IV) phenytoin cannot be given rapidly due to its risk for cardiac arrhythmias. Fosphenytoin can be given at triple the rate of phenytoin and can be given intramuscularly. The MRI findings for a patient who was in SE are shown.

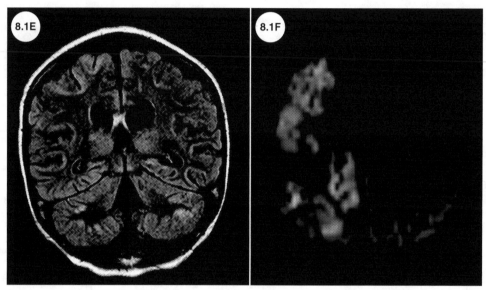

Images 8.1E and 8.1F: Coronal FLAIR and axial diffusion-weighted images demonstrate hyperintensity and multiple areas of restricted diffusion, primarily in the cortical ribbon of the right hemisphere.

▪ Epilepsia partialis continua refers to a persistent focal motor seizure, typically involving the hand, foot, or face.

▪ The mainstay of treatment is AEDs. These are summarized in **Table 8.1.2**.

▪ Women of childbearing age should have a pregnancy test prior to the initiation of any AED and clinicians must be aware that many AEDs lower the effectiveness of birth control medications. Most AEDs are teratogenic, though the vast majority of women have uncomplicated pregnancies. The risk of having uncontrolled seizures during pregnancy is considered more dangerous than the effects of medications, and the continued use of medications is suggested for most patients. All women in whom pregnancy is a possibility should be placed on high doses of folate to help minimize the risk of neural tube defects.

▪ Patients with epilepsy do not necessarily need to be on lifelong medications. Patients who have been seizure-free on medications for several years and have a normal neurological examination, MRI, and EEG may no longer need AEDs, and considering the side effects of these medications, attempts to lower or stop these medications are a reasonable action in many patients. Medications should be gradually lowered over the course of 3 to 4 months. The highest risk for seizure recurrence is in the first 3 months after medication discontinuation.

▪ There is some controversy over whether patients with a single seizure and no family history of seizures should be treated in the context of a normal neurological examination, EEG, and MRI. Most neurologists would not initiate treatment in such patients unless they had a second seizure.

▪ Approximately 30% of patients have seizures that are refractory to medical treatments. In these patients, surgical removal of epileptogenic foci can dramatically reduce or even eliminate seizures. Surgical removal of the temporal lobe is the most common surgical procedure in epilepsy and results in freedom from seizures in about 80% of patients, and a drastic reduction in seizure frequency in almost all patients. In this procedure, intracranial electrodes are implanted to

Table 8.1.2 Antiepileptic Medications

Medication	Indications	Common/Concerning Side Effects
Carbamazepine (Tegretol)	Partial seizures	Can worsen absence, myotonic, and atonic seizures; hyponatremia, vertigo, headache, ataxia, blood dyscrasias
Oxcarbazepine (Trileptal)	Partial seizures	Can lead to hyponatremia, but does not affect the levels of other medications
Lacosamide (Vimpat)	Poorly controlled partial-onset seizures	
Phenytoin (Dilantin)	Partial seizures, generalized tonic–clonic seizures, tonic and atonic seizures	Gum hyperplasia, osteoporosis, hirsutism, rash with chronic use; ataxia, nystagmus, and confusion at high levels
Lamotrigine (Lamictal)	Effective in juvenile myoclonic epilepsy and Lennox–Gastaut syndrome	Stevens–Johnson syndrome, especially if started at high doses; must be raised slowly to prevent rash
Levetiracetam (Keppra)	Partial-onset, myoclonic, or tonic–clonic seizures	Depression, psychosis
Eslicarbazepine (Aptiom)	Partial-onset seizures as monotherapy or adjunctive therapy	Dizziness, nausea, headache, and sedation
Rufinamide (Banzel)	Adjunctive treatment of seizures associated with Lennox–Gastaut syndrome in children 4 years and older and adults	Sedation
Tiagabine (Gabitril)	Adjunctive treatment for partial seizures	Sedation and cognitive slowing
Gabapentin (Neurontin)	Focal and partial seizures; neuropathic pain	Dizziness, fatigue, depression
Phenobarbital	Used primarily in children in developing countries or to treat status epilepticus; used for all seizure types except absence	Sedation and behavioral changes
Pregabalin (Lyrica)	Partial-onset seizures, neuropathic pain	Poor memory, poor coordination, dry mouth, visual disturbances, and weight gain
Topiramate (Topamax)	Monotherapy in partial or mixed seizures, drop attacks in Lennox–Gastaut syndrome	Nephrolithiasis, weight loss, cognitive slowing especially at higher doses
Zonisamide (Zonegran)	Adjunctive treatment in partial seizures	Nephrolithiasis, weight loss
Vigabatrin (Sabril)	Infantile spasms due to tuberous sclerosis and adjunctive therapy for adult patients with refractory complex partial seizures	Sedation, visual loss
Felbamate (Felbatol)	Partial and generalized seizures associated with Lennox–Gastaut syndrome	Potentially fatal aplastic anemia and liver failure
Clobazam (Onfi)	Lennox–Gastaut syndrome in children older than 2; tonic–clonic, complex partial, and myoclonic seizures	Tolerance and rebound seizures when discontinued
Valproate (Depakote)	Primary generalized epilepsies including absence, myoclonic, and tonic–clonic seizures	Weight gain, pancreatitis, neural tube defects in pregnancy, hepatic toxicity in young children; interacts with many other antiepileptic drugs
Perampanel (Fycompa)	Refractory partial seizures	Neuropsychiatric dysfunction, violent thoughts
Ethosuximide (Zarontin)	Used only in absence seizures	

try to localize the epileptogenic tissue. Functional studies such as PET and single photon emission computed tomography (SPECT) are used to help further localize the epileptic focus. Careful brain mapping of the proposed area of resection is required prior to any epilepsy surgery to ensure that patients are not left with severe language or cognitive deficits after the surgery. A Wada test is an injection of sodium amobarbital, a barbiturate, directly into one of the carotid arteries. This effectively sedates a single hemisphere of the brain allowing for memory and language functioning to be tested in each hemisphere. This helps ensure that eloquent brain areas are not removed. Additionally, electrocorticographic mapping on awake patients can be performed at the time of the operation to better delineate the function of exact brain areas prior to their potential resection.

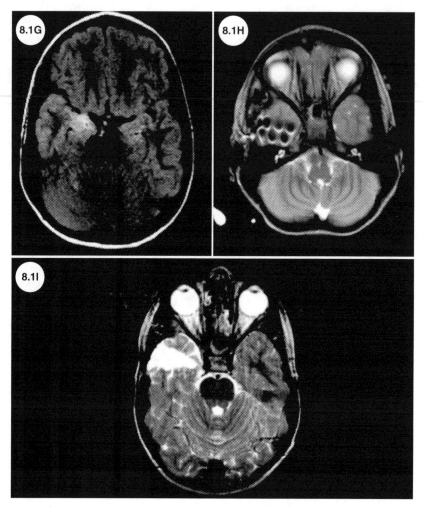

Image 8.1G: Axial FLAIR image demonstrates hyperintensity of the right medial temporal lobe.
Image 8.1H: Axial T2-weighted image demonstrates intracranial electrodes used to determine the seizure focus.
Image 8.1I: Axial T2-weighted image demonstrates postoperative changes after a partial right temporal lobectomy.

- In patients for whom cortical areas cannot be removed without potentially devastating neurological impairment, a surgical technique known as multiple subpial transections is used to prevent seizure spread. It involves making a number of small incisions into the cerebral cortex with the hopes of disrupting epileptic circuits in the brain without impairing the function of the brain areas. This technique is most commonly employed in seizures that originate in brain areas responsible for language or motor function, which cannot be removed without significant neurological impairment. This surgical procedure is useful in seizure syndromes such as Landau–Kleffner syndrome, where surgery cannot be performed without potentially devastating the patient.

- In some patients with epilepsy refractory to medications, surgical lesions can be made in the corpus callosum to prevent seizures spreading from one hemisphere to the other. It is used almost exclusively in patients with generalized epilepsy with drop attacks.

- Vagus nerve stimulation involves implanting an electrode on the midcervical portion of the vagus

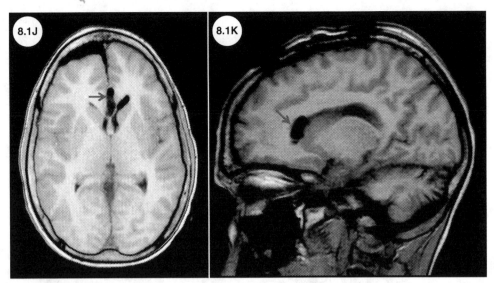

Images 8.1J and 8.1K: Axial and sagittal T1-weighted images demonstrate anterior corpus callosotomy (red arrows).

nerve, which then sends intermittent electrical impulses through the nerve. VNS is recommended in patients with bilateral temporal seizure foci.

References

1. Proposal for revised classification of epilepsies and epileptic syndromes. Commission on classification and terminology of the International League Against Epilepsy. *Epilepsia.* 1989;30:389.

2. Berg AT, Berkovic SF, BrodieMJ, et al. Revised terminology and concepts for organization of seizures and epilepsies: report of the ILAE Commission on Classification and Terminology, 2005–2009. *Epilepsia.* 2010;51:676.

3. Abosch A, Bernasconi N, Boling W. Factors predictive of suboptimal seizure control following selective amygdalohippo-campectomy. *J Neurosurg.* 2002;97(5):1142–1151.

4. Engel J Jr, McDermott MP, Wiebe S, et al. Early surgical therapy for drug-resistant temporal lobe epilepsy: a randomized trial. *JAMA.* March 2012;307(9):922–930.

8.2 Frontal Lobe Epilepsy

Case History

A 26-year-old presented with nocturnal hypermotor seizures with confusion and disorientation. Brain MRI showed an abnormal lesion.

Diagnosis: Frontal Lobe Epilepsy Due to Focal Cortical Dysplasia

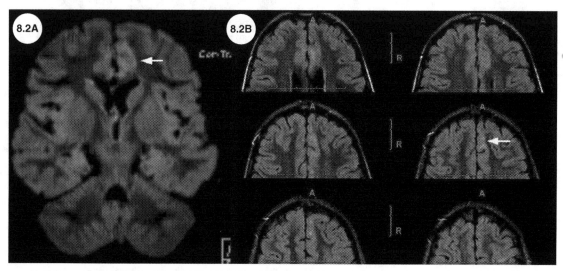

Images 8.2A and 8.2B: Serial axial FLAIR MRI of the frontal lobes (8.2A) and coronal FLAIR MRI (8.2B) demonstrating subtle gray–white blurring and FLAIR hyperintensity in the left anterior cingulate gyrus and adjacent left medial frontal gyrus from a pathologically proven cortical dysplasia (image courtesy of Timothy Shepherd, MD).

Introduction

- Frontal lobe epilepsy is the second most common focal epilepsy after TLE. Patients tend to have stereotyped, hypermotor seizures typically during their sleep that are short-lasting (<30 seconds) compared to temporal lobe seizures; these are commonly confused with nonepileptic seizures (NES). Prominent motor manifestations, complex automatisms, and quick secondary generalization are common features of focal seizures with brief impairment of consciousness. Fencing posturing, speech arrest, eye deviation, facial grimacing, kicking, laughing, or other vocalizations are more common in frontal lobe seizures.

- **Neuronal migrational disorders:** Heterotopias are neuronal migrational disorders (NMDs) where gray matter gets arrested as neurons migrate from periventricular regions toward pia during embryonic stages.

- Heterotopias can either be focal, nodular, or multifocal (as in tuberous sclerosis) or preferentially involve one hemisphere as in hemimegalencephaly. Subcortical band heterotopias (SBHs) are typically periventricular, bilateral nodular collections of gray matter with relatively smooth margins, which gives the appearance of a double cortex. Pachygyria is abnormal tissue in the right location with abnormal sulcation and gyration of the mantle, which is typically thicker than 8 mm. Polymicrogyria (PMG) is either two- or four-layered cortex, which is less than 5 to 7 mm in thickness.

- Focal cortical dysplasias (FCDs) are classified into three categories (types I, II, and III) and further divided into various subtypes (**Table 8.2.1**) in a fully myelinated brain.

- Other important NMDs include lissencephaly, which is characterized by smooth brain surface, and abnormal gyration, which varies between agyria and pachygyria (Image 8.2C).

Table 8.2.1 Classification of Focal Cortical Dysplasias

Types	Features
Type I	Ia: abnormal vertical alignment of neurons Ib: abnormal horizontal alignment Ic: horizontal and vertical malalignment
Type II	IIa: dysmorphic neurons without balloon cells IIb: dysmorphic neurons with balloon cells
Type III	IIIa: HS IIIb: glioneural tumors (eg, ganglioglioma, DNET) IIIc: vascular malformations (CCMs, AVMs, telangiectasias, meningioangiomatosis) IIId: prenatal or perinatal ischemic injury, TBI, scars due to inflammatory or infectious lesions

AVMs, arteriovenous malformations; CCMs, cerebral cavernous malformations; DNETs, dysembryoplastic neuroepithelial tumors; HS, hippocampal sclerosis; TBI, traumatic brain injury.

■ Lissencephaly with posteriorly predominant gyral abnormalities is caused by mutations in the *LIS1* gene. Anteriorly predominant lissencephaly in heterozygous males and SBH in heterozygous females are caused by mutations of the *XLIS* (double cortex gene on chromosome X).

■ Schizencephaly is another rare form of MCD, which is characterized by the presence of a transcortical cleft, which can extend from ventricles to the pia with open or fused lips, and often PMG is seen on the lips of the schizencephaly (Image 8.2D).

■ Hemimegalencephaly is the unilateral hamartomatous excessive growth of all or part of one cerebral hemisphere at different phases of embryonic development. MRI in these cases reveals an enlarged hemisphere with increased white matter volume, cortical thickening, agyria, pachygyria, PMG, or lissencephaly and blurring of the gray–white matter junction. Often, a large, ipsilateral irregularly shaped ventricle may be seen.

Clinical Presentation

■ Most FCD types present with intractable seizures with or without mild to severe learning disabilities.

■ Bilateral perisylvian PMG due to mutation in *MECP2* gene can present with dysarthria, pseudobulbar palsy, spastic quadriparesis, learning disability, epilepsy, and intractable seizures. Complex partial seizures and drop attacks are the most common seizure types.

Hypotonia, microcephaly, IS, and learning disabilities are seen in lissencephaly. Severe forms such as Miller–Dieker syndrome due to deletion or mutations of the *LIS1* gene on chromosome 17 characterized by facial dysmorphic features can have various seizure types and even premature death. Type I (classic) lissencephaly typically presents with marked hypotonia and paucity of movement. Type II lissencephaly is associated with muscular-dystrophy-like syndromes and includes *Walker–Warburg syndrome, Fukuyama syndrome*, and *muscle–eye–brain (MEB) disease*.

Radiographic Appearance and Diagnosis

■ FCD type I may be characterized by subtle blurring of the gray–white junction with typically normal cortical thickness, moderately increased white matter signal hyperintensities on T2/FLAIR images, and decreased signal intensity on T1-weighted images.

■ FCD type IIA cortical dysplasias are characterized by marked blurring of the gray–white junction on T1 and T2-FLAIR images due to hypo- or dysmyelination of the subcortical white matter with or without cortical thickening. Here, the increased white matter signal changes on T2-weighted and FLAIR images frequently taper toward the ventricles (aka the *transmantle sign*), which marks the involvement of radial glial neuronal bands. This radiologic feature differentiates FCD from low-grade tumors. Type II lesions are more commonly seen outside the temporal lobe with predilection for the frontal lobes.

■ Type III FCD is typically associated with another principal lesion such as hippocampal sclerosis, tumor, a vascular malformation, or another acquired pathology during early life.

■ Magnetization prepared rapid acquisition gradient echo (MP-RAGE) sequence can yield high-resolution T1-weighted images for more stable abnormalities of cortical thickness.

■ High-resolution 3D T1-weighted volumetric imaging provides superior gray–white contrast, which is critical to identify subtle cortical malformations in patients with epilepsy. Higher magnetic strengths (3 or 7 Tesla) can detect very subtle cortical dysplasias.

■ Increased signal change is more obvious on T2-weighted images, and FLAIR. Proton density reveals blurring of interphase between gray matter and white matter.

■ MRI in Lissencephaly shows thickened cortex, diminished white matter, and vertical sylvian fissures, giving a typical figure 8 appearance of the brain (Image 8.2C).

■ The histological features of FCD include disruption of cortical lamination; giant neurons, dysplastic "balloon cells" in white matter; excess of neurons in the white matter, causing blurring of the interface between the gray matter and white matter.

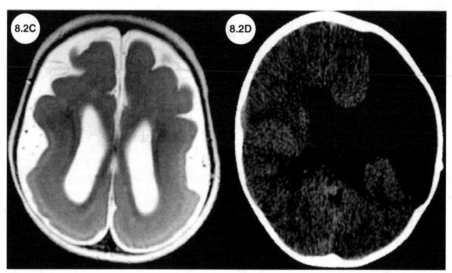

Images 8.2C and 8.2D: Brain MRI T2-weighted image (8.2C) shows overall paucity of gyri with thickened and flattened appearance. Pattern is more posteriorly affected suggesting LIS1 mutation, and CT head noncontrast axial Images 8.2D) show open lip schizencephaly in the left frontotemporoparietal regions (image credit courtesy Sarah Milla, MD).

Treatment

■ Treatment of the epilepsy associated with cortical dysplasia is often frustrating, but surgical approaches based on accurately defining epileptogenic regions are proving increasingly successful.

■ AEDs are used to treat seizures but more than 60% to 70% of patients have medically intractable seizures due to FCD.

■ A complete resection of the epileptogenic zone is required to achieve seizure freedom after the epilepsy surgery.

■ Corpus callosotomy and VNS are other options in diffuse or bilateral dysplasias.

■ Functional hemispherectomy is another option for patients with hemimegalencephaly.

■ Genetic diagnosis is important for accurate counseling of families.

References

1. Taylor DC, Falconer MA, Bruton CJ, et al. Focal dysplasia of the cerebral cortex in epilepsy. *J Neurol Neurosurg Psychiatry.* 1971;34:369–387.
2. Palmini A, Najm I, Avanzini G, et al. Terminology and classification of the cortical dysplasias. *Neurology.* 2004;62:S2–S8.
3. Barkovich AJ, Kuzniecky RI. Neuroimaging of focal malformations of cortical development. *J Clin Neurophysiol.* 1996;13:481–494.
4. Barkovich J, Kuzniecky RI, Jackson GD, et al. A developmental and genetic classification for malformations of cortical development. *Neurology.* 2005;65:1873–1887.
5. Tassi L, Colombo N, Garbelli R, et al. Focal cortical dysplasia: neuropathological subtypes, EEG, neuroimaging and surgical outcome. *Brain.* 2002;125(8):1719–1732.

8.3 Limbic Encephalitis

Case History

A 23-year-old female presented with a cluster of seizures. She was otherwise healthy. She had been acting oddly for the past two weeks. She was thinking that her neighbors were spying on her. She was found missing two days prior to her presentation in the emergency room. The patient was diaphoretic on exam and appeared paranoid about hospital staff.

Diagnosis: Limbic Encephalitis

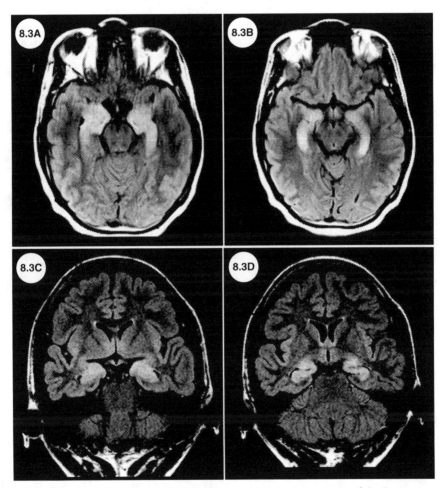

Images 8.3A–8.3D: Axial and coronal FLAIR MRIs demonstrate hyperintensity of the hippocampi bilaterally in a patient with limbic encephalitis.

Introduction

■ Limbic encephalitis (LE) is an inflammatory disorder of the limbic system (**Illustration 8.3.1**).

■ Two major etiologies of LE are recognized: infectious and autoimmune. In cases of infectious LE, viral agents such as herpes simplex are most often implicated. Autoimmune LE can be further divided into paraneoplastic and nonparaneoplastic forms of the disease.

Clinical Presentation

■ Variable but most commonly include memory loss, personality changes, psychiatric symptoms

The Limbic System

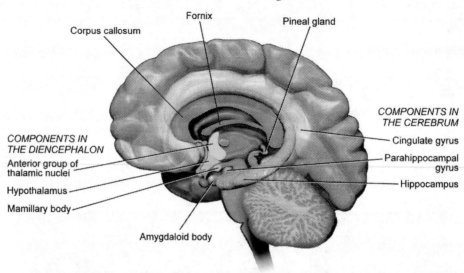

Illustration 8.3.1: Components of the limbic system.

Source: Blausen.com. Blausen gallery 2014. *Wikiversity Journal of Medicine.* 2014. doi:10.15347/wjm/2014.010. ISSN20018762.

ranging from depression to frank psychosis, involuntary movements, and seizures.

- Several cancer types have been associated with paraneoplastic encephalomyelitis and LE.

  - Underlying tumor is small cell lung cancer in approximately 75% of cases

  - Other tumors include seminoma and other testicular tumors, thymoma, breast cancer, Hodgkin lymphoma, uterine or other gynecological tumors

  - Tumor frequently undiagnosed at the time the neurological syndrome develops

  - The type of associated autoantibody varies with tumor type. Small cell lung cancer usually associated with anti-Hu or CRMP5 antibodies in serum and cerebrospinal fluid (CSF)

- The clinical presentation varies depending on the areas involved as listed in the following:

  - Temporolimbic regions: LE

  - Brainstem: opsoclonus–myoclonus

  - Cerebellum: cerebellar degeneration

  - Retina: melanoma-associated retinopathy (MAR), carcinoma-induced retinopathy (CAR)

  - Spinal cord: myelopathy

  - Dorsal root ganglia: sensory neuronopathy

- Neuromuscular junction: Lambert-Eaton myasthenic syndrome

- Peripheral nerve and muscle: dermatomyositis

- Multiple levels: encephalomyelitis

Radiographic Appearance and Diagnosis

- Brain MRI: Hyperintensities of the medial temporal lobes on T2-weighted images may or may not be present with or without Gd-enhancement. The MRI may be normal in a substantial number of patients.

- Paraneoplastic LE is associated with the production of various antibodies in association with a tumor. The most common tumors involved are tumors of the lung (specifically small cell tumors), thymus, breast, ovaries, and testis. In young females, ovarian teratomas are frequently implicated. The most commonly implicated antibodies are anti-Ma2, anti-amphiphysin, anti-CV2/CRMP5, LGI-1, and anti-NMDA receptor (**Table 8.3.1**).

- Nonparaneoplastic LE is often associated with antibodies against the *voltage-gated potassium channel*.

- EEG: nonspecific, focal, or generalized slowing, epileptiform activity, periodic lateralized epileptiform discharges (PLEDs).

- CSF: may be normal or abnormal, modest protein elevation less than 100 is most common, mild lymphocytic pleocytosis.

- Exclude metabolic and toxic encephalopathies.

- Paraneoplastic and autoimmune biomarkers (ie, "paraneoplastic panel" on CSF and serum; see **Table 8.3.1**).

- Pan-CT: chest, abdomen, and pelvis; scrotal ultrasound to rule out testicular tumors; mammogram.

Table 8.3.1 Various Antibodies Encountered in Patients With Autoimmune Encephalitis

Antibody Panel	Neuronal Antibodies Panel
ANA Anti-dsDNA Rnp/Smith-Ab SS-A and SS-B ANCA (c-ANCA, p-ANCA) ACLA	Anti-Hu Anti-Yo Anti-Ri Anti Ma2 Anti-CV2/CRMP5 Anti-NMDA Anti-amphiphysin Anti-LGI-I Anti-CASPR-2 Anti-GAD65 Anti-AMPA Anti-GABA-A, GABA-B Anti-IgLON5 encephalopathy Anti-glycine (α-I subunit)

Treatment

- Although controlled trials are lacking, immunosuppressive therapies including intravenous immunoglobulin (IVIG), plasmapheresis, and steroids are commonly used.

- Cyclophosphamide or rituximab is used if these therapies are not efficacious.

- Symptomatic treatment includes antipsychotics and antiseizure medications. NueDexta (dextromethorphan/quinidine) can be used for the treatment of pseudobulbar affect.

References

1. Anderson NE, Barber PA. Limbic encephalitis—a review. *J Clin Neurosci*. September 2008;15(9):961–971.
2. Toledano M, Pittock SJ. Autoimmune epilepsy. *Semin Neurol*. June 2015;35(3):245–258.
3. Heine J, Prüss H, Bartsch T, Ploner CJ, Paul F, Finke C. Imaging of autoimmune encephalitis—relevance for clinical practice and hippocampal function. *Neuroscience*. May 2015;309:68–83. pii: S0306-4522(15)00479-0.
4. Ramanathan S, Mohammad SS, Brilot F, Dale RC. Autoimmune encephalitis: recent updates and emerging challenges. *J Clin Neurosci*. May 2014;21(5):722–730.
5. Armangue T, Leypoldt F, Dalmau J. Autoimmune encephalitis as differential diagnosis of infectious encephalitis. *Curr Opin Neurol*. June 2014;27(3):361–368.
6. Dalmau J, Graus F, Rosenblum MK, Posner JB. Anti-Hu—associated paraneoplastic encephalomyelitis/sensory neuronopathy. A clinical study of 71 patients. *Medicine (Baltimore)*. 1992;71:59.
7. Gultekin SH, Rosenfeld MR, Voltz R, et al. Paraneoplastic limbic encephalitis: neurological symptoms, immunological findings and tumour association in 50 patients. *Brain*. 2000;123(Pt. 7):1481.
8. Basu S, Alavi A. Role of FDG-PET in the clinical management of paraneoplastic neurological syndrome: detection of the underlying malignancy and the brain PET-MRI correlates. *Mol Imaging Biol*. 2008;10:131.
9. Alamowitch S, Graus F, Uchuya M, et al. Limbic encephalitis and small cell lung cancer. Clinical and immunological features. *Brain*. 1997;120(Pt. 6):923.
10. Shimazaki H, Ando Y, Nakano I, Dalmau J. Reversible limbic encephalitis with antibodies against the membranes of neurones of the hippocampus. *J Neurol Neurosurg Psychiatry*. 2007;78:324.
11. Blausen.com. Blausen gallery 2014. *Wikiversity Journal of Medicine*. 2014. doi:10.15347/wjm/2014.010. ISSN 20018762.

8.4 Status Epilepticus

Case History

A 36-year-old was transferred from another hospital for continuous generalized seizures.

Diagnosis: Convulsive Status Epilepticus

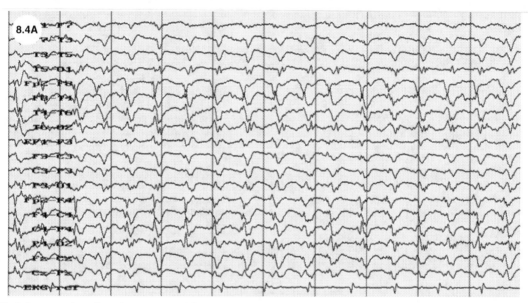

Image 8.4A: EEG clips (bipolar montage) show convulsive status epilepticus; note 2–2.5 Hz generalized spike- and slow-wave discharges in an unresponsive patient.

Introduction

1. Definition and epidemiology:
   a. Status epilepticus (SE) is a condition resulting either from the failure of the mechanisms responsible for seizure termination or from the initiation of mechanisms, which lead to abnormally prolonged seizures (after time point t1). Here t1 is considered 5 minutes and SE can have long-term consequences (after time point t2; the second time point is 30 minutes) including neuronal death, neuronal injury, and alteration of neuronal networks, depending on the type and duration of seizures.
   b. The proposed diagnostic classification system of SE contains four axes:
      - Axis 1—**Semiology**: forms of SE with prominent motor systems, those without prominent motor systems, and currently indeterminate conditions

- Axis 2—**Etiology**: known and unknown causes
- Axis 3—**EEG correlates**: name of pattern, morphology, location, time-related features, modulation, and effect of intervention
- Axis 4—**Age**: neonatal, infancy, childhood, adolescent and adulthood, and elderly
   c. There are approximately 20 SE cases per 100,000 people in the United States yearly, with higher incidence in early childhood (<5 years) and in the elderly (>65 years). SE occurs most commonly in children less than a year of age (135–156 in 100,000/year).

2. Subgroup:
   a. By seizure phenotype, SE is classified to three main subtypes. The most commonly reported form (~50%) is generalized convulsive SE (GCSE). Convulsive SE is clinically

obvious initially; however, after 30 to 45 minutes of continuous seizures clinical signs may become subtle or absent. The only sign may be twitching of eyes or fingers, or autonomic manifestation such as tachycardia, papillary dilatation, or hypertension. In such cases, a continuous electroencephalogram (EEG) would be the only way to monitor seizure activities.

b. Focal motor SE (FMSE), or epilepsy partialis continua, is a continuous muscle twitching without generalization, which is frequently seen in a single limb or a side of the face. This subtype is relatively uncommon, and how aggressively one needs to treat FMSE largely depends on the clinical context.

c. The last subtype, non-convulsive SE (NCSE), represents a heterogeneous group of nonmotor seizures. It includes primary generalized SE (eg, absence SE), secondary generalized SE, and complex partial SE. Since their clinical presentation varies widely, ranging from somnolent to comatose status, the only way to diagnose NCSE is electroencephalogram (EEG). For this reason, NCSE is likely under-recognized, particularly in critically ill patients with impaired mental status. Five to ten percent of comatose patients in the intensive care unit (ICU), and up to 34% of neurological ICU patients may be in NCSE if examined by EEG. In patients with severe anoxic-ischemic encephalopathy, NCSE is associated with poor neurological outcome.

d. The refractory status is when it does not break with using first- and second-line AEDs such as lorazepam, diazepam, and IV load of phenytoin and phenobarbital. The super-refractory SE is when even IV anesthetics such as propofol, Versed, and pentobarbital fail to control seizures.

3. Etiology:

a. The most common risk factor of SE is a prior history of epilepsy (22%–26%). However, more than half of SE occurs in people without prior seizures. In adults, most common causes of SE are cerebrovascular accidents (25%), change in medications (18%–20%), alcohol/substance withdrawal (10%–13%), and less frequent causes include anoxia, metabolic derangement, infection, trauma, and tumor, in a descending order. In contrast, one-third of pediatric SE cases are due to infection fever (ie, prolonged febrile convulsion [PFC]), followed by low AED levels.

4. Mortality:

a. The prognosis of SE is greatly dependent on age, etiology, promptness of treatments, and complications that occur in its course. Short-term mortality, measured as death rate during hospitalization for SE or within 30 days of SE, ranges from 8% to 22% across all age groups. Most of these early deaths occur in those with acute symptomatic etiology.

b. Although long-term mortality of SE is not as well studied as short-term outcomes, a population-based cohort study showed that among survivors of the initial 30 days after their first SE, over 40% died in the next 10 years. This is approximately threefold higher mortality compared to the general population. However, serious medical complications during the hospitalization, irreversible neurological damage, and functional deterioration on discharge likely contribute to the long-term outcome.

c. Children have a much lower mortality rate (3%–15%) than adults (15%–22%), which is probably due both to their physiologic resilience and to the nature of etiology in this age group. For example, PFCs carry a low mortality rate, rarely last longer than 2 hours, and are generally more responsive to treatments than GCSEs of other etiologies. Etiologies that cause severe persistent systemic disturbances such as anoxia are less common in children yet carry similar mortality as when it occurs in adults.

5. Morbidity:

a. Prolonged seizures: Morbidity and mortality rates of SE appear to have crude correlation to its etiology. In the past, NCSE has been thought to be a benign condition. However, recent studies indicate that even NCSE is associated with significant complications.

b. Unremitting seizure activities result in cardiorespiratory, autonomic, and metabolic complications as well as irreversible neuronal injury. Prolonged convulsive seizures may lead to hypothermia, acidosis, rhabdomyolysis, renal failure, trauma, and pulmonary aspiration. Prolonged seizure activities lasting as little as 30 to 60 minutes may result in irreversible neuronal damage secondary to excitotoxicity, apoptosis, synaptic reorganization, and impaired protein and DNA synthesis. Seizures lasting longer than 1 hour are predictive of poor outcome.

c. Certain regions of the brain are more likely to be affected by SE than others. They include hippocampal complex, amygdala, thalamus, and cerebellar pyramidal cells, all of which have abundant receptors for excitatory neurotransmitters and are therefore more prone to excitotoxicity and other mechanisms of insult. Some victims of SE suffer from irreversible dysfunction in memory, balance, affect, and cognition. PFCs, considered benign in the past, are thought to result in acute hippocampal injury and MTS, later leading to development of temporal epilepsy. A causal association, however, is still being argued, since genetic predisposition is an important cause both for febrile seizures and MTS.

d. Since SE often requires an intensive level of care and prolonged hospitalization, there are additional complications associated with treatment. Adverse effects of anticonvulsant drugs, drug–drug interactions, ventilator-associated pneumonia, and other nosocomial infections are just a few examples.

Treatment

■ SE is a true neurological and medical emergency, requiring prompt recognition and initiation of treatments. Many old and newer anticonvulsant drugs have been studied for their effectiveness in SE. Most commonly used agents are summarized in **Table 8.4.1**.

■ In general, IV benzodiazepines are the first-line agents for GCSE in adults. Lorazepam is a preferred agent to diazepam and midazolam because of its better water solubility and hence a longer serum half-life (4–6 hours). About 65% of GCSE can be terminated with the initial benzodiazepine therapy.

■ If seizures continue after the administration of lorazepam, IV phenytoin or fosphenytoin is the next choice of agent. Although not as widely available, fosphenytoin has advantages over phenytoin in that it can be infused three times faster, can be administered intramuscularly, and has a better side-effect profile. Following a loading dose, an additional smaller dose (ie, 25%–50% of the initial dose) of phenytoin or fosphenytoin can be given.

■ For continuing seizures, a loading dose of IV phenobarbital may be administered, followed by a second dose (ie, 25%–50% of the initial dose).

■ If this fails to break SE, general anesthesia may be the next line of agent. The first-, second-, and third-line agents used in SE are listed in **Table 8.4.1**.

■ Alternatively, newer agents with broad spectrum, such as IV valproic acid or levetiracetam, can be used at this point, depending on past experiences, drug availability, and personal preferences.

■ At any point during the treatment, an emergency intubation may be necessary. If the patient has

Table 8.4.1 Treatment of Status Epilepticus

I/V Lorazepam	0.1 mg/kg (4–8 mg loading dose; not more than 8 mg/24 h)
I/V Phenytoin	Loading dose: 20 mg/kg IV Maximum infusion rate: 50 mg/min
I/V Fosphenytoin	Loading dose: 20 mg/kg IV Maximum infusion rate: 150 mg/min
I/V Valproate	Loading dose: 20 mg/kg IV, higher doses 30–60 mg/kg can be used Infusion rate: 5 mg/kg/min
I/V Phenobarbital	Loading dose: 15 mg/kg to 20 mg/kg Maximum rate: 50 mg/min to 100 mg/min
Midazolam (Versed) I/M, nasal, buccal	0.2 mg/kg (nasal/buccal faster than IM)
Continuous IV midazolam Infusion*	Bolus dose: 0.2 mg/kg, repeat boluses of 0.2 mg/kg to 0.4 mg/kg every 5 min until seizures stop, up to a maximum total loading dose of 2 mg/kg Initial infusion rate: 0.1 mg/kg/h Maintenance: 0.05 mg/kg/h–2.9 mg/kg/h (continuous IV rate should be increased by 20%)

(continued)

Table 8.4.1 Treatment of Status Epilepticus (*continued*)

Continuous IV propofol infusion*	Bolus dose: 1 mg/kg Repeat 1 mg/kg to 2 mg/kg boluses q 3–5 min until seizures stop, up to 10 mg/kg Initial infusion rate: 2 mg/kg/h Continuous infusion rate: 1 mg/kg/h to 15 mg/kg/h Do not exceed >5 mg/kg/h for >48 h
Continuous IV pentobarbital infusion*	Loading dose: 5 mg/kg, repeat 5 mg/kg boluses until seizures stop. Maximum bolus rate: 25 mg/min to 50 mg/min (based on blood pressure) Initial infusion rate: 1 mg/kg/h Maintenance rate: 0.5 mg/kg/h to 10.0 mg/kg/h

*All continuous infusions should be kept on a steady dose for 12 to 24 hours and slow withdrawal of infusions is recommended over 24 hours. If seizures return, try even slower withdrawal.

seizures continuing over an hour on presentation, has severe systemic derangement, or develops SE while in the ICU, the treating physician can immediately proceed with continuous infusion of general anesthetic agents such as propofol, midazolam, or phenobarbital.

- If patients with known epilepsy develop SE, it is often due to a low serum level of their AEDs, and the administration of their home medications may be necessary unless one is absolutely sure of their compliance.

- For absence SE, first-line agents such as sodium valproate, ethosuximide, and benzodiazepines are effective. Other agents such as zonisamide, levetiracetam, lamotrigine, lacosamide, and topiramate can also be helpful. On the other hand, phenytoin, carbamazepine, oxcarbazepine, and tiagabine can exacerbate absence seizures and should be avoided. Out of the third-generation AEDs (perampanel, eslicarbazepine, lacosamide), only lacosamide is available in the IV form and is being used off-label in SE.

References

1. Brenner RP. EEG in convulsive and nonconvulsive status epilepticus. *J Clin Neurophysiol.* September–October 2004;21(5):319–331.
2. Kaplan PW. The EEG of status epilepticus. *J Clin Neurophysiol.* June 2006;23(3):221–229.

8.5 | Infantile Spasms

Case History

A 5-month-old baby girl brought to a clinic for complaints of unusual movements is observed to have clusters of stereotyped posturing with eye-rolling, neck and hip flexion, and bilateral arm extension shortly after waking not associated with feeding; afterwards she is often more fussy or subdued than usual. There are no neurocutaneous abnormalities noted on exam.

Diagnosis: Infantile Spasms

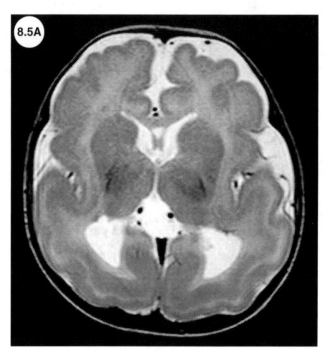

Image 8.5A: Axial T2 MRI demonstrating lissencephalpy (one of many structural abnormalities potentially associated with infantile spasms).

Introduction

- Infantile spasms (IS) are the most common early-onset epileptic encephalopathy. Epilepsy is more common in infancy than any other time in childhood, and epileptic spasms are the most common single type of seizure. IS may present as a component of West syndrome, a clinical triad consisting of epileptic spasms, hypsarrhythmia on EEG, and developmental delay or regression.

- There are many potential underlying causes of IS. The majority (~60%) of cases are due to structural or metabolic etiologies; the rest are either linked to other genetic defects or as-of-yet unknown causes (categorized as idiopathic).

Clinical Presentation

- IS typically present as clusters of stereotyped brief seizures, which can include flexion or extension of the arms, legs, torso, and head.

  - Clusters often occur upon awakening or around sleep–wake transitions.

  - Spasms consist of a sharp jerk followed by up to ~1 to 2 seconds of tonic posturing.

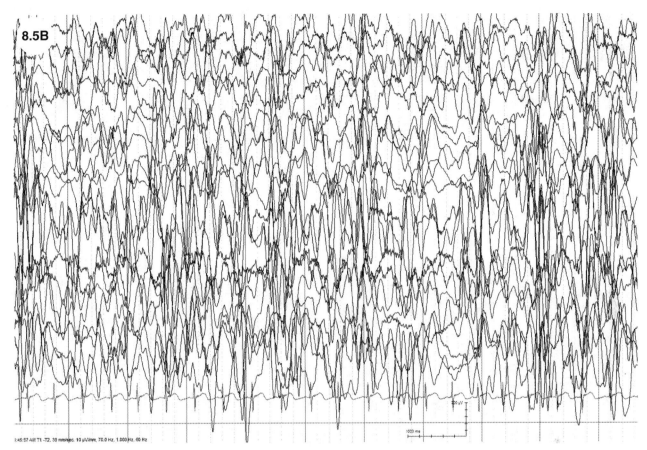

Image 8.5B: Background hypsarrhythmia; note the high voltage (>200 mV), lack of anterior to posterior organization, and multifocal epileptic activity. This is an interictal period with no spasms.

- Overall incidence of ~2 to 3 per 10,000 live births, with onset typically between 3 to 7 months of age (~93% before 2 years of age).

- Patients may have a known neurological diagnosis or syndromic findings including (but not limited to):
  - Tuberous sclerosis
  - Down syndrome
  - Autism
  - Intellectual disability

- The most common causes of IS include:
  - Hypoxic-ischemic encephalopathy (~10%)
  - Chromosomal anomalies (~8%)
  - CNS malformation (~8%)
  - Perinatal stroke (~8%)
  - Tuberous sclerosis (~7%)
  - Periventricular leukomalacia or hemorrhage (~5%)
  - Immune-mediated (rare)
  - Other rare neurometabolic or genetic syndromes

- Regardless of cause, neurodevelopmental outcome is generally poor.
  - The most important factor in long-term outcome is early and effective control not only of spasms but hypsarrhythmia as well.
  - Patients with an underlying identified structural or metabolic etiology tend to be more refractory to treatment.

- A significant portion of infants go on to have long-term epilepsy.
  - In most cases epileptic spasms eventually resolve with time.
  - Spasms are often replaced with new (or multiple) seizure types.
  - A significant proportion may evolve to LGS.

Radiographic Appearance and Diagnosis

- The very first step in diagnosis is typically EEG or video EEG monitoring, to both characterize the paroxysmal episodes concerning for epileptic spasms and also assess the background for potential hypsarrhythmia.

  - Hypsarrhythmia (**Image 8.5B**) is a chaotic high voltage multifocal epileptic interictal background seen between spasms; less typical findings may be referred to as modified or atypical hypsarrhythmia.

- Clinical epileptic spasms are typically associated with high-amplitude epileptic activity followed by diffuse attenuation known as an "electrodecremental response" during which the very abnormal-appearing background hypsarrhythmia is replaced with a more suppressed background (**Image 8.5C**).

- Consider potential supplementation for metabolic abnormalities or vitamin deficiencies (pyridoxine, for example), which may lead to rapid improvement in the EEG.

- Neuroimaging is recommended for any infant presenting with epilepsy, including IS.

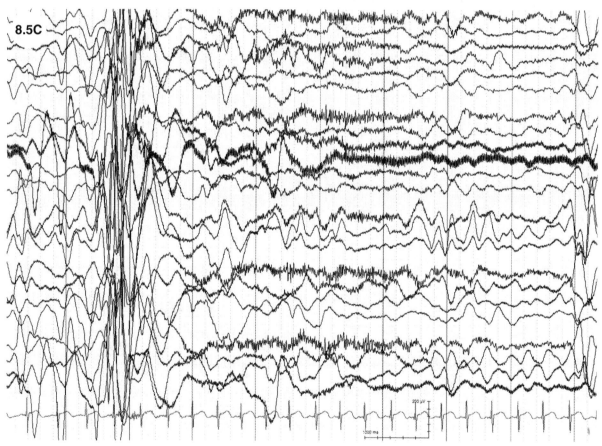

Image 8.5C: Electroclinical infantile spasm with onset ~2 seconds in with high-amplitude generalized epileptic activity followed by diffuse attenuation and slowing; same patient and scale as in Image 8.5B.

- MR is typically the most appropriate initial imaging modality, though in urgent or extenuating circumstances ultrasound or CT imaging may be considered.

- Once feasible, MR brain imaging should be obtained.

- Subsequent imaging for further workup (including potential surgical evaluation) may include functional magnetic resonance imaging (fMRI), PET, magnetoencephalogram (MEG), or SPECT

  - Electroencephalography–functional magnetic resonance imaging (EEG–fMRI) has demonstrated epileptiform discharges associated with occipitally predominant positive blood oxygen level dependent

(BOLD) signal changes in the cerebral cortex while high-amplitude slow-wave activity in hypsarrhythmia is associated with BOLD signal changes in the brainstem, putamen, and thalamus.

- Early PET studies have shown areas of focal cortical hypometabolism and subcortical hypermetabolism (in the putamen and brainstem) associated with hypsarrhythmia. Expansion of glucose hypometabolism may be seen on PET with persistent epilepsy.

- Potential causes identifiable on imaging considered sufficient for diagnosis include:

  - Tuberous sclerosis
  - Evidence of prior hyoxic ischemic encephalopathy (HIE) or other cerebrovascular event
  - Clear underlying structural abnormalities

- Genetic evaluation for any infantile-onset epileptic encephalopathy without identified cause (including IS) should be undertaken with access to genetic counseling by trained personnel, as diagnosis of specific underlying neurometabolic causes may alter specific treatments and outcomes.

  - Primary and secondary level investigations should include serum glucose, hematologic screening, liver function tests, ammonia, urinalysis, serum lactate and pH, arterial gases, plasma electrolytes including anion gap measurement, and CSF analysis including glucose (with comparison to plasma to rule out hypoglycorrhachia).

  - Tertiary and quaternary level investigations should include any additional amino or organic acidopathy testing as well as specific enzymatic studies (which may require biopsies) or genetic screening including more broad sequencing and analysis.

  - Specific metabolic conditions associated with IS include biotinidase deficiency, Menkes disease, mitochondrial respiratory chain diseases, amino acidopathies, and organic acidurias.

Treatment

- The shorter the interval between spasm onset and commencement of treatment, the better the potential developmental outcome, with the potential for meaningful improvement not only in seizures but in cognition and behavior.

- Barring a specific diagnosis with alternative primary treatment, ACTH historically has been considered preferable for the short-term control of spasms (initially studied in high doses).

  - Low-dose ACTH appears to be as effective as high-dose ACTH yet has a more tolerable side-effect profile.

  - Oral steroids (in particular, the prednisolone dosing in **Table 8.5.1**) are probably also

Table 8.5.1 Treatments With Dosing for Infantile Spasms With Corresponding Side Effects

Treatment	Typical U.S. Dosing Range	Potential Side Effects
High-dose ACTH	~75–150 IU/m²/day for ~2 weeks followed by a gradual taper	Depression of the immune system, hypertension, behavior change/irritability, increased appetite/weight gain, sleep disturbance, potential adrenal suppression requiring taper
Low-dose ACTH	~ 20–40 IU/day (also with potential taper)	Theoretically similar to high-dose ACTH but to a significantly lesser degree of magnitude
Oral steroids	Preferred: Prednisolone ~40–60 mg/day Other options: —Prednisone 2 mg/kg/day —Methylprednisolone 20mg/kg/day IV for 3 days followed by a steroid taper	Dose-dependent depression of the immune system, hypertension, behavior change/irritability, increased appetite/weight gain, sleep disturbance, potential adrenal suppression requiring taper
Vigabatrin	~50–150 mg/kg/day	Symptomatic and asymptomatic visual field defects (loss of peripheral vision); sedation or other behavioral changes; abnormalities on MRI imaging

(continued)

Table 8.5.1 Treatments With Dosing for Infantile Spasms With Corresponding Side Effects (*continued*)

Treatment	Typical U.S. Dosing Range	Potential Side Effects
Topiramate	Typically ~5–9 mg/kg/day but described in infants up to ~24 mg/kg/day	Appetite and weight loss, confusion/impaired cognition/sedation, glaucoma, renal calculi
Valproate	~30 mg/kg/day reportedly effective; dosing to achieve therapeutic levels may range from ~15 to 60 mg/kg/day	Hepatotoxicity (particularly if concern for underlying neurometabolic disease), hyperammonemia, sedation, pancreatitis, encephalopathy, thrombocytopenia
Ketogenic diet	High fat, adequate protein, low carbohydrate diet (delivered in variable ratios).	Constipation, hyperlipidemia, dehydration, renal calculi, slowed growth/weight gain, bone fractures

ACTH, adrenocorticotropic hormone.

effective for short-term control, and should certainly be considered if ACTH is not feasible.

■ Vigabatrin is also effective for short-term control of spasms; it is typically considered second-line following ACTH/steroids with the exception of patients with tuberous sclerosis.

　■ In patients with tuberous sclerosis, vigabatrin is considered first-line treatment.

■ Patients are typically re-evaluated frequently (initially at ~2-week intervals) to assess response to treatment, both with regard to epileptic spasms and background hypsarrhythmia.

■ Third- or fourth-line therapies include topiramate or valproate, particularly in infants with severe or static neurological insults without prior evidence of regression.

　■ Additional subsequent treatment options for refractory cases include benzodiazepines, levetiracetam/other antiepileptics, immunomodulatory agents as warranted (IVIG, plasmapheresis), epilepsy surgery—for appropriate candidates—or ketogenic diet (KD).

References

1. Wilmhurst JM, Gaillard WD, Vinayan KP, et al. Summary of recommendations for the management of infantile seizures: Task force report for the ILAE commission of pediatrics. *Epilepsia*. 2015;56(8):1185–1197.
2. Galanopoulou AS, Moshé SL. Pathogenesis and new candidate treatments for infantile spasms and early life epileptic encephalopathies: a view from preclinical studies. *Neurobiology of Disease*. 2015;79:135–149.
3. Widjaja E, Go C, McCoy B, Snead OC. Neurodevelopmental outcome of infantile spasms: a systematic review and meta-analysis. *Epilepsy Research*. 2015;109:155–162.
4. Nieh SE, Sherr EH. Epileptic encephalopathies: new genes and new pathways. *Neurotherapeutics*. 2014;11:796–806.
5. Siniatchkin M Capovilla G. Functional neuroimaging in epileptic encephalopathies. *Epilepsia*. 2013;54(Suppl. 8):27–33.
6. Riikonen R. Recent advances in the pharmacotherapy of infantile spasms. *CNS Drugs*. 2014;28:279–290.
7. Pavone P, Striano P, Falsaperla R, Pavone L, Ruggieri M. Infantile spasms syndrome, West syndrome and related phenotypes: what we know in 2013. *Brain & Development*. 2014;36:739–751.
8. Hancock EC, Osborne JP, Edwards SW. Treatment of infantile spasms (Review). *The Cochrane Library*. 2013;6:1–69.
9. Wanigasinghe J, Arambepola C, Ranganathan SS, Sumanasena S, Attanapola G. Randomized, single-blind, parallel clinical trial on efficacy of oral prednisolone versus intramuscular corticotropin on immediate and continued spasm control in West syndrome. *Pediatric Neurology*. 2015;53:193–199.

8.6 Lennox–Gastaut Syndrome

Case History

A 4-year-old boy with history of IS presents for evaluation of ongoing seizures. His mother reports that he has frequent seizures throughout the day and night. Most seizures are very brief jerks, sometimes resulting in falls. He also has periods of staring lasting seconds to sometimes a minute. His other medical history includes speech and gross motor delay. He has had several AED trials without improvement in his seizures.

Diagnosis: Lennox–Gastaut Syndrome

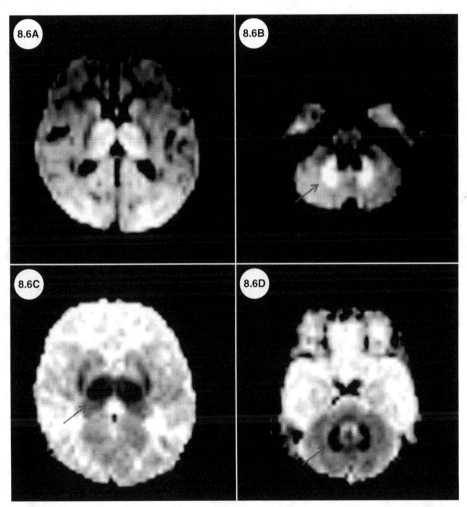

Images 8.6A–8.6D: Brain MRI axial diffusion-weighted and apparent diffusion coefficient (ADC) images showing diffusion positive lesions in thalami (8.6A), cerebellar tonsils (8.6B), and drop-out signal in the corresponding regions on ADC (8.6C and 8.6D).

Introduction

Lennox–Gastaut Syndrome (LGS) is a childhood epileptic encephalopathy characterized by a triad:

- Multiple seizure types, which are often refractory to treatment
- Interictal slow spike and wave pattern (2.5 Hz) with overall slow background

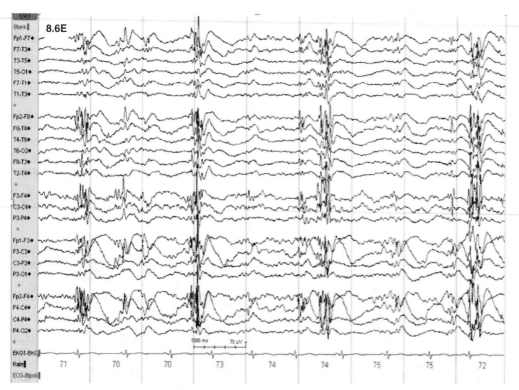

Image 8.6E: Bipolar montages showing generalized polyspikes/spikes and slow waves, which are maximal in the frontal and frontocentral regions.

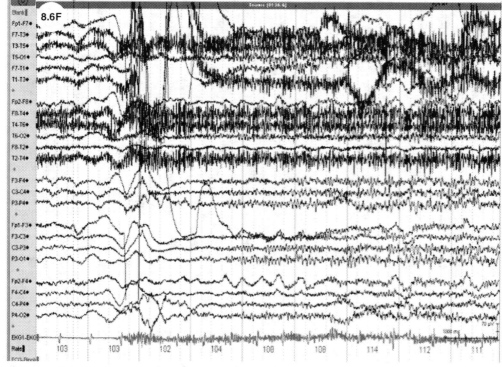

Image 8.6F: Bipolar montage shows low-amplitude 15–20 Hz fast activity in the parasagittal regions admixed with muscle artifacts during a tonic seizure. Patient had stiffening of the whole body, which lasted for about 15 seconds; the red bar represents the clipped segment of the seizure onset.

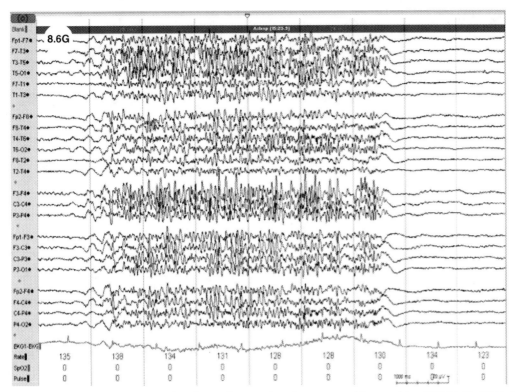

Image 8.6G: Bipolar montage shows a brief run of generalized paroxysmal fast activity (GPFA) 10–20 Hz lasting approximately 6 seconds without any clinical correlate during sleep.

■ Cognitive decline

Clinical Presentation

- ■ Patients with LGS have multiple seizure types including IS; drop attacks are a common presentation caused by tonic, atonic, or less commonly, myoclonic seizures (see **Table 8.6.1**). The majority of patients have at least one episode of SE or nonconvulsive status. GTCs and focal seizures can occur, but are not as frequent as other seizure types.

- ■ Comorbid conditions may include behavioral, psychiatric, or sleep disorders.

- ■ The etiology can be idiopathic, or develop from prior brain insults or structural lesions.

- ■ The onset varies in childhood from 2 to 6 years, and is more common in males.

Table 8.6.1 Common Seizure Types and Ictal Patterns (Most Common to Least Common)

Seizure Type	Ictal Pattern	Semiology
Tonic	Low voltage, fast activity (~10 Hz)	Stiffening of trunk, extremities, or whole body; often during sleep
Atypical absence	Slow spike and slow wave <2.5 Hz	Not completely unaware, lasts longer than typical absence, hyperventilation does not provoke them
Atonic	High voltage, bisynchronous spikes	Loss of tone
Myoclonic	Bisynchronous spike and wave	Single movement or clusters

Treatment

- ■ Most patients are refractory to medical treatment. Typically patients are treated with broad-spectrum medications because of multiple seizure types, focal as well as generalized. Narrow-spectrum drugs such as carbamazepine can be more effective to treat complex partial seizures bearing in mind that it may worsen other generalized seizure types. Polytherapy is commonly employed and AEDs with least drug-to-drug interactions or synergistic efficacy are chosen (see **Table 8.6.2**). Topiramate, felbamate, lamotrigine, valproate, and rufinamide are all approved as adjunctive therapy in LGS. Levetiracetam, zonisamide, and clonazepam show some evidence of efficacy also.

Table 8.6.2 Commonly Used AEDs in Patients With LGS

AED	Mechanism of Action	Common Side Effects
Valproate	Increases GABA	Thrombocytopenia, hepatic failure, teratogenic, hyperammonemia, encephalopathy
Benzodiazepines (especially clobazam)	Potentiates GABA	CNS depression including drowsiness
Lamotrigine	Inhibits glutamate and Na+ channels	Rash including SJS
Felbamate	Broad spectrum	Aplastic anemia, hepatic failure, loss of appetite, headache, insomnia
Topiramate	Broad spectrum	Paresthesia, somnolence, anorexia, loss of appetite, oligohydrosis, increased risk of kidney stones, cognitive side effects
Rufinamide	Unknown, in vitro affects sodium inactivation	Vomiting, pyrexia, rash

CNS, central nervous system; GABA, γ-aminobutyric acid; SJS, Stevens-Johnson syndrome.

■ Other treatment options include vagal nerve stimulator (VNS), corpus callosotomy, and KD.

■ Corpus callosotomy is commonly done in patients with drop attacks or partial seizures with secondary generalization. **Table 8.6.3** summarizes the types of disconnection surgeries done in patients with LGS. Outcome is thought to be slightly better with total callosotomy. Adverse effects usually improve with time, and happen in both types of callosotomy.

■ **Dietary therapy:** The principle of special diet is to change the milieu of brain, which relies on

Table 8.6.3 Types of Corpus Callosotomy

% Corpus Callosotomy	Rational	Outcome	Adverse Effects
Anterior 2/3rds to 4/5ths	Spares the splenium of the corpus callosum for passage of visual information	Reduction in seizure frequency, improved overall function	Disconnection syndrome, alien hand syndrome
Total (90%)	Further reduction of epileptic spread	Further reduction in seizure frequency, improved overall function	Disconnection syndrome, alien hand syndrome, language impairment, memory loss, new seizures, new deficits

carbohydrates to fats as its primary source of energy. There are multiple theories on how ketosis exerts its antiseizure effects. About 50% of patients notice more than 50% of reduction in their seizures and up to 30% notice 90% of strict protein, calorie, and especially carbohydrate restriction in the setting of a high fat diet is needed for ketosis, and can be difficult to maintain. In 10% of patients with intractable epilepsy, staying on this diet for months or years can result in a sustained seizure freedom, and allow for withdrawal of AEDs. Side effects include weight loss, acidosis, kidney stones (5%), growth slowing, poor bone health, risk of dehydration, and dyslipidemia. **Table 8.6.4** summarizes various types of special diets that are used in clinical practice. Some are more stringent like classic KD while others such as low glycemic index treatment (LGIT) are more flexible in carbohydrate and fat intake. KG diet is contraindicated in patients with carnitine deficiency, porphyrias, beta-oxidation disorders, or pyruvate carboxylase deficiency.

Table 8.6.4 Ketogenic Diet and Its Variants

Ketogenic Diet (KD) Type	How It Works	What Is Restrictive	Starting the Diet	Adverse Effects and Downfalls*
Classic KD	Fat to protein ratio 3:1 or 4:1	Calories/Protein	Inpatient monitoring of glucose/ketones and family teaching	Hyperlipidemia, kidney stones, poor growth, osteopenia, requires blood monitoring
Modified Atkins diet (MAD)	10–15 g/day carbs; 20 g/day in older patients	Carbohydrates	Outpatient	Some need to advance to classic KD for better seizure control
Medium chain triglyceride (MCT) diet	MCT substituted for long chain triglycerides used in classic KD	Calories/Protein	Outpatient, start slow to decrease GI upset	Gastrointestinal (GI) upset
Low glycemic index treatment (LGIT)	40–60 g/day	Carbohydrates, specifically glycemic index of carbs <50	Outpatient	Does not produce ketone bodies

*Similar side effects for all diets, but decreased in MAD/LGIT/MCT.

The **vagus nerve stimulator** (VNS) is a device that provides intermittent electrical stimulation of the left vagus nerve, which is effective in reducing seizures, and received Food and Drug Administration (FDA) approval in 1997. The stimulator is similar to a cardiac pacemaker and is surgically implanted subcutaneously. The right vagus nerve is not stimulated because of its rich innervation to the sinoatrial node of the heart. The mechanism by which stimulation reduces seizures is not well established. Adverse effects are generally mild and include hoarseness, throat pain, or a feeling of dyspnea during stimulation. The cost of the device and its implantation may be limiting factors. Clinical trials demonstrate that less than 5% of patients become seizure-free with VNS placement but approximately one-third of patients experience a clinically significant decrease in their seizure frequency. The device may have value for generalized epilepsies, especially LGS and specifically atonic seizures. Many centers will try a VNS prior to a callosotomy for intractable atonic seizures. VNS has a responder rate of 40% (ie, 40% of patients have a 50% or more decrease in their seizures).

References

1. Al-Banji M, Zahr DK, Jan MM. Lennox-Gastaut syndrome management update. *Neurosciences.* July 2015;20(3):207–212.
2. Arzimanoglou A, Guerrini R, Aicardi J. Lennox-Gastaut syndrome. In: *Aicardi's Epilepsy in Children.* Philadelphia, PA: Lippincott Williams & Wilkins, 2004:38–50.
3. Asadi-Pooya AA, Sharan A, Nei M, Sperling MR. Corpus callosotomy. *Epilepsy and Behavior.* August 2008;13(2):271–278.
4. Guerrini R, Pellock JM. Chapter 11. Age-related epileptic encephalopathies. In: *Handbook of Clinical Neurology.* 2012;107:179–193.
5. Malmgren K, Rydenhag B, Hallböök T. Reappraisal of corpus callosotomy. *Curr Opin Neurol.* April 2015;28(2):175–181.
6. Montouris GD, Wheless JW, Glauser TA. The Efficacy and tolerability of pharmacologic treatment options for Lennox-Gastaut Syndrome. *Epilepsia.* 2014;55(Suppl. 4):10–20.
7. Werz MA, Pita, IL. Chapter 7. Lennox-Gastaut syndrome. *Epileptic Syndromes.* Saunders; 2010:33–41.
8. Winesett SP, Bessone SK, Kossoff EH. The ketogenic diet in pharmacoresistant childhood epilepsy. *Expert Rev Neurother.* June 2015;15(6):621–628.

8.7 | Childhood Absence Epilepsy

Case History

A 6-year-old female presented with frequent brief episodes of staring.

Diagnosis: Childhood Absence Epilepsy

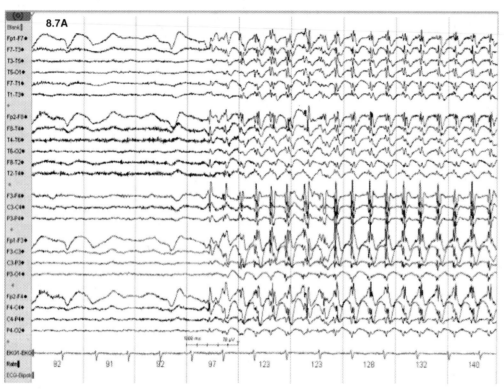

Image 8.7A: EEG tracing with bipolar montage shows generalized regular and symmetrical spikes/polyspikes and slow waves maximal in the frontal and frontocentral regions.

Introduction

■ Absence seizures (see **Table 8.7.1**) comprise 2% to 15% of childhood epilepsy, which is 2 to 5 times more common in girls. About 15% to 40% of patients with these epilepsies have a family history of epilepsy.

■ Onset is typically between 4 and 10 years of age.

■ Most patients have normal neurological examinations and normal cognition.

■ Childhood absence epilepsy is caused by abnormalities in T-type calcium channels, which are responsible for rhythmic depolarizing activity in the thalamic neurons.

■ Inherited in autosomal-dominant pattern with incomplete penetrance chromosomes 20q, 16p13.3, and 8q24.3.

■ A mutation in the GABA (A) receptor gene *GABRB3* has been found in Mexican families with childhood absence epilepsy. Mutations showed hyperglycosylation in vitro, with reduced GABA-evoked current density from whole cells. Expression of this gene in the developing brain may help explain an age-related onset and remission in childhood absence epilepsy.

Table 8.7.1 Classification of Absence Seizures

Absence	Typical: 3 Hz spike and slow wave Atypical: Slow 2–2.5 Hz spike and slow wave
Absence with special features	Myoclonic absence Eyelid myoclonia Jeavons syndrome

Clinical Presentation

■ The episodes are characterized by very brief episodes of sudden behavioral arrest, blank stare, and motionless state with loss of awareness. Loss of postural tone, automatisms, and eye flutter, or eyelid myoclonia can be seen. About 3% may experience GTCs.

■ The staring spells start and end abruptly and last for 5 to 10 seconds and up to hundreds of seizures can occur per day.

■ Patients have no preceding aura and no postictal phase unlike complex partial seizures, which are typically characterized by auras and can have postictal symptoms.

■ Seizures can be provoked by hyperventilation in approximately 90% of children.

■ Absence of SE is characterized by sustained impairment of consciousness associated with generalized 3 Hz spike and waves. Patients often exhibit facial twitching, eye blinking, staring, and automatisms.

Electrographic Appearance and Diagnosis

■ EEG shows classic 3 Hz generalized spike- and slow-wave pattern. Otherwise, these patients have normal posterior dominant rhythm. The epileptiform discharges are generalized in distribution but typically have maximal field in frontal and frontocentral regions (see EEG in **Image 8.7A**).

■ The epileptiform discharges are typically provoked by hyperventilation.

Treatment

■ Primary drugs of choice are ethosuximide, valproic acid, and lamotrigine.

■ Initial trial with ethosuximide (T-type calcium channel blocker) because of fewer incidences of side effects.

■ Treatment is usually with IV lorazepam or valproic acid.

■ Duration of therapy is variable, although the general rule is to taper off therapy after 2 years of seizure freedom.

■ About 80% of patients outgrow this form of epilepsy. Children with early onset have the best prognosis with complete remission 2 to 6 years after onset.

■ Onset of absence seizures before age 3 years is associated with neurodevelopmental abnormalities and other seizure types such as atonic or myoclonic epilepsy, can be refractory to treatment, and carry a poorer prognosis.

■ Refractory absences resistant to medical treatment may be associated with SCNA1 mutation and glucose transporter defect type 1. Rufinamide or KD may be effective in patients with absence and atypical absences associated with LGS.

References

1. Fong GC, Shah PU, Gee MN, et al. Childhood absence epilepsy with tonic-clonic seizures and electroencephalogram 3-4-Hz spike and multispike-slow wave complexes: linkage to chromosome 8q24. *Am J Hum Genet*. October 1998;63(4):1117–1129.
2. Wallace RH, Marini C, Petrou S, et al. Mutant GABA(A) receptor gamma2-subunit in childhood absence epilepsy and febrile seizures. *Nat Genet*. May 2001;28(1):49–52.

8.8 | Rasmussen's Encephalitis

Case History

An 8-year-old boy presented with medically intractable partial epilepsy. Over the next several months, he developed gradual loss of language skills and was found to have weakness of the right side of his body.

Diagnosis: Rasmussen's Encephalitis

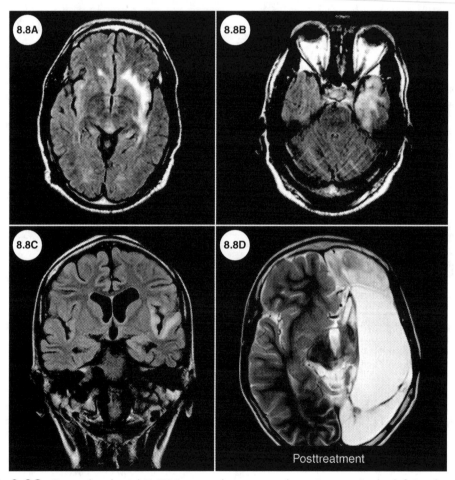

Images 8.8A–8.8C: Coronal and axial FLAIR images demonstrate hyperintensty in the left insular cortex and temporal lobe; **Image 8.8D** shows left modified hemispherectomy.

Introduction

■ Rasmussen's encephalitis (RE) develops from a region of inflammation that is localized to one cerebral hemisphere. However, very young children (<2 years), adolescents, and young adults can have bilateral involvement. Lobar and brainstem variants have also been described.

■ It affects children younger than 10 years, with the average age of onset being 6 years. In around 10% of cases of RE, the disease starts after the age of 12 to 13 years, with onsets occurring as late as in mid-30s.

■ It is thought to be due to either a chronic viral infection or an autoimmune response against glutamate receptors.

- Typically, the central cortex is implicated early in the disease and involves other areas gradually.

Clinical Presentation

- Patients suffer from either simple or complex partial seizures. Recurrent focal motor seizures, termed epilepsia partialis continua, are common, and often do not respond to AEDs.

- Patients eventually develop motor, sensory, or language dysfunction due to progressive nature of the disease, which becomes evident on serial neuroimaging. Symptoms progress over the course of 1 year.

- In very young children less than 2 years of age, adolescents, and adults, bilateral cerebral hemispheres may be involved.

Radiographic Appearance and Diagnosis

- MRI shows hyperintensity on T2-weighted images in the affected hemisphere. There is no enhancement with the addition of contrast, though there may be restricted diffusion on diffusion-weighted images.

- During the acute stage, inflammation is evident as FLAIR signal hyperintensity, disproportionately involving the gray matter. In the chronic stage, this inflammation resolves and atrophy ensues.

- There is progressive atrophy of the cerebral hemisphere.

- In 10% of the patients, the changes can be seen bilaterally.

- A brain biopsy may be needed to make the diagnosis in equivocal cases.

Treatment

- The mainstay of treatment is glucocorticoids, IVIG, plasmapheresis, and immunosuppressive therapy (rituximab, tacrolimus, natalizumab) in an attempt to control the inflammation.

- In some patients, seizures are refractory to aforementioned treatments and standard antiepileptic medications.

- Excision techniques such as anatomical hemispherectomy and hemidecortication or disconnection techniques such as functional hemispherectomy and hemispherotomy are effective in controlling seizures with RE (see **Table 8.8.1**).

Table 8.8.1 Various Excision and Disconnection Epilepsy Surgeries

Surgical Technique	Comments
Anatomic hemispherectomy	Removal of hemisphere sparing ipsilateral basal ganglia and thalamus; carries greatest intraoperative risks; blood loss is managed by early occlusion of vascular supply (ACA, MCA, PCA)
Functional hemispherectomy (Rasmussen)	Extensive cortical resection in temporal and central cortex (frontal/parietal) with disconnection of residual frontal and occipital cortex by transecting white matter fibers
Hemispherotomy	Disconnecting the hemisphere with minimal brain tissue removal; approaches can be vertical and peri-insular (lateral)
Hemidecortication	Removal of the whole hemisphere with sparing of the white matter; avoids opening of the lateral ventricle

ACA, anterior cerebral artery; MCA, middle cerebral artery; PCA, posterior cerebral artery.

References

1. Ciliberto M, Powers AK, Limbrick DL, Titus J, Munro B, Smyth MD. Palliative functional hemispherotomy in patients with bilateral seizure onset. *J Neurosurg Pediatr.* 2012;9: 381–388.
2. Limbrick DD, Narayan P, Johnston JM, Ojemann JG, Park TS, Smyth MD. Outcomes following hemispherotomy: the St. Louis Children's Hospital experience. (Abstract) *Child's Nervous System.* 2007;23(9):1062.
3. Limbrick DD, Narayan P, Powers AK, et al. Hemispherotomy: efficacy and analysis of seizure recurrence. *J Neurosurg Pediatr.* 2009;4:323–332.
4. Narayan P, Isik U, Trevathan E, et al. Functional hemispherectomy for epilepsy in childhood: Institutional experience [Platform presentation]. Salt Lake City, UT: Joint Pediatric Section; 2003.

CHAPTER 9
INFECTIOUS DISEASES

9.1 | HIV Dementia Complex

Case History

A 45-year-old man with untreated HIV infection presented with 4 months of cognitive slowing. On examination, he was disheveled and sat passively in the chair. He did not know the date or location and was unperturbed by his failures.

Diagnosis: HIV Dementia Complex

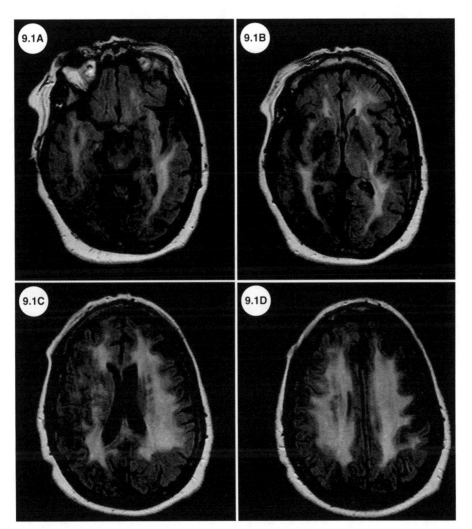

Images 9.1A–9.1D: Axial fluid-attenuated inversion recovery (FLAIR) images demonstrate extensive periventricular and subcortical white matter hyperintensities in a patient with HIV.

Introduction

■ Direct infection of the central nervous system (CNS) with HIV presents with a dementia that progresses over several months, termed HIV dementia complex (HIVD). The likelihood of developing HIVD is inversely related to the CD4 count, and dementia is considered a late feature of HIV infection. It is now most commonly found in patients with resistance to or nonadherence to highly active antiretroviral therapy (HAART).

- It is part of a spectrum of cognitive disorders seen in patients with HIV, which are collectively termed HIV-associated neurocognitive disorders.

Clinical Presentation

- Patients present with personality changes, psychomotor retardation, and a subcortical dementia, characterized by difficulty sustaining attention, executive function abnormalities, and slow processing speed. Language and memory functions are relatively unimpaired. By definition, activities of daily living must be impaired.

- This presentation may mimic infections with cytomegalovirus, progressive multifocal leukoencephalopathy (PML), and neoplastic processes, lymphoma in particular. However, these are much more likely to present with focal neurological deficits compared to HIVD.

Radiographic Appearance and Diagnosis

- The radiographic appearance of HIVD typically shows symmetric, confluent white matter hyperintensities on T2-weighted images without mass effect or enhancement. Significant, diffuse atrophy is common.

- There is no specific test for HIVD, but it is important to evaluate patients for other opportunistic infections and other causes of dementia.

Treatment

- There is no specific treatment for HIVD beyond starting HAART therapy. The overall prognosis is poor.

References

1. Brew BJ, Chan P. Update on HIV dementia and HIV-associated neurocognitive disorders. *Curr Neurol Neurosci Rep.* August 2014;14(8):468.
2. Manji H, Jäger HR, Winston A. HIV, dementia and antiretroviral drugs: 30 years of an epidemic. *J Neurol Neurosurg Psychiatry.* October 2013;84(10):1126–1137.
3. Kelly CM, Miller AR, Aji B, Solomon T. HIV dementia: a diagnosis to keep in mind. *Br J Hosp Med (Lond).* July 2012;73(7):410–411.
4. Steinbrink F, Evers S, Buerke B, et al. Cognitive impairment in HIV infection is associated with MRI and CSF pattern of neurodegeneration. *Eur J Neurol.* March 2013;20(3):420–428.

9.2 HIV-Associated Vacuolar Myelopathy

Case History

A 56-year-old woman with a history of untreated HIV developed paraparesis with severe burning and tingling.

Diagnosis: HIV-Associated Vacuolar Myelopathy

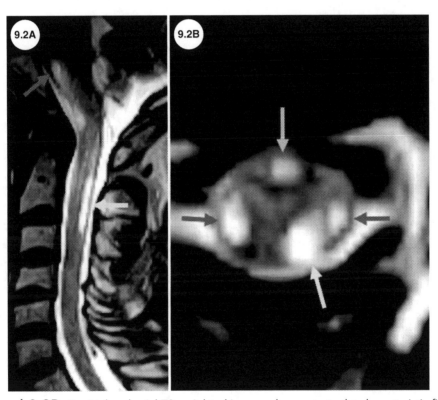

Images 9.2A and 9.2B: Sagittal and axial T2-weighted images demonstrate the characteristic findings of HIV-myelopathy. The red arrows point to lateral corticospinal tracts, the yellow and red arrows point to the dorsal columns, and the blue arrow points to the anterior corticospinal tract.

Introduction

■ HIV-associated vacuolar myelopathy (VM) occurs during the late stages of HIV infection, when CD4+ counts are very low. It is thought that HIV impairs the vitamin-B12-dependent transmethylation pathway.

Clinical Presentation

■ Patients present with gradual paraparesis, stiffness, sensory loss, imbalance, and bowel/ bladder dysfunction. The arms are usually spared. Pain, due to involvement of the dorsal columns, is common. It often occurs in conjunction with other AIDS-defining illnesses.

Radiographic Appearance and Diagnosis

■ MRI is the preferred imaging modality. Spinal cord atrophy is the most common finding. The thoracic cord is most commonly affected, but the entire cord is vulnerable. In some patients, there is vacuolization of the corticospinal tract and dorsal columns, resembling the myelopathy produced by B12 deficiency. Other patients may have more diffuse signal abnormality.

Treatment

■   There is no known treatment, nor is there evidence that antiretroviral therapy can improve symptoms or slow progression. Supportive care includes antispasticity agents, management of sphincter dysfunction, pain management, and rehabilitation.

References

1. Di Rocco A, Simpson DM. AIDS-associated vacuolar myelopathy. *AIDS Patient Care STDS*. June 1998;12(6):457–461.
2. Di Rocco A. Diseases of the spinal cord in human immunodeficiency virus infection. *Semin Neurol*. 1999;19(2): 151–155.
3. Di Rocco A, Bottiglieri T, Werner P, et al. Abnormal cobalamin-dependent transmethylation in AIDS-associated myelopathy. *Neurology*. March 2002;58(5):730–735.

9.3 Herpes Simplex Encephalitis

Case History

A healthy 23-year-old man presented with confusion and agitation for 3 days. He was disoriented with weakness of his left arm, of which he was unaware. He had a seizure in the emergency department.

Diagnosis: Herpes Encephalitis

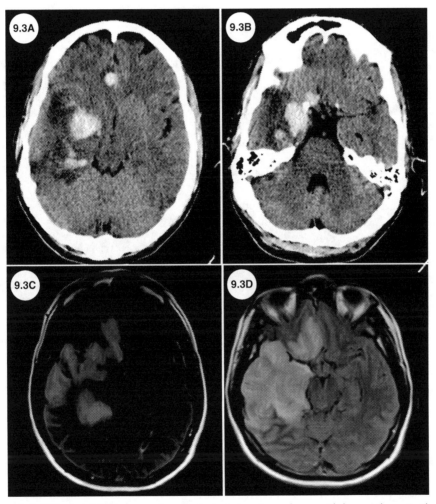

Images 9.3A and 9.3B: Axial CT images demonstrate extensive edema with hemorrhage in the right temporal and frontal lobes in a patient with HSV encephalitis. **Images 9.3C and 9.3D:** Axial FLAIR images demonstrate hyperintensity and necrosis of the right temporal lobe.

Introduction

- The most common cause of viral encephalitis in the United States is infection with herpes simplex virus 1 (HSV-1). The presumed route of infection is reactivation of latent virus within the trigeminal ganglion.

Clinical Presentation

- Patients present with rapid-onset encephalitis. This includes seizures, headaches, and changes in cognition or personality. Fever is common.

Radiographic Appearance and Diagnosis

- HSV has a predilection for the limbic system. CT shows asymmetric hemorrhagic necrosis of the inferior frontal and temporal lobes. This finding is absent early in the disease course, however, and initial CT may be completely normal. On MRI T2-weighted images, there is hyperintensity of the affected areas, both cortex and white matter. With the addition of contrast there may be a variety of patterns, including enhancement of the meninges, cortex, or focal enhancement, often ring-shaped. Restricted diffusion is common as well.

- Cerebrospinal fluid (CSF) is hemorrhagic with a leukocytosis ranging from 5 to 1,000 cells/mm^3. Initially these are monocytes, but a lymphocytic predominance develops over time. There may be mild elevations of the protein and opening pressure and a normal or mildly decreased glucose. The diagnosis can be confirmed by HSV polymerase chain reaction (PCR).

- An electroencephalogram (EEG) may show periodic lateralizing epileptiform discharges, generalized slowing, or focal temporal lobe spikes.

Treatment

- It is treated with intravenous (IV) acyclovir. Treatment should begin as soon as the illness is suspected, as mortality approaches 75% in untreated patients. Survivors are often left with permanent deficits, with less than 5% of patients making a complete neurological recovery. Renal function must be carefully monitored in patients on acyclovir.

References

1. Safain MG, Roguski M, Kryzanski JT, Weller SJ. A review of the combined medical and surgical management in patients with herpes simplex encephalitis. *Clin Neurol Neurosurg.* November 2014;128C:10–16.
2. Kennedy PG, Steiner I. Recent issues in herpes simplex encephalitis. *J Neurovirol.* August 2013;19(4):346–350.

9.4 Ramsay Hunt Syndrome

Case History

A 45-year-old woman developed a painful rash on her right ear, followed by hearing loss and a facial palsy on that side.

Diagnosis: Herpes Zoster Oticus

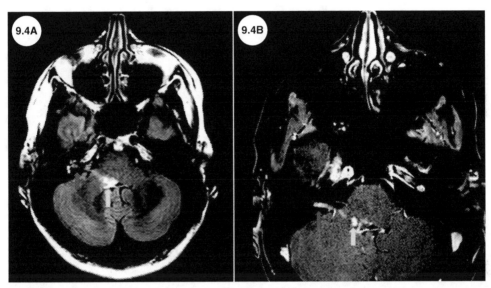

Images 9.4A and 9.4B: Axial FLAIR and postcontrast T1-weighted images demonstrate hyperintensity and enhancement of the seventh and eighth cranial nerves (red arrow) and geniculate ganglion (yellow arrow) on the right.

Introduction

■ Herpes zoster oticus (Ramsay Hunt syndrome) is caused by reactivation of the varicella zoster virus (VZV) in the geniculate ganglion of the facial nerve.

Clinical Presentation

■ It presents with a painful, vesicular rash of the external acoustic meatus and tympanic membrane, ipsilateral peripheral facial weakness, and loss of taste. The pain precedes the rash by several hours or days. There may be hearing loss, tinnitus, ataxia, or vertigo in some cases.

Radiographic Appearance and Diagnosis

■ MRI may reveal hyperintensity and enhancement of the facial nerve, geniculate ganglion, and even the facial nerve nucleus in the pons. Similar findings may be seen in Bell's palsy, though some enhancement of the facial nerve can be a normal finding.

■ Patients will have red, oozing blisters typical of a shingles rash over their ears, within the ears, and in their ear canals.

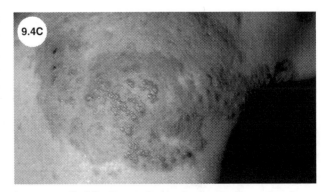

Images 9.4C: The typical rash of varicella zoster virus is shown on a thoracic dermatome.

Treatment

- Prednisone and acyclovir may hasten recovery if started within the first three days of symptom onset. Older patients and those with more severe facial weakness have a worse prognosis.

- Vaccination against VZV helps prevent the condition.

References

1. Shin DH, Kim BR, Shin JE, Kim CH. Clinical manifestations in patients with herpes zoster oticus. *Eur Arch Otorhinolaryngol.* July 2016;273(7):1739–1743.
2. Kuo CY, Lin YY, Wang CH. Painful rash of the auricle: herpes zoster oticus. *Ear Nose Throat J.* December 2014; 93(12):E47.

9.5 Progressive Multifocal Leukoencephalopathy

Case History

A 54-year-old man with HIV presented with confusion, apathy, and weakness of his left arm for 3 months. He had not taken his HIV medications in several years.

Diagnosis: Progressive Multifocal Leukoencephalopathy

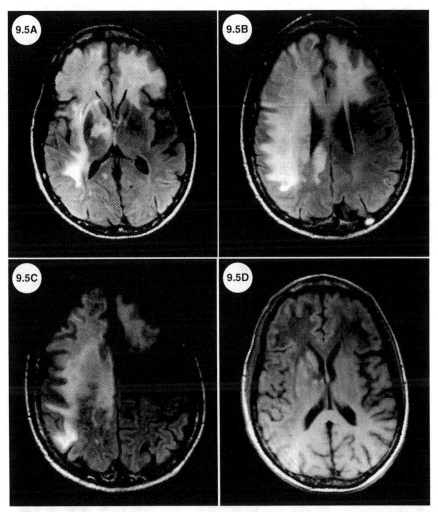

Images 9.5A–9.5C: Axial FLAIR images demonstrate confluent white matter lesions in the frontal lobes bilaterally, and throughout the temporal and parietal lobes on the right, without mass effect. **Image 9.5D:** The lesions are hypointense on the T1-weighted image.

Introduction

- Progressive multifocal leukoencephalopathy (PML) is a devastating infection of oligodendrocytes caused by the JC virus, a papovavirus.

- PML most commonly occurs in patients with late-stage AIDS (CD4 < 100) or immunosuppressed patients, such as multiple sclerosis (MS) patients treated with the monoclonal antibody natalizumab.

Clinical Presentation

- PML of the CNS presents with subacute onset of focal neurological defects, such as weakness, sensory or visual loss, aphasia, personality changes, or cognitive decline. Most patients experience significant decline over several months. Less commonly, patients may present with a seizure.

Radiographic Appearance and Diagnosis

- The MRI typically shows asymmetric involvement of the white matter, often involving the subcortical U-fibers. The lesions are hyperintense on T2-weighted images and hypointense on T1-weighted images, without mass effect. Although enhancement may occur with the administration of contrast, it is not typical. Diffusion restriction is common.

- In patients treated with natalizumab, the lesions of PML can initially be indistinguishable from MS lesions. Over time, the lesions of PML grow to be more confluent or may develop a "milky-way" pattern of multiple punctate lesions. There may be uneven restricted diffusion on diffusion-weighted images (DWIs). The diagnosis is

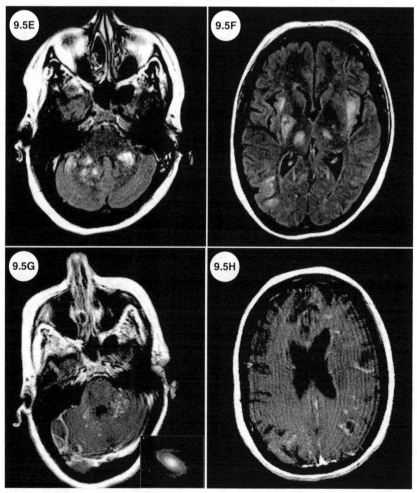

Images 9.5E–9.5H: Axial FLAIR and postcontrast T1-weighted images demonstrate multifocal white matter hyperintensities in the cerebellum, thalami, insula, and cortex characteristic of PML in a patient treated with natalizumab. The lesions enhance with contrast, and the characteristic "milky-way" appearance (red arrows) is seen in the cerebellum.

confirmed by detecting the JC virus via PCR in the spinal fluid, though the result may be negative early in the disease course depending on the sensitivity of the test used. There is no direct treatment for PML, but with early detection patients with MS may have a favorable outcome.

■ It is confirmed by detection of the JC virus via PCR in the CSF, though false negatives may occur. In certain cases, a biopsy is required to definitively make the diagnosis.

Treatment

■ There is no direct treatment, but reconstitution of the immune system with HAART therapy in AIDS patients may be helpful. Immune reconstitution inflammatory syndrome (IRIS) is an inflammatory responsive that can occur in HIV patients with reconstitution of the immune system after the initiation of HAART. Patients with low CD4 counts who have not received prior HAART therapy are at the greatest risk. It occurs in about 20% of patients. Patients present with visual deficits, confusion, personality changes, cognitive deficits, weakness, ataxia, and seizures. Even with the initiation of HAART, the outcome is generally poor, and the disease is often fatal within 1 year.

Pretreatment Images

■ MS patients treated with natalizumab have an improved prognosis depending on how far

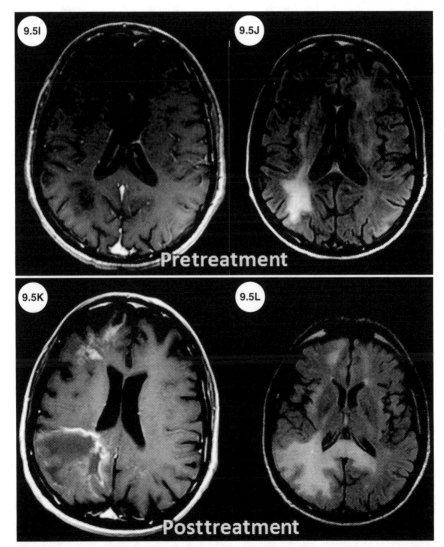

Images 9.5I and 9.5J: Postcontrast axial T1-weighted and FLAIR images showing white matter lesions consistent with PML in the right occipitoparietal and left frontal lobes. **Images 9.5K and 9.5L:** Postcontrast axial T1-weighted and FLAIR images demonstrating large areas of enhancement in the right frontal, parietal, and occipital lobes with significant edema after the initiation of HAART therapy.

advanced their disease is at the time of diagnosis. Of the approximately 600 cases thus far, 20% have been fatal, and some have made a full recovery.

References

1. Berger JR. Progressive multifocal leukoencephalopathy. *Handb Clin Neurol.* 2014;123:357–376.
2. Ferenczy MW, Marshall LJ, Nelson CD, et al. Molecular biology, epidemiology, and pathogenesis of progressive multifocal leukoencephalopathy, the JC virus-induced demyelinating disease of the human brain. *Clin Microbiol Rev.* July 2012;25(3):471–506.
3. Serana F, Chiarini M, Sottini A, et al. Immunological biomarkers identifying natalizumab-treated multiple sclerosis patients at risk of progressive multifocal leukoencephalopathy. *J Neuroimmunol.* December 2014;277(1–2): 6–12.
4. Baldwin KJ, Hogg JP. Progressive multifocal leukoencephalopathy in patients with multiple sclerosis. *Curr Opin Neurol.* June 2013;26(3):318–323.

9.6 | Tuberculous Meningitis

Case History

A 28-year-old man from India developed cranial nerve deficits and soon became encephalopathic.

Diagnosis: Tuberculous Meningitis

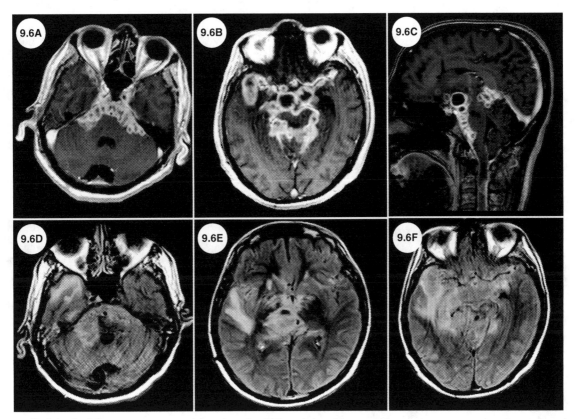

Images 9.6A–9.6C: Postcontrast axial and sagittal T1-weighted images demonstrate extensive ring-enhancing lesions in the basal meninges in a patient with tuberculosis, representing tuberculomas. **Images 9.6D–9.6F:** Axial FLAIR images show significant edema and mass effect associated with the lesions.

Introduction

■ Infection with *Mycobacterium tuberculosis* occurs from person to person by infected respiratory droplets. It is not common in Western countries except in the setting of an immunocompromised state, especially in patients with AIDS. The most common route of infection of the CNS is hematogenous spread from a systemic source. Approximately 10% of patients develop neurological complications.

Clinical Presentation

■ It most commonly affects the basal meninges, manifesting with cranial neuropathies, primarily of the abducens nerve, and altered mental status. Other presentations include seizures, vasculitis with subsequent infarction, hydrocephalus, and focal neurological deficits if there are tuberculomas within the brain.

■ Patients with tuberculous meningitis are categorized by stage on presentation, based upon mental status and focal neurological signs as follows:

1. **Stage I:** Patients are lucid with no focal neurological signs or evidence of hydrocephalus.
2. **Stage II**: Patients exhibit lethargy and confusion. They may have mild focal signs, such as cranial nerve palsy or hemiparesis.
3. **Stage III**: Represents advanced illness with delirium, stupor, coma, seizures, multiple cranial nerve palsies, and/or dense hemiplegia.

■ Myelopathy can occur due to infection of the vertebral body (Pott disease) or due to direct infection of the spinal canal and spinal cord with tuberculomas in the absence of any lesion to the bone. There can be both intraspinal granulomatous tissue, which compresses the cord from the outside, or intramedullary tuberculomas. Pott disease arises from the vertebral body, usually in the thoracic or lumbar spine, which then invades the epidural space. Patients present with the subacute onset of severe, localized pain and fever. Myelopathic signs develop if there is compression of the spinal cord.

Radiographic Appearance and Diagnosis

■ CNS tuberculosis most commonly causes a basal meningitis with enhancing lesions and resultant mass effect and edema in the brain, as seen in **Images 9.6A–9.6F**.

■ Tuberculomas may be found throughout the brain parenchyma as well.

■ Within the spine, there can be both intraspinal granulomatous tissue that compresses the cord from the outside, as well as intramedullary tuberculomas.

■ In Pott disease, the thoracolumbar spine is involved in 80% to 90% of cases, but any area of the spinal axis may be affected.

■ The CSF typically reveals highly elevated protein, often greater than 1,000 mg/dL, a low glucose, and a lymphocytic pleocytosis, though this may not be evident in patients with compromised immune systems. The elevation of the protein may be high enough to cause obstruction of CSF flow and hydrocephalus. Acid-fast bacilli and PCR are usually positive in the CSF.

■ The diagnosis is often evident due to pulmonary symptoms or tuberculosis elsewhere in the body.

Treatment

■ Treatment begins with an "intensive phase," which includes isoniazid, rifampin, pyrazinamide, and a fourth drug, either a fluoroquinolone or an injectable aminoglycoside, given daily for 2 months. This is followed by a regimen of isoniazid and rifampin alone. For HIV-negative patients glucocorticoid therapy is often added. Patients with hydrocephalus or symptoms of

Image 9.6G: Gross pathology demonstrates a thick basal exudate in a patient with tuberculosis (image credit Yale Rosen).

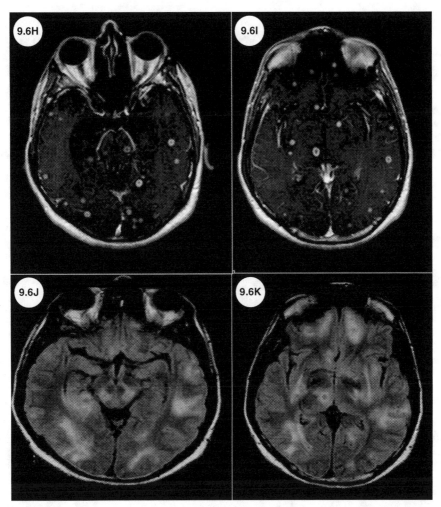

Images 9.6H–9.6K: Postcontrast axial T1-weighted and FLAIR images demonstrate innumerable ring-enhancing lesions throughout the brainstem and brain with surrounding edema and mass effect from tuberculomas.

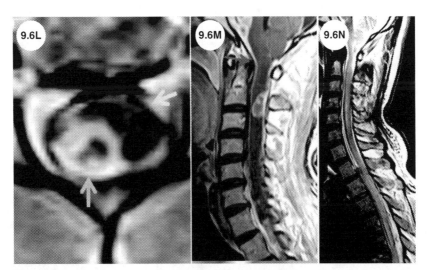

Images 9.6L and 9.6M: Postcontrast axial and sagittal T1-weighted images of the cervical spine demonstrate thin linear enhancement of the meninges (red arrow) and a larger lesion at C2 with cord compression. On the axial image, the spinal cord is indicated by the yellow arrow, while the large tubercular lesion is indicated by the blue arrow.
Image 9.6N: Sagittal T2-weighted image demonstrates hyperintensity throughout the cervical cord.

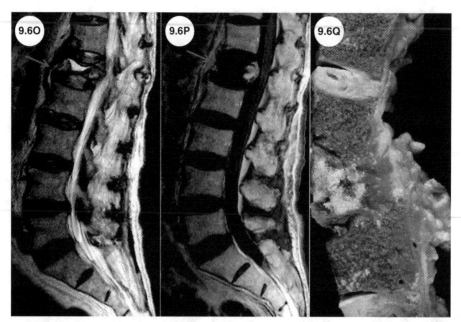

Images 9.6O and 9.6P: Sagittal T2-weighted and postcontrast T1-weighted images demonstrate a severe compression fracture of the L1 vertebral body with retropulsion of bone into the spinal canal indenting the tip of the conus medullaris in a patient with Pott disease. **Image 9.6Q:** Gross pathology of Pott disease (image credit Dr. Yale Rosen).

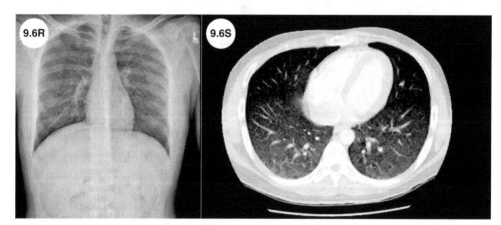

Images 9.6R and 9.6S: Chest radiograph and axial CT image demonstrate miliary tuberculosis.

increased intracranial pressure (ICP) may require surgical decompression of the ventricular system.

■ The illness is universally fatal in 1 to 2 months without treatment, and fatal in about 25% of those with treatment. Immunocompromised patients fare worse.

■ For patients with Pott disease, the same antitubercular treatment is indicated as for tuberculous meningitis, though neurosurgical debridement and stabilization of the spine may be required in patients with acute neurological deterioration, spinal deformity with instability, resistance to drug therapy, or paravertebral abscess.

References

1. Bernaerts A, Vanhoenacker FM, Parizel PM, et al. Tuberculosis of the central nervous system: overview of neuroradiological findings. *Eur Radiol.* August 2003;13(8):1876–1890.
2. Sahu SK, Giri S, Gupta N. Longitudinal extensive transverse myelitis due to tuberculosis: a report of four cases. *Postgrad Med.* October–December 2014;60(4):409–412.
3. Sanei Taheri M, Karimi MA, Haghighatkhah H, Pourghorban R, Samadian M, Delavar Kasmaei H. Central nervous system tuberculosis: an imaging-focused review of a reemerging disease. *Radiol Res Pract.* 2015;2015:202806.
4. Mondol BA, Siddiqui MR, Mohammad QD, Saha NC, Hoque MA, Uddin MJ. Tuberculosis of the central nervous system. *Mymensingh Med J.* April 2010;19(2):312–322.

9.7   Bacterial Meningitis

Case History

A 4-week-old infant presented with lethargy and a fever.

Diagnosis: Infant With Meningitis

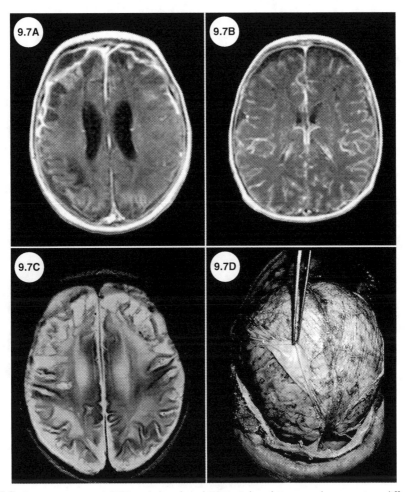

Images 9.7A–9.7C: Postcontrast axial T1-weighted and T2-weighted images demonstrate diffuse pial enhancement and bilateral, frontal, subdural empyemas in an infant with a group B streptococcal meningitis. **Image 9.7D:** Gross pathology of bacterial meningitis (image credit Centers for Disease Control and Prevention [CDC]).

Introduction

■ Most cases of bacterial meningitis result from the hematogenous spread of bacteria from an upper respiratory tract infection to the choroid plexus (**Table 9.7.1**). Blood cultures reveal the causative organism in many cases. Alternatively, bacteria can directly enter the subarachnoid space from infections of the nasopharynx, dental abscesses, or following trauma or neurosurgical manipulation. The extension of an infectious agent into the ependymal cells or ventricles is termed ventriculitis.

Clinical Presentation

■ It most commonly presents with the rapid onset of stiff neck, fever, headache, and altered mental

Table 9.7.1 Causes of Meningitis by Risk Group

Risk and/or Predisposing Factor	Bacterial Pathogen
Neonate	Group B streptococci E coli L monocytogenes
Childhood–50 years	S pneumoniae N meningitidis H influenzae → Vaccine now exists
Age older than 50 years	S pneumoniae N meningitidis L monocytogenes Aerobic gram-negative bacilli
Immunocompromised state	S pneumoniae N meningitidis L monocytogenes Aerobic gram-negative bacilli
CSF shunts/neurosurgery	Staphylococcus aureus Coagulase-negative Staphylococci Aerobic gram-negative bacilli, including Pseudomonas aeruginosa
Skull fracture	S pneumoniae H influenzae Group A streptococci

status. Focal neurological deficits, primarily hearing loss and seizures, occur as well. Infants may present with lethargy, poor feeding, and hypothermia as opposed to fever.

Radiographic Appearance and Diagnosis

- Imaging studies are not of paramount importance in the acute situation unless a mass lesion is suspected that may preclude a lumbar puncture. However, an MRI will typically show meningeal enhancement, and in cases of cerebral edema, there will be sulcal effacement. Other later complications may include hydrocephalus, subdural empyema, and infarction.

- The typical CSF findings are a leukocytosis (100 to 10,000 WBCs/mL), lowered glucose (<40% of serum glucose), an elevated protein (100–500 mg/dL), and an elevated opening pressure. CSF studies should be sent for gram stain, which is positive in about 60% of cases, and culture, which is positive in about 75% of cases.

Treatment

- Treatment for bacterial meningitis should begin as soon as the illness is suspected, even before a lumbar puncture is performed. All patients should be treated empirically with a third-generation cephalosporin with the addition of ampicillin in neonates and patients older than 50. Corticosteroid therapy has also been shown to reduce morbidity from meningitis, such as deafness, though primarily in high-income countries.

- With prompt treatment, the mortality rate is approximately 20%, though many survivors still have significant morbidity.

References

1. Brouwer MC, McIntyre P, Prasad K, van de Beek D. Corticosteroids for acute bacterial meningitis. *Cochrane Database Syst Rev.* September 2015;9:CD004405.
2. Oliveira CR, Morriss MC, Mistrot JG, Cantey JB, Doern CD, Sánchez PJ. Brain magnetic resonance imaging of infants with bacterial meningitis. *J Pediatr.* July 2014;165(1): 134–139.

9.8 | Intracerebral Abscess

Case History

A 54-year-old man presented with headaches and left-sided weakness.

Diagnosis: Intracerebral Abscess

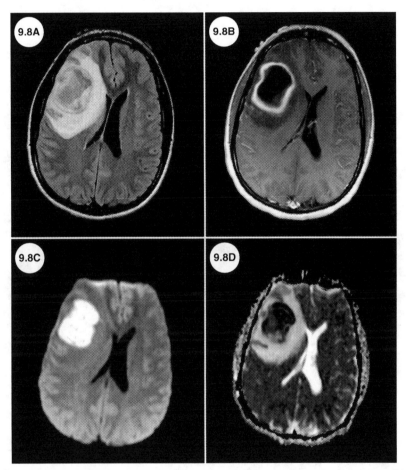

Images 9.8A and 9.8B: Axial FLAIR and postcontrast T1-weighted images demonstrate a large ring-enhancing lesion in the right frontal lobe with mass effect on the lateral ventricle and significant edema. **Images 9.8C and 9.8D:** DWI and apparent diffusion coefficient map demonstrate restricted diffusion of the lesion. The abscess is in the early encapsulation stage.

Introduction

- Brain abscesses most commonly result from direct infection from an adjacent site. Frontal lobe abscess typically result from a primary infection in the sinuses, while temporal lobe abscess commonly result from a middle ear infection or mastoiditis. In these cases of contiguous spread, the result is a single abscess.

- In cases of hematogenous spread, the most common primary infection is pulmonary, followed by endocarditis. In such cases, multiple abscesses may result.

- Most abscesses contain multiple organisms, and the most common pathogens are *Streptococcus* species, *Bacteroides*, *Enterobacteriaceae*, and other anaerobic bacteria. In cases of head trauma, *Staphylococcal* species are most commonly implicated.

Clinical Presentation

■ Abscesses present with headaches, seizures, nausea and vomiting, and focal neurological deficits. Fever and neck pain are not common. Abscesses may rupture into the ventricles, causing a sudden and drastic deterioration.

Radiographic Appearance and Diagnosis

■ T1-weighted images typically show central hypodensity with ring enhancement. T2-weighted images may show edema around the lesion, depending on its stage. There is often intense restricted diffusion on DWI.

■ There are four stages to abscess formation:

1. **Early cerebritis:** There is little mass effect and minimal enhancement.
2. **Late cerebritis:** Characterized by the development of a necrotic center. Early abscesses, as shown in **Images 9.8E–9.8H**, are associated with a significant amount of edema and intense enhancement.
3. **Early encapsulation:** There is a well-defined mass with intense ring enhancement. This is shown in **Images 9.8A–9.8D**.
4. **Late encapsulation:** Mature abscesses have a collagen capsule, with less cerebritis and edema. The length of time required to form a mature abscess varies from weeks to months.

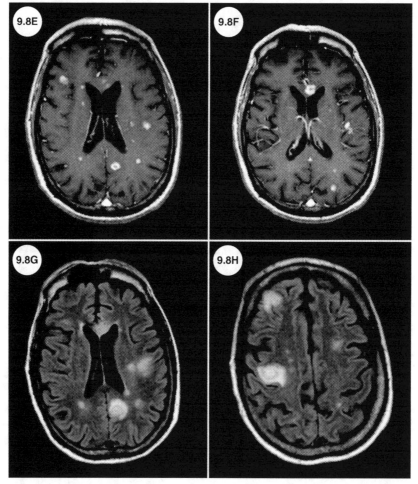

Images 9.8E and 9.8F: Postcontrast axial T1-weighted images demonstrate innumerable ring-enhancing lesions in the white matters. The presence of multiple abscesses suggests hematogenous spread from a systemic source.
Images 9.8G and 9.8H: Axial FLAIR images demonstrate edema representing an intense inflammatory response. The intense edema and inflammatory response indicate that these are early in their formation.

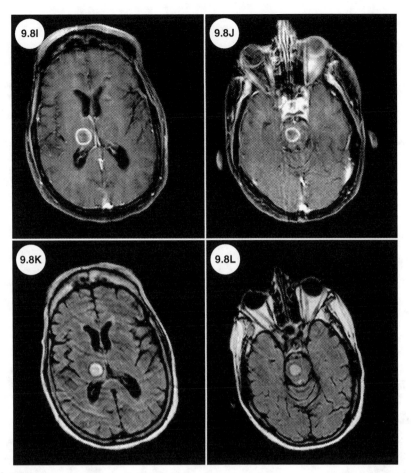

Images 9.8I and 9.8J: Postcontrast axial T1-weighted images demonstrate ring-enhancing lesions in the right thalamus and pons, with characteristic findings of late encapsulation. **Images 9.8K and 9.8L:** Axial FLAIR images demonstrate minimal hyperintensity of these later stage abscesses.

■ The diagnosis is made based on clinical and radiographic features. It is not always possible to distinguish abscesses from neoplasms, and a biopsy may be required to make the diagnosis. CSF analysis and blood cultures are typically of little diagnostic value.

Treatment

■ Empiric therapy is with vancomycin, metronidazole, and a third-generation cephalosporin for 6 to 8 weeks. Antibiotics are most effective if given prior to encapsulation. In mature abscesses, cases with increased ICP, or abscesses near the ventricles, surgical drainage may be indicated to prevent rupture of the abscess into the ventricle. Clinical improvement precedes radiographic improvement.

References

1. Sáez-Llorens X, Nieto-Guevara J. Brain abscess. *Handb Clin Neurol.* 2013;112:1127–1134.
2. Muzumdar D, Jhawar S, Goel A. Brain abscess: an overview. *Int J Surg.* 2011;9(2):136–144.
3. Hakan T. Management of bacterial brain abscesses. *Neurosurg Focus.* 2008;24(6):E4.

9.9 | Spinal Epidural Abscess

Case History

A 36-year-old man with a history of IV heroin use presented with leg weakness, fever, and low back pain. On examination he was weak in both legs with saddle anesthesia.

Diagnosis: Spinal Epidural Abscess

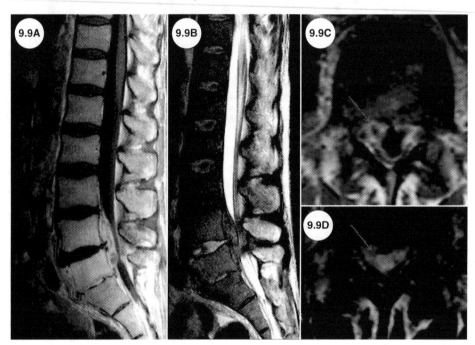

Images 9.9A–9.9D: Postcontrast sagittal and axial T1-weighted images demonstrate an enhancing lesion of the lumbar spine (red arrows) with compression of the cauda equina.

Introduction

■ Spinal epidural abscess (SEA) is an infection in the spinal epidural space leading to injury of the spinal cord or cauda equina directly by mechanical compression and indirectly by vascular compromise. Most SEAs occur in the thoracic area.

■ The infectious agent in SEAs is *Staphylococcus aureus* about 50% of the time. However, *Streptococcus*, gram-negative bacilli, anaerobes, fungi, and tuberculosis (in endemic areas) can also present with epidural abscess. The most common route of infection is hematogenous spread from infection elsewhere in the body, though about one-third of cases are due to direct spread from an adjacent infection. About one-third of cases have a history of trauma to the back, sometimes quite minor in nature. Patients with compromised immune systems, IV drug use, and skin infections are at the highest risk.

Clinical Presentation

■ The classic presentation is a triad of fever, back pain/tenderness, and neurological deficits. The following staging system has been described:

1. **Stage 1:** Focal neck or back pain at the level of the spine affected

2. **Stage 2:** Radicular pain and paresthesias

3. **Stage 3:** Motor weakness, sensory deficits, and bladder/bowel dysfunction

4. **Stage 4:** Progression to paralysis

Radiographic Appearance and Diagnosis

■ MRI best delineates both the longitudinal and paraspinal extension of the abscess and may help differentiate infection from other etiologies. It will reveal an enhancing lesion with compression of the underlying neural tissue. Pus will be hyperintense on T2-weighted images and hypointense on T1-weighted images with restricted diffusion. Diskitis and osteomyelitis occur in 80% of patients and may be demonstrated on CT images as well as MRI.

■ The responsible pathogen is commonly identified in blood cultures. Serum studies reveal a leukocytosis in two-thirds of patients and typically an elevated erythrocyte sedimentation rate (ESR), though these findings are not specific for SEA. A lumbar puncture is relatively contraindicated if an SEA is suspected, but may be essential to exclude meningitis.

Treatment

■ Emergency surgical decompression of the spinal cord with drainage of the abscess is the mainstay of treatment. Neurological deficits may progress rapidly and are permanent if they last over 24 hours.

■ Empiric antibiotic coverage effective against methicillin-resistant staphylococcus aureus (MRSA) is recommended. The combination of antistaphylococcal penicillin, third-generation cephalosporin, and aminoglycoside is prescribed for postsurgical infection. Culture results guide definitive therapy.

References

1. Connor DE Jr, Chittiboina P, Caldito G, Nanda A. Comparison of operative and nonoperative management of spinal epidural abscess: a retrospective review of clinical and laboratory predictors of neurological outcome. *J Neurosurg Spine.* July 2013;19(1):119–1127.
2. Patel AR, Alton TB, Bransford RJ, Lee MJ, Bellabarba CB, Chapman JR. Spinal epidural abscesses: risk factors, medical versus surgical management, a retrospective review of 128 cases. *Spine J.* February 2014;14(2):326–330.
3. Arko L, Quach E, Nguyen V, Chang D, Sukul V, Kim BS. Medical and surgical management of spinal epidural abscess: a systematic review. *Neurosurg Focus.* August 2014;37(2):E4.

9.10 | Neurocysticercosis

Case History

A 40-year-old man from India presented with two seizures over the course of one day. The patient denied any prior seizure history as well as any head trauma or family history of seizures. He had a normal neurological exam.

Diagnosis: Neurocysticercosis

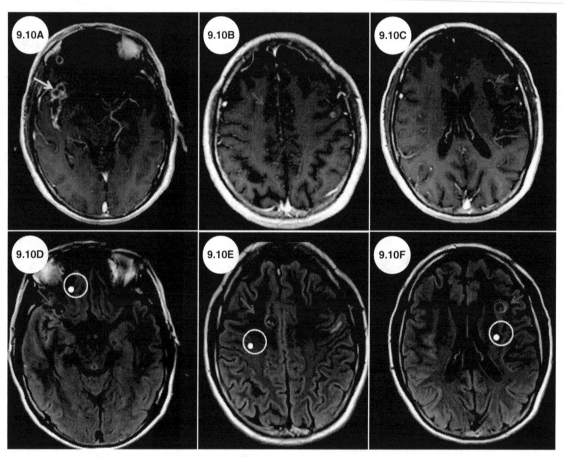

Images 9.10A–9.10C: Postcontrast axial T1-weighted images demonstrate round, peripherally enhancing lesions with a central hyperintensity (red arrows) in the brain parenchyma and the Sylvian fissure on the right (yellow arrow).
Images 9.10D–9.10F: Axial FLAIR images demonstrate cystic lesions with a central hyperintensity (red arrows) representing the scolex, the "hole with dot" sign of the vesicular stage of neurocysticercosis.

Introduction

■ Neurocysticercosis is caused by infection with *Taenia solium*, the pork tapeworm. It is the most common parasitic infection of the CNS and is common in India, Mexico, and South America, as well as parts of Asia, Africa, and Eastern Europe.

■ Initial human infection occurs due to the consumption of infected pork. The cystericerci embed in the stomach and the eggs are excreted in the feces. Ingestion of *T. solium* eggs then occurs via the fecal–oral route. The larvae attach to and invade the intestine where they migrate throughout the body (**Illustration 9.10.1**).

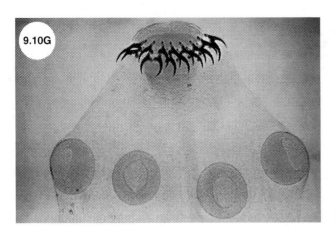

Image 9.10G: The scolex (head) of *Taenia solium* with its four suckers and two rows of hooks (image credit CDC).

Clinical Presentation

■ Symptoms most frequently arise when the cyst dies within the brain parenchyma, triggering an inflammatory reaction. It is the most common cause of acquired epilepsy in endemic areas, and seizures are the most common presentation

(70%–90% of patients). It is common in the United States in immigrants from endemic areas.

■ With a large lesion burden, there may be significant mass effect and edema, producing focal neurological deficits, headache, encephalopathy, hydrocephalus, and meningismus.

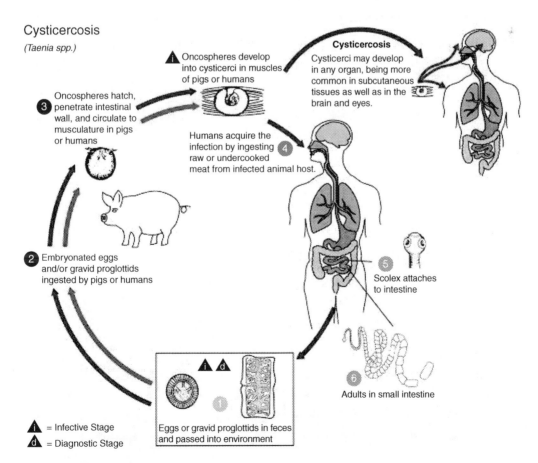

Illustration 9.10.1: Life cycle of *Taenia solium* (Illustration credit CDC).

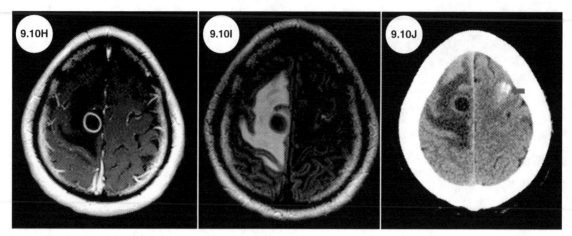

Images 9.10H–9.10J: Postcontrast axial T1-weighted, FLAIR, and noncontrast axial CT images demonstrate a ring-enhancing lesion in the right frontal lobe with an intense inflammatory reaction from neurocysticercosis in the colloidal stage. On the noncontrast axial CT image, an older, calcified lesion is also seen (red arrow).

Imaging Characteristics and Diagnosis

■ There are four stages to the life cycle, though more than one state may exist in a single patient at the same time.

1. **Vesicular stage:** There is a thin vesicular wall and a viable scolex in the middle. As seen in the aforementioned case, a visible scolex in the center of a hole produces the "hole with dot" sign. There is minimal if any enhancement with the addition of contrast. Lesions are most common at the gray–white junction. **Images 9.10A–9.10F** are from the vesicular stage.

2. **Colloidal stage:** There is a thick vesicular wall with a degenerating scolex and an intense inflammatory reaction with edema and marked enhancement of the cyst wall.

3. **Granular stage:** There is a thick vesicular wall and the scolex has degenerated. The edema and enhancement have decreased.

4. **Calcified stage:** The parasite has transformed into calcified nodules. At this stage, the cysts are dead. There will be no edema

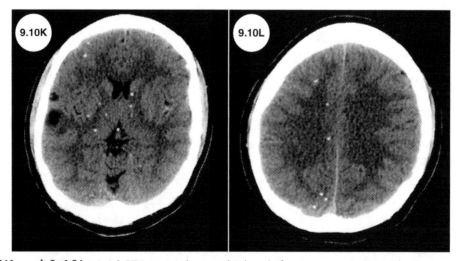

Images 9.10K and 9.10L: Axial CT images show multiple calcifications consistent with neurocysticercosis in the calcified state.

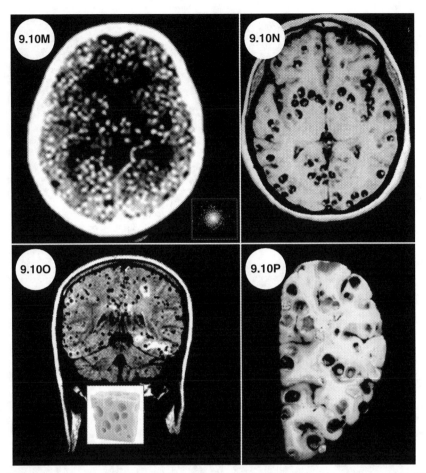

Images 9.10M–9.10O: Postcontrast T1-weighted, precontrast T1-weighted, and coronal FLAIR images demonstrate innumerable cysts in a patient with neurocysticercosis. On postcontrast imaging the lesions have a "starry-night" appearance, and on other sequences the brain has a "Swiss-cheese" appearance (images courtesy of Dr. Rajan Jain). **Image 9.10P:** Gross pathology of neurocysticercosis.

Source: Image 9.10P from Andrea Sylvia Winkler. Epilepsy and neurocysticercosis in sub-Saharan Africa. In: Sibat HF, ed. *Novel Aspects on Cysticercosis and Neurocysticercosis*; 2013. ISBN: 978-953-51-0956-3. doi:10.5772/53289. www.intechopen.com/books/novel-aspects-on-cysticercosis-and-neurocysticercosis/epilepsy-and-neurocysticercosis-in-sub-saharan-africa

or enhancement on postcontrast imaging. On CT, the dead parasites will present as small, punctate calcifications.

- With a large lesion burden, the brain is said to resemble "Swiss cheese," with a so-called "starry-night" appearance on postcontrast images.

- Cysts can form within the ventricular system as well, most commonly within the fourth ventricle or the subarachnoid space. This pattern is termed racemose (**grape-like**) neurocysticercosis. This can lead to ventricular obstruction and hydrocephalus. The cysts are isodense to CSF and there may be enhancement of the cyst wall and edema of the adjacent brain tissue. The scolex is typically not visible.

- Involvement of the spinal canal and cord may cause a myelopathy. As with the brain, lesions can be either intramedullary or extramedullary, compressing the cord from the outside.

Treatment

- Albendazole is used to kill the parasite, and corticosteroids are often used to minimize the inflammatory reaction. Not all patients need treatment as the majority of cysts show spontaneous resolution. Treatment should be initiated only once a patient is medically stable in terms of seizures, edema, and intracranial hypertension. Once the calcified state is reached, no antiparasitic treatment is needed, though patients may still suffer from seizures.

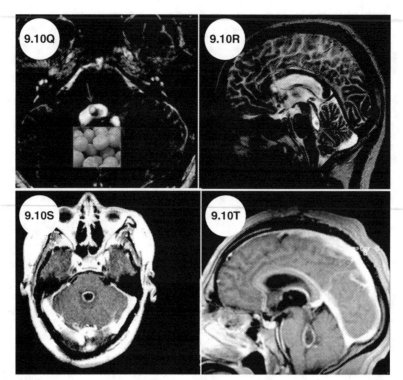

Images 9.10Q and 9.10R: Axial constructive interference in steady state and postcontrast sagittal T2-weighted images demonstrate racemose ("grape-like") neurocysticercosis (red arrow) of the fourth ventricle. The fourth ventricle is significantly dilated. **Images 9.10S and 9.10T:** Postcontrast axial and sagittal T1-weighted images demonstrate a ring-enhancing cyst in the fourth ventricle.

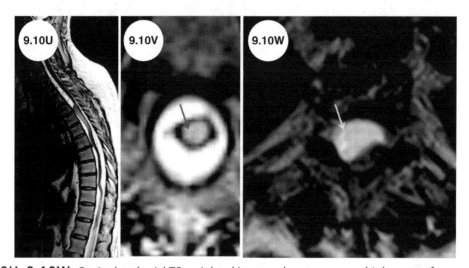

Images 9.10U–9.10W: Sagittal and axial T2-weighted images demonstrate multiple cysts of neurocysticercosis within the spinal cord (red arrow) and within the spinal canal (yellow arrow) compressing the spinal cord.

■ In patients with intraventricular cysts, surgical removal of the cyst may be required. Shunting of the ventricular system may be required to treat hydrocephalus.

References

1. Garcia HH, Nash TE, Del Brutto OH. Clinical symptoms, diagnosis, and treatment of neurocysticercosis. *Lancet Neurol.* December 2014;13(12):1202–1215.

2. Lerner A, Shiroishi MS, Zee CS, Law M, Go JL. Imaging of neurocysticercosis. *Neuroimaging Clin N Am.* November 2012;22(4):659–676.

3. Sotelo J. Clinical manifestations, diagnosis, and treatment of neurocysticercosis. *Curr Neurol Neurosci Rep.* December 2011;11(6):529–535.

4. Andrea Sylvia Winkler. Epilepsy and neurocysticercosis in sub-Saharan Africa. In: Sibat HF, ed. *Novel Aspects on Cysticercosis and Neurocysticercosis*; 2013. ISBN: 978-953-51-0956-3. doi:10.5772/53289. http://www.intechopen.com/books/novel-aspects-on-cysticercosis-and-neurocysticercosis/epilepsy-and-neurocysticercosis-in-sub-saharan-africa

9.11 | Toxoplasmosis

Case History

A 46-year-old woman with HIV presented with headaches, generalized weakness, and visual disturbances. The patient had been noncompliant with HAART therapy and had a CD4 count of 88. On exam, she was confused, diffusely weak, and had trouble visually identifying common objects.

Diagnosis: Toxoplasmosis

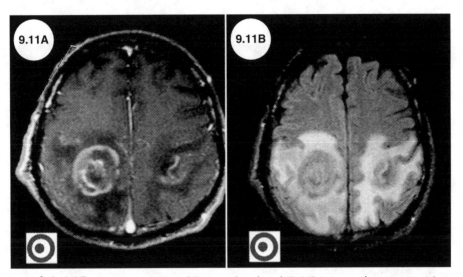

Images 9.11A and 9.11B: Postcontrast axial T1-weighted and FLAIR images demonstrate ring-enhancing lesions with significant edema in the frontal and parietal lobes bilaterally. They demonstrate the "eccentric target" sign characteristic of toxoplasmosis.

Introduction

- Toxoplasmosis is caused by the intracellular parasite *Toxoplasma gondii*. Cysts are ingested through undercooked meat, soil, cat feces, or contaminated water. It is a common parasite, though only symptomatic in immunocompromised patients. In some areas, over 95% of people have shown evidence of infection, and over 60 million people in the United States are infected.

- Cats are its definitive hosts, and humans can be infected by consuming food contaminated with cat feces or eating undercooked meat of animals with tissue cysts. It can also be transmitted transplacentally, from the mother to her fetus.

- CNS toxoplasmosis is seen most commonly in late-stage AIDS (CD4 < 200) or other

immunosuppressed patients. In patients with AIDS, toxoplasmosis is the most frequent cause of an intracranial mass lesion.

Clinical Presentation

- Patients present with fever, decreased mental status, focal neurological deficits, headaches, or seizures. Cysts can also form in skeletal and heart muscle and in the eyes.

Radiographic Appearance and Diagnosis

- The lesions are hyperintense on T2-weighted images, often with a large amount of mass effect and edema. They enhance with the administration of contrast in a solid or ring-shaped pattern. The lesions often have an "eccentric target" appearance.

■ The majority of effected AIDS patients have multiple lesions, most commonly in the basal ganglia, thalami, or gray–white junction.

■ Distinguishing between toxoplasmosis and primary CNS lymphoma (PCNSL) is difficult. Both present with multiple masses that may have solid or ring-like enhancement. CT scans can be helpful in differentiating toxoplasmosis from

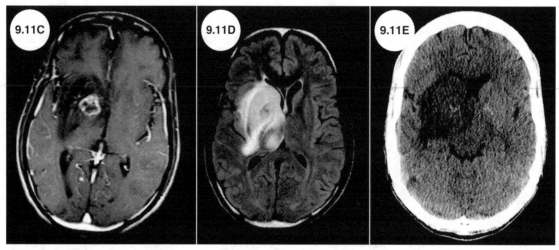

Images 9.11C and 9.11D: Postcontrast axial T1-weighted and FLAIR images demonstrate a ring-enhancing lesion in the right basal ganglia with significant edema and resultant mass effect. **Image 9.11E:** Axial CT image demonstrates hypodensity in the area of the lesion. This hypodensity on CT supports the diagnosis of toxoplasmosis.

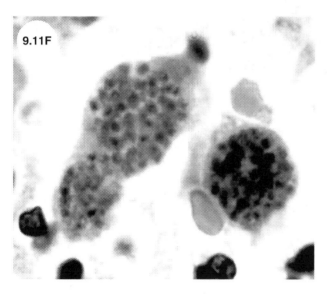

Image 9.11F: Histology of a pseudocyst containing bradyzoites (image credit Yale Rosen).

PCNSL. The lesions of toxoplasmosis are typically hypodense, while lymphomas are typically hyperdense due to increased cellularity.

■ Toxoplasma IgG should be sent when evaluating any intracranial mass in an HIV positive patient. In patients who test negative for toxoplasma IgG antibodies, the diagnosis of PCNSL is favored, though toxoplasmosis is not ruled out. In patients who test positive for toxoplasma IgG antibodies, both toxoplasmosis and PCNSL are possibilities.

Treatment

■ Patients with suspected toxoplasmosis should receive empiric treatment with trimethoprim–sulfamethoxazole (TMP–SMX) and folinic acid. Treatment should continue for 6 weeks or until there is no enhancement on MRI. Over 90% of patients with toxoplasmosis respond to treatment. If the lesions do not diminish on repeat imaging within 1 to 2 weeks, a brain biopsy to evaluate for PCNSL is indicated.

Pretreatment Images

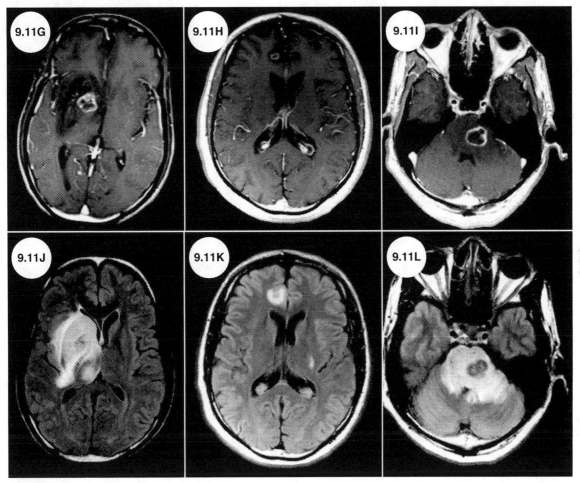

Images 9.11G–9.11I: Postcontrast axial T1-weighted images demonstrate ring-enhancing lesions in the right basal ganglia, right frontal lobe, and in the pons. **Images 9.11J–9.11L:** Axial FLAIR images demonstrate significant edema and mass effect.

Posttreatment Images

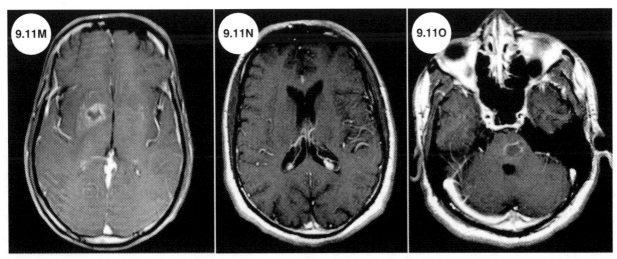

Images 9.11M–9.11O: Postcontrast axial T1-weighted images demonstrate decreased enhancement and size of the lesion after treatment.

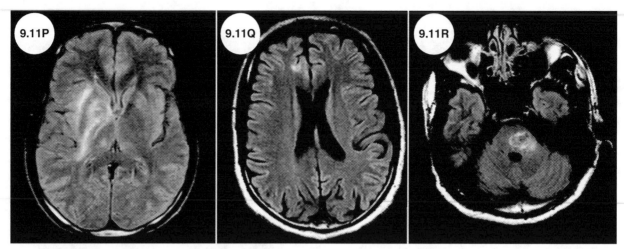

Images 9.11P–9.11R: Axial FLAIR images demonstrate marked decline in edema and mass effect.

References

1. Saadatnia G, Golkar M. A review on human toxoplasmosis. *Scand J Infect Dis*. November 2012;44(11):805–814.
2. Masamed R, Meleis A, Lee EW, Hathout GM. Cerebral toxoplasmosis: case review and description of a new imaging sign. *Clin Radiol*. May 2009;64(5):560–563.
3. Ramsey RG, Gean AD. Neuroimaging of AIDS. I. Central nervous system toxoplasmosis. *Neuroimaging Clin N Am*. May 1997;7(2):171–186.
4. Offiah CE, Turnbull IW. The imaging appearances of intracranial CNS infections in adult HIV and AIDS patients. *Clin Radiol*. May 2006;61(5):393–401.

9.12 | Aspergillosis

Case History

A 45-year-old man with untreated HIV infection presented after a seizure. His friend reported 4 weeks of cognitive slowing and generalized malaise.

Diagnosis: Aspergillosis

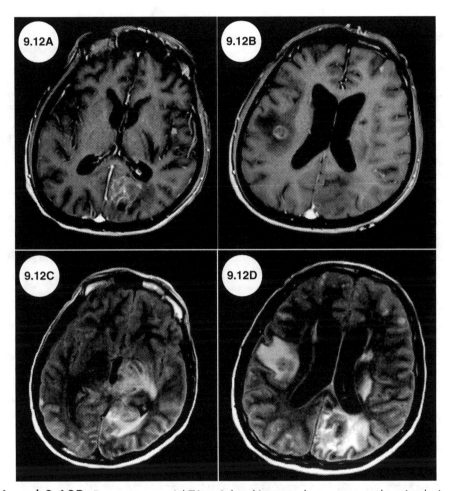

Images 9.12A and 9.12B: Postcontrast axial T1-weighted images demonstrate enhancing lesions (red arrows) in the left occipital and right frontal lobes. **Images 9.12C and 9.12D:** Axial FLAIR images demonstrate significant edema associated with the lesions.

Introduction

■ Aspergillosis is an infection caused by *Aspergillus*, a ubiquitous fungus. CNS infection can cause a necrotizing vasculitis, which presents with hemorrhagic abscesses in the ependymal region.

Clinical Presentation

■ It most commonly presents with pulmonary symptoms, such as cough or dyspnea. In the CNS, the most common features are cognitive changes, focal neurological deficits, and seizures.

The symptom onset is usually dramatic and rapidly progressive. Affected patients are typically immunocompromised.

Radiographic Appearance and Diagnosis

▪ Lesions are commonly seen in the cerebral hemispheres, thalami, basal ganglia, and corpus callosum. The lesions are hypointense on T2-weighted images, although there may be hyperintense edema surrounding the lesions. There is frequently minimal or no contrast enhancement or edema, due to the immunosuppressed status of the patient. Enhancement is more prominent in immunocompetent patients and is often ring-shaped.

▪ Hemorrhage is seen in about 25% to 50% of patients, and this is best visualized on CT scans.

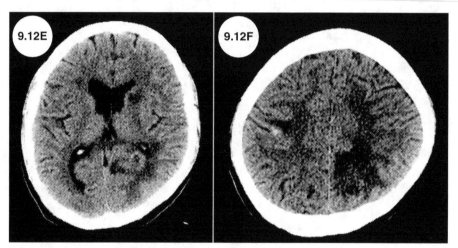

Images 9.12E and 9.12F: Axial CT scans demonstrate small areas of hemorrhage (red arrows) in hypodense lesions.

▪ It can also cause a necrotizing vasculitis, which can lead to subsequent infarction.

▪ The distinction between this fungal infection and metastatic disease may be difficult, but the combination of punctate calcification and ring-enhancing lesions favors infections.

▪ The diagnosis is confirmed via a biopsy, showing the characteristic *Aspergillus* hyphae branching at a 45 degree angle. As many patients with suspected aspergillosis are too ill to tolerate such an invasive procedure, detecting *Aspergillus* via PCR in the CSF is highly suggestive.

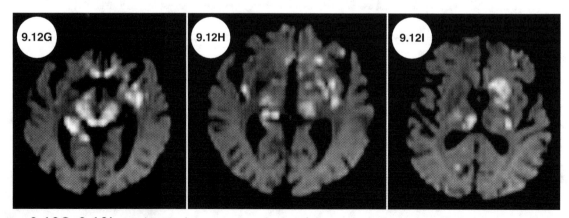

Images 9.12G–9.12I: Axial DWIs demonstrate multiple infarctions in the brainstem, thalami, and basal ganglia bilaterally in a patient with aspergillosis.

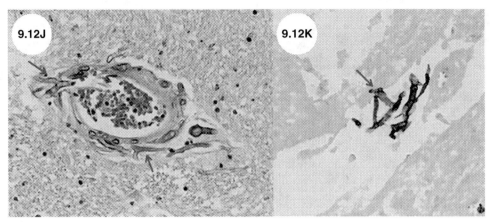

Image 9.12J: Luxol fast blue hematoxylin and eosin (H&E) stain shows *Aspergillus* hyphae invading a blood vessel wall (red arrows). **Image 9.12K:** Grocott methenamine silver stain demonstrates the characteristic branching at a 45 degree angle.

Treatment

▦ Voriconazole is more effective than amphotericin B in the treatment of invasive aspergillosis, though only about 35% of patients respond. Without treatment, the mortality rate is near 100%.

References

1. DeLone DR, Goldstein RA, Petermann G, et al. Disseminated aspergillosis involving the brain: distribution and imaging characteristics. *AJNR Am J Neuroradiol.* October 1999;20(9):1597–1604.
2. Yamada K, Shrier DA, Rubio A, et al. Imaging findings in intracranial aspergillosis. *Acad Radiol.* February 2002;9(2): 163–1671.
3. Ruhnke M, Kofla G, Otto K, Schwartz S. CNS aspergillosis: recognition, diagnosis and management. *CNS Drugs.* 2007;21(8):659–676.
4. Reinwald M, Buchheidt D, Hummel M, et al. Diagnostic performance of an Aspergillus-specific nested PCR assay in cerebrospinal fluid samples of immunocompromised patients for detection of central nervous system aspergillosis. *PLoS One.* 2013;8(2):e56706.

9.13 | Creutzfeldt–Jakob Disease

Case History

A 65-year-old man presented with rapid-onset dementia. On exam, he knew his name, but not his age or the location. He thought he was in his office, though he had not worked in several months. He had a profound startle response to any unexpected noise.

Diagnosis: Creutzfeldt–Jakob Disease

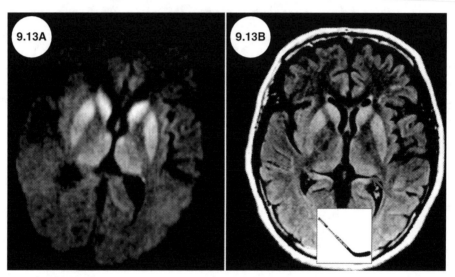

Images 9.13A and 9.13B: Diffusion-weighted and FLAIR axial images demonstrate restricted diffusion and hyperintensity in the caudate, putamen, and thalamus in a patient with CJD. The hyperintensity of the pulvinar and dorsomedial thalamic nuclei of the thalamus (red arrow) creates the "hockey stick" sign.

Introduction

■ Creutzfeldt–Jakob disease (CJD) is due to a conformational change of a prion protein that leads to a toxic gain of function. It is sporadic 90% of the time and typically occurs in patients over the age of 60. There are familial forms (fatal familial insomnia), infectious forms (mad cow disease or variant CJD), and iatrogenic forms, via infected surgical equipment or corneal transplants. Kuru is a spongiform encephalopathy formerly seen in New Guinea due to consumption of human brain tissue.

■ It is very rare, affecting only 1 in 1 million people.

Clinical Presentation

■ It presents as a rapid-onset dementia with dramatic personality changes and psychiatric symptoms usually over the course of 3 to 4 months.

It is associated with startle myoclonus, ataxia, weakness, and sensory deficits.

Diagnosis and Radiographic Appearance

■ As seen in **Images 9.13A and 9.13B**, hyperintensity on T2-weighted images of the pulvinar and dorsomedial thalamic nuclei creates the "hockey stick" sign. The "pulvinar" sign refers to bilateral hyperintensities of the pulvinar nuclei of the thalamus. Hyperintensity and diffusion restriction of the cortical ribbon are also common. This is an early sign and initially asymmetric. In more advanced disease, the white matter will be affected as well.

■ The CSF may show 14-3-3 protein, though this is not specific for CJD. The EEG may show periodic, generalized, high-amplitude sharp waves.

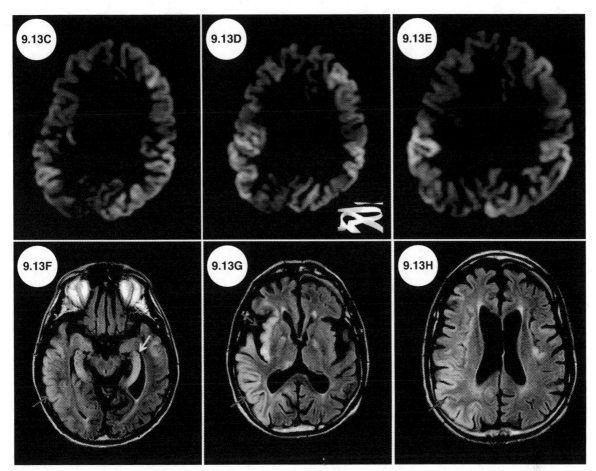

Images 9.13C–9.13E: Axial DWIs demonstrate restricted diffusion in the cortex of a patient with CJD.
Images 9.13F–9.13H: Axial FLAIR images demonstrate diffuse hyperintensity of the cortex (red arrows), mostly on the right, and bilateral hippocampi (yellow arrow).

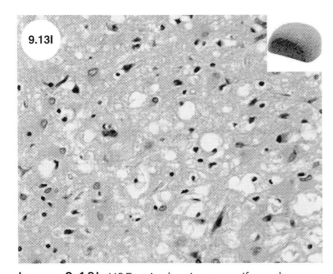

Image 9.13I: H&E stain showing spongiform changes in the cortex and loss of neurons in a case of variant CJD (image credit Sherif Zaki, MD, PhD; Wun-Ju Shieh, MD, PhD, MPH).

■ Neuronal death leads to a spongiform appearance of the brain on pathological examination.

Treatment

■ There is no treatment, and it is universally fatal within a year.

References

1. Vitali P, Maccagnano E, Geschwind MD, et al. Diffusion-weighted MRI hyperintensity patterns differentiate CJD from other rapid dementias. *Neurology.* 2011;76: 1711–1719.
2. Lee J, Hyeon JW, Kim SY, Hwang KJ, Ju YR, Ryou C. Review: Laboratory diagnosis and surveillance of Creutzfeldt-Jakob disease. *J Med Virol.* January 2015;87(1):175–186.
3. Wang LH, Bucelli RC, Patrick E, et al. Role of magnetic resonance imaging, cerebrospinal fluid, and electroencephalogram in diagnosis of sporadic Creutzfeldt-Jakob disease. *J Neurol.* February 2013;260(2):498–506.

CHAPTER 10

NEURODEGENERATIVE DISEASES

10.1　Alzheimer's Disease

Case History

A 72-year-old woman was brought in by her family. The patient herself said that she felt well, but her family said that she had been "forgetting everything" recently. For example, she would purchase the same products at the grocery store, forgetting that she had bought them only several days earlier. She had also become paranoid, feeling that someone was moving her glasses and wallet. She had no awareness of her deficits.

Diagnosis: Alzheimer's Disease

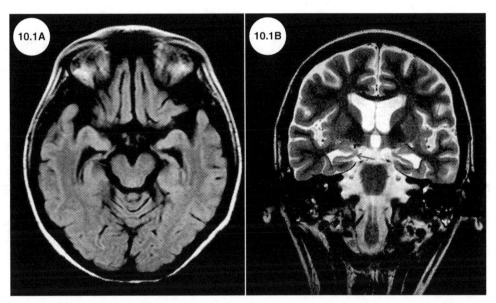

Images 10.1A and 10.1B: Axial fluid-attenuated inversion recovery (FLAIR) and coronal T2-weighted images demonstrate severe atrophy of the hippocampi (red arrow) with compensatory dilatation of the temporal horns of the lateral ventricles.

Introduction

- Alzheimer's disease (AD) is the most common type of dementia, accounting for about 66% of cases. The incidence and prevalence increase with age, and most individuals are diagnosed when they are over 60 years old. AD is slightly more common in women than in men, with a relative risk of 1.5.

- While 75% of cases have no clear etiology, approximately 25% are clearly familial, with two or more family members affected. In addition to specific genes, an association has been found with the apolipoprotein E epsilon 4 (ApoE e4) genotype, which mediates neuronal cholesterol transport.

Clinical Presentation

- There are four stages of the disease: predementia, early, moderate, and advanced. In predementia, patients have difficulty with short-term memory, but functioning is not impaired. In early dementia, symptom progression interferes with some level of functioning, but patients remain mostly independent. In moderate disease, patients are unable to perform most routine activities of daily living. In the advanced stage, patients are entirely dependent on caregivers for even their most basic needs.

- Patients are often brought in by caretakers or family members with complaints of memory loss or loss of daily function. The hallmark of AD is impairment of declarative memory (memory for facts and events), which relies on medial temporal structures. More specifically, episodic memory (remembrance of events and contexts) is impaired, while semantic memory (vocabulary and concepts) is preserved until later in the disease course.

- Language and visuospatial skills tend to be affected earlier than executive function and behavior in AD. Procedural memory and motor skills, which rely on the subcortical system, are spared until the late stages. Reduced verbal fluency, including word-finding difficulty, reduced vocabulary, circumlocution and anomia on confrontation, are typically found at presentation in patients with AD. This progresses to reduced spontaneous speech, agrammatism, paraphasic errors, and ultimately impaired comprehension. Repetition is typically maintained until late in the disease course. Visuospatial impairment, such as misplacing items and difficulty navigating in unfamiliar or familiar territory, is often the presenting symptom of a patient with AD. Visual agnosia (inability to recognize objects) and prosopagnosia (inability to recognize faces) are late-stage phenomena.

- Impairment in executive function is often subtle during the early stages. Later in the disease, individuals have difficulty completing complex tasks and demonstrate poor judgment and planning. Behavioral and personality changes also occur late in the disease course. Patients may become disinhibited, agitated, or demonstrate frank psychosis.

- Posterior cortical atrophy (Benson's syndrome) is a variant of AD in which patients present with progressive impairment of visuospatial and visuoperceptual capabilities. Initially, patients may only complain of blurred vision or difficulty reading. Eventually, patients develop apraxia, alexia, inability to recognize objects and faces (prosopagnosia), difficulty processing complex visual scenes (simultanagnosia), and trouble navigating through space. Eventually, patients develop symptoms of typical AD. Depression and anxiety are common as well. The disease tends to present at an earlier age (50–60 years).

Radiographic Appearance and Diagnosis

- The diagnosis of AD is primarily a clinical one. Most clinicians use a bedside mental status exam to screen for the presence of dementia. The Montreal Cognitive Assessment is the most sensitive bedside test. It assesses multiple cognitive domains including short-term memory recall, visuospatial abilities, multiple aspects of executive functions, language ability, orientation to time and place, concentration, and working memory. It is important to screen for reversible causes of dementia, which occur in a small minority of cases.

- As seen in **Images 10.1A and 10.1B**, the hallmark of AD on MRI is atrophy of the hippocampus, entorhinal cortex, and temporoparietal lobes. In later stages of the disease, there is global cortical atrophy, and compensatory dilatation of the ventricles may be apparent.

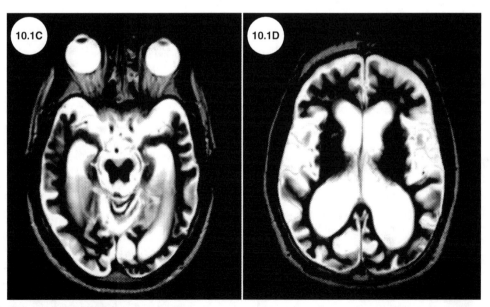

Images 10.1C and 10.1D: Axial T2-weighted images demonstrate severe, generalized cortical atrophy with compensatory dilatation of the ventricular system in a patient with advanced AD.

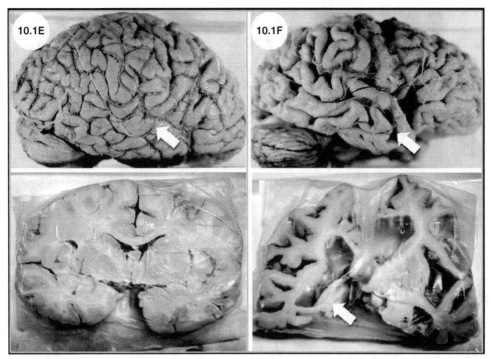

Images 10.1E and 10.1F: Gross specimens of a normal brain (10.1E) and a patient with Alzheimer's disease (10.1F) demonstrate diffuse atrophy, hydrocephalus ex vacuo, and atrophy of the hippocampus (white arrows).

Source: Soto-Rojas LO, de la Cruz-López F, Torres MAO, et al. (2015). Neuroinflammation and alteration of the blood-brain barrier in Alzheimer's Disease. In: Zerr I, ed. *Alzheimer's Disease - Challenges for the Future.* http://www.intechopen.com/books/ howtoreference/alzheimer-s-disease-challenges-for-the-future/neuroinflammation-and-alteration-of-the-blood-brain-barrier-in-alzheimer-s-disease.

- In posterior cortical atrophy, there is atrophy of the posterior parts of the brain out of proportion to the frontal and temporal lobes.

- PET scanning uses an injected radioactive tracer to quantify cerebral blood flow, metabolism, and receptor binding. Patients with AD have glucose hypometabolism in the temporal and parietal lobes. The degree of decreased glucose metabolism correlates with the severity of dementia.

- AD can only be confirmed on histopathology, something which is rarely done in practice. On histological examination, the characteristic

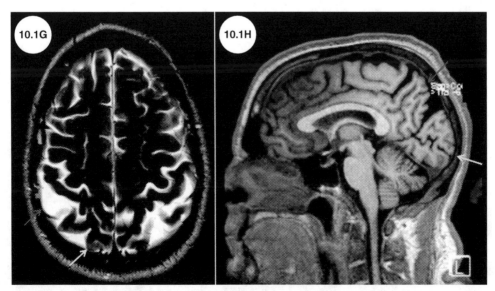

Images 10.1G and 10.1H: Axial T2-weighted and sagittal T1-weighted images demonstrate atrophy of the parietal (red arrows) and occipital lobes (yellow arrows) in a patient with posterior cortical atrophy.

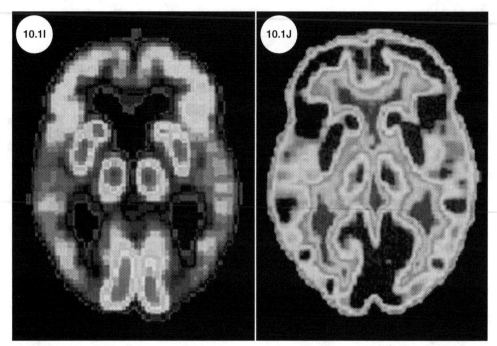

Image 10.1I: PET scan demonstrates hypometabolism of the temporal lobes. **Image 10.1J:** A normal PET scan is presented for comparison (image credit Health and Human Services Department, National Institutes of Health, National Institute on Aging).

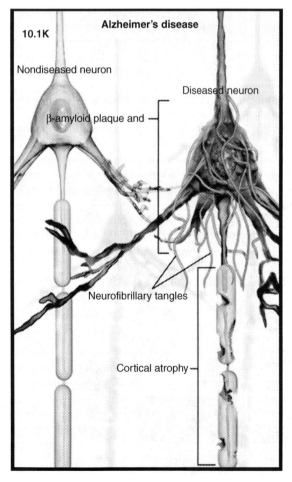

Image 10.1K: Illustration demonstrating the pathological changes in AD (image credit Bruce Blausen; https://commons. wikimedia.org/wiki/File:Blausen_0017_AlzheimersDisease.png).

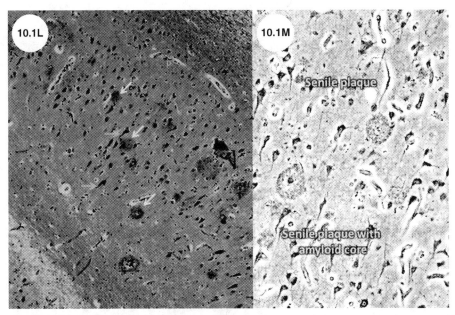

Images 10.1L and 10.1M: Bielschowsky silver stain and Golgi stain demonstrating plaques (yellow arrows) and neurofibrillary tangles (blue arrows) in a patient with AD. Image 10.1L courtesy of Dr. Seema Shroff, Fellow, Neuropathology, NYULMC.

findings are amyloid plaques and neurofibrillary tangles. Plaques are insoluble deposits of beta-amyloid peptide and cellular material outside of neurons. Neurofibrillary tangles are aggregates of hyperphosphorylated tau protein that accumulate within neurons and cause disintegration of microtubules intracellularly.

Treatment

■ There is no cure for AD. Cholinesterase inhibitors and memantine, a noncompetitive N-methyl-D-aspartate receptor (NMDA) receptor antagonist, show modest benefits in the areas of cognition, behavior, and activities of daily living in moderate–severe AD. Nonpharmacological interventions, such as those that focus on patient and caregiver safety, are often the most essential, but challenging, interventions. Management of depression and behavioral disturbances with psychotropic medications may be helpful. However, the side effects of atypical antipsychotic drugs mostly outweigh their benefits.

References

1. Trinh NH, Hoblyn J, Mohanty S, Yaffe K. Efficacy of cholinesterase inhibitors in the treatment of neuropsychiatric symptoms and functional impairment in Alzheimer disease: a meta-analysis. *JAMA.* January 2003;289(2): 210–216.
2. Braskie MN, Thompson PM. A focus on structural brain imaging in the Alzheimer's disease neuroimaging initiative. *Biol Psychiatry.* April 2014;75(7):527–533.
3. Weiner MW, Veitch DP, Aisen PS, et al. 2014 Update of the Alzheimer's Disease Neuroimaging Initiative: A review of papers published since its inception. *Alzheimers Dement.* June 2015;11(6):e1–e120.
4. Schneider LS, Tariot PN, Dagerman KS, et al. Effectiveness of atypical antipsychotic drugs in patients with Alzheimer's disease. *N Engl J Med.* October 2006;355(15):1525–1538.
5. Wang J, Yu JT, Wang HF, et al. Pharmacological treatment of neuropsychiatric symptoms in Alzheimer's disease: a systematic review and meta-analysis. *J Neurol Neurosurg Psychiatry.* January 2015;86(1):101–119.
6. Soto-Rojas LO, de la Cruz-López F, Torres MAO, et al. (2015). Neuroinflammation and alteration of the blood-brain barrier in Alzheimer´s Disease. In: Zerr I, ed. *Alzheimer's Disease - Challenges for the Future.* http://www.intechopen.com/books/howtoreference/alzheimer-s-disease-challenges-for-the-future/neuroinflammation-and-alteration-of-the-blood-brain-barrier-in-alzheimer-s-disease.

10.2 Frontotemporal Dementia

Case History

A 56-year-old man was fired from his job due to inappropriate behavior. He had started berating junior workers for mild offenses and made inappropriate sexual references with female colleagues. His appearance and personal hygiene deteriorated.

Diagnosis: Frontotemporal Dementia

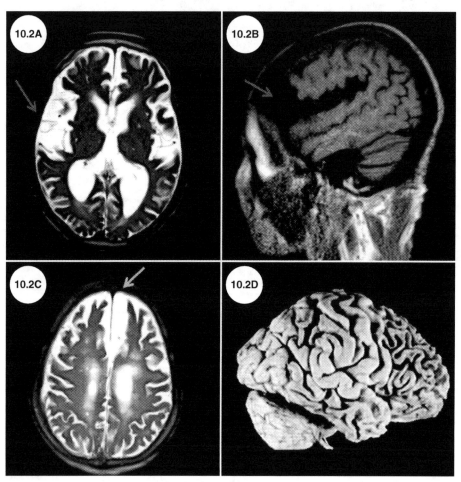

Images 10.2A–10.2C: Axial T2-weighted and sagittal T1-weighted images demonstrate significant atrophy of the frontal and temporal lobes with relative sparing of the occipital and parietal lobes. The Sylvian fissures are markedly widened (red arrows) as is the space between the frontal lobes (blue arrow). **Image 10.2D:** The findings are evident on gross pathology.

Introduction

■ Frontotemporal dementia (FTD), also known as Pick's disease, is a dementing process that targets the frontal and temporal lobes. It accounts for 3% to 16% of all dementias. The average age of onset is between 50 and 60 years, and is

therefore more prevalent than AD in individuals under 60 years.

■ About 10% are due to a genetic mutation, inherited in an autosomal-dominant pattern. Another 30% to 40% of cases have a family history significant for dementia or a psychiatric disorder, suggesting that there may be other genetic or environmental factors that influence the development of FTD.

Clinical Presentation

- There are two major subtypes of FTD: a behavioral and a language variant.

Behavioral Variant (bvFTD)

- The pathology of bvFTD begins in the orbitofrontal cortex, anterior insula, and anterior cingulate cortex before spreading to dorsolateral frontal lobe regions. Patients exhibit disinhibition, apathy, and loss of interest early in the disease course. Classic characteristics include childishness, excessive hoarding of items, inappropriate familiarity with strangers, wandering, absence of embarrassment, perseverative routines, preoccupation with promptness and time, neglect of personal hygiene, loss of interest in family, and loss of empathy/warmth for others. Patients lack insight into their disabilities.

- Some patients exhibit motor habits as well, including hand rubbing, rocking, or sniffing. They may exhibit oral dyskinesia-like movements. Unlike AD, patients perform well in visuospatial tasks and learning new information.

- The median age of survival is 6 to 8 years after onset.

Primary Progressive Aphasia (PPA)

- There are three subtypes of PPA.

Progressive Nonfluent Aphasia (PNFA)

- PNFA is associated with degeneration in the left peri-Sylvian region. Patients develop agrammatism, word-finding difficulty, and speech apraxia (difficulty with the sequencing of syllables). Speech is slow, with a telegraphic quality. The use of nouns is relatively preserved, but use of tense and prepositions is often incorrect. Patients also make phonemic errors, such as saying "lair" instead of "chair." Patients are aware of their errors, and make many attempts to correct their speech.

- Comprehension is intact, even at the later stages of the disease when patients can no longer speak. Similarly, spatial skills and episodic memory are relatively preserved.

- Median duration of survival after onset is 11 to 12 years.

Semantic Variant (SV)

- SV is characterized by bilateral, asymmetric anterior temporal lobe atrophy. This area is responsible for integration of visual, auditory, verbal, and somatosensory information. On the right, it is specialized for visual stimuli, whereas the left is specialized for verbal stimuli. The presentation differs based on which side is predominantly involved.

- In right-sided atrophy, patients present with the inability to recognize well-known faces (prosopagnosia). They can demonstrate a loss of empathy and disinhibition, and this can be difficult to distinguish from bvFTD.

- In left-sided atrophy, patients present with a fluent-type aphasia. They lose the ability to recognize the meaning of words, but have intact fluency, articulation, phonation, and syntax. Naming becomes progressively more impaired, so that patients may initially be able to place "golden retriever" as "dog," then only as "animal," and finally only as "thing."

- Individuals are aware of their deficits and may present independently for evaluation.

- The median duration of survival after onset is 8 to 12 years.

Logopenic Progressive Aphasia (LPA)

- Similar to PNFA, speech is often slow and halting in LPA. Fluency and articulation of the words are maintained, however, and the halting nature of speech is derived solely from extreme word-finding difficulty.

- A number of other disorders may overlap with FTD, including amyotrophic lateral sclerosis (ALS), corticobasal degeneration (CBD), and progressive supranuclear palsy (PSP).

Radiographic Appearance and Diagnosis

- There is no diagnostic test that firmly establishes the diagnosis. MRI is the most sensitive imaging modality in the evaluation of a patient with suspected FTD, though it may be normal early in the disease course.

- bvFTD is associated with focal atrophy in bilateral frontal lobes and anterior temporal lobes. PNFA is associated with atrophy in the left inferior frontal, insular, and peri-Sylvian regions. SV is associated with atrophy in the left anterior temporal region, which later spreads to the amygdala, hippocampus, and right anterior temporal regions.

- Single photon emission computed tomography (SPECT) scanning may demonstrate hypoperfusion in the frontal and temporal lobes, while PET imaging will show hypometabolism in the same areas with or without involvement of the basal ganglia.

- Laboratory evaluations and a psychiatric assessment are important to rule out reversible causes of dementia that may mimic FTD.

Treatment

- Treatment is directed at controlling symptoms. Selective serotonin reuptake inhibitors may be useful in decreasing disinhibited behavior, overeating, and repetitive behavior. Low-dose trazodone or an atypical antipsychotic may be helpful in diminishing agitation and disinhibition. Patients with FTD are often exquisitely sensitive to the motor side effects of antipsychotics, however, and display high rates of parkinsonian symptoms.

References

1. Pressman PS, Miller BL. Diagnosis and management of behavioral variant frontotemporal dementia. *Biol Psychiatry*. April 2014;75(7):574–581.
2. Bott NT, Radke A, Stephens ML, Kramer JH. Frontotemporal dementia: diagnosis, deficits and management. *Neurodegener Dis Manag*. 2014;4(6):439–454.
3. Cardarelli R, Kertesz A, Knebl JA. Frontotemporal dementia: a review for primary care physicians. *Am Fam Physician*. December 2010;82(11):1372–1377.

10.3 | Huntington's Disease

Case History

A 56-year-old man presented with chorea and irritability. His mother died at 62 from a similar illness.

Diagnosis: Huntington's Disease

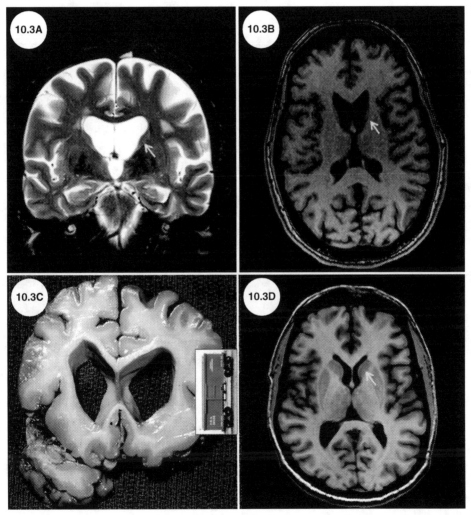

Images 10.3A and 10.3B: Coronal T2-weighted and axial T-weighted images demonstrate atrophy of the head of the caudate (yellow arrows). **Image 10.3C:** Gross specimen demonstrates the same findings, creating the appearance of "boxcar ventricles." **Image 10.3D:** Normal MRI for comparison showing the head of the caudate indenting the frontal horn of the lateral ventricle (yellow arrow).

Introduction

■ Huntington's disease (HD) is the most common inherited form of chorea. It is a trinucleotide repeat disorder of the DNA base sequence CAG on chromosome 4 with an autosomal-dominant inheritance pattern. It shows anticipation, meaning that it presents earlier in successive generations. Patients with less than 35 repeats will not have symptoms, while patients with 35 to 40 repeats may have some symptoms. Patients with over 40 repeats will always develop the disease. For unclear reasons, patients who inherit the disease from their fathers develop symptoms earlier.

■ It occurs in 5 to 10 per 100,000 persons.

Clinical Presentation

■ HD is marked by psychosis and choreiform movements that develop around age 40. Patients with symptoms prior to this have a higher number of CAG repeats. Patients initially develop facial twitching and grimacing, finger twitching, and a slight turning of the trunk that may initially be confused with simple restlessness. Over time, these movement abnormalities evolve into overt choreiform movements. Patients develop motor impersistence, such as an inability to keep the tongue protruded (serpentine tongue) or to maintain a tight handgrip (milkmaid grip). Other findings include dystonia, bulbar dysfunction (dysarthria and dysphagia), myoclonus, ataxia, and postural instability.

■ Patients also develop cognitive dysfunction marked by poor concentration and memory with preservation of language. Patients are often aware of this decline, and depression, not infrequently leading to suicide, is common in HD. In later stages, patients may develop delusions and become frankly psychotic.

■ The Westphal variant occurs in about 5% of patients. It occurs in patients younger than 20 and is marked by seizures in addition to dementia, ataxia, and parkinsonism.

Radiographic Appearance and Diagnosis

■ On imaging, atrophy of the caudate nucleus leads to enlargement of the frontal horns of the lateral ventricles, creating "boxcar ventricles." This can be quantified by measuring the frontal horn width *and intercaudate distance*. There may also be atrophy of the putamen and global cortical atrophy.

■ The diagnosis is confirmed through genetic testing. Given the implications for family members, this should only be done with appropriate genetic counseling.

Treatment

■ There is no direct treatment, and patients experience a relentless deterioration leading to death after about 15 years. Younger patients have a more rapid course.

■ High potency, typical antipsychotics or the dopamine-depleting agent tetrabenazine are useful in the treatment of disabling chorea. Treatment of depression and protection against suicide are key facets of managing the disease.

References

1. Kumar A, Kumar Singh S, Kumar V, Kumar D, Agarwal S, Rana MK. Huntington's disease: an update of therapeutic strategies. *Gene*. February 2015;556(2):91–97.
2. Ha AD, Fung VS. Huntington's disease. *Curr Opin Neurol*. 2012 Aug;25(4):491–498.
3. Kim SD, Fung VS. An update on Huntington's disease: from the gene to the clinic. *Curr Opin Neurol*. August 2014;27(4):477–483.

10.4 | Parkinson's Disease

Case History

A 74-year-old man developed tremors and stiffness of his left arm. On examination he had a resting tremor and cogwheel rigidity in his left arm, a shuffling gait, and a decreased blink rate.

Diagnosis: Parkinson's Disease

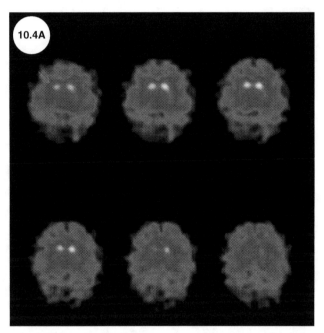

Image 10.4A: DaTscan reveals decreased tracer localization in the right middle and posterior putamen in a patient with Parkinson's disease. The normal side is shaped like a comma; the abnormal side is like a period.

Introduction

■ Parkinson's disease (PD) affects over 1 million patients in the United States. It affects 1% of the population over the age of 55, though disease onset can occur as young as 35. The vast majority of the cases are sporadic, but about 5% are inherited.

■ Pathologically, PD is due to the idiopathic degeneration of dopamine-producing neurons in the substantia nigra pars compacta. Patients do not become symptomatic until 60% to 80% of neurons are lost. There is also loss of neurons in other central nervous system (CNS) areas, and even in the peripheral nervous system (**Illustration 10.4.1**).

Clinical Presentation

■ The four core motor symptoms are tremor, rigidity, bradykinesia, and postural instability/gait abnormalities. Symptoms are unilateral at onset

---

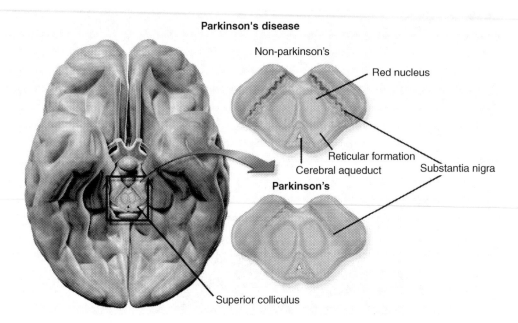

Illustration 10.4.1: An illustration of the pathology of Parkinson's disease.

Source: Blausen gallery 2014. *Wikiversity Journal of Medicine.* 2014. doi:10.15347/wjm/2014.010. ISSN 20018762.

but typically spread to the contralateral side as the disease progresses.

■ Nonmotor symptoms include autonomic dysfunction, sleep disorders (such as REM behavior sleep disorder), sensory abnormalities (such as anosmia), and neuropsychiatric symptoms. Depression is most common, but psychosis, slowness of thought (bradyphrenia), and frank dementia may also be present. Some of the nonmotor features of PD can precede the onset of motor symptoms by many decades.

Radiographic Appearance and Diagnosis

■ PD is a clinical diagnosis made when patients have bradykinesia and one of the other core motor features—tremor, rigidity, or postural instability—for which there is no other cause.

■ Adjunctive tests may be used to help support a diagnosis of PD in unclear cases. DaTscans involve an intravenous (IV) injection of ioflupane iodine-123 and detection of its uptake by dopamine transporters on SPECT imaging. In patients with PD, there is decreased uptake of contrast in the basal ganglia due to depletion of dopamine.

■ In patients who display classic features of PD and are responding well to treatment, there is no need to pursue a DaTscan. DaTscans cannot

distinguish PD from other disorders with parkinsonism, such as multiple system atrophy (MSA), PSP, or CBD.

■ On pathological examination, loss of pigmentation in the substantia nigra is evident.

■ Affected neurons exhibit Lewy bodies, which are intracytoplasmic inclusions composed of alpha-synuclein and ubiquitin. Lewy neuritis are aggregates of alpha-synuclein found in diseased axons.

■ A wide variety of other neurodegenerative disorders, medications, or toxins may mimic idiopathic PD. Clues that a patient may be suffering from a disease other than idiopathic PD include:

     Restriction of vertical gaze

     Onset of illness before the age of 40

     Symmetrical symptom onset

     Significant autonomic dysfunction

     Lack of response to medications used to treat PD

     Rapid progression of disability including early-onset dementia and prominent falls

     Facial dystonia from levadopa

     Upper and/or lower motor neuron signs

     Obstructive sleep apnea/excessive snoring

     Inspiratory stridor during daytime or sleep (laryngeal dystonia)

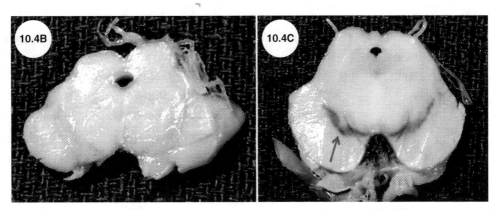

Image 10.4B: Gross image of substantia nigra in Parkinson's disease. **Image 10.4C:** Gross image of normal substantia nigra (red arrow) (image courtesy of Roberta J. Seidman, MD).

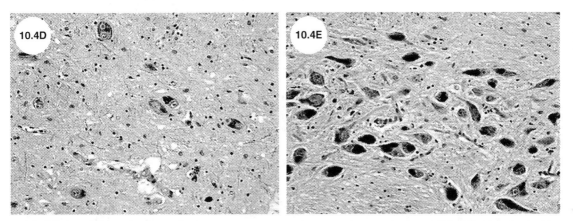

Image 10.4D: Histological image of substantia nigra in Parkinson's disease. **Image 10.4E:** Histological image of normal substantia nigra.

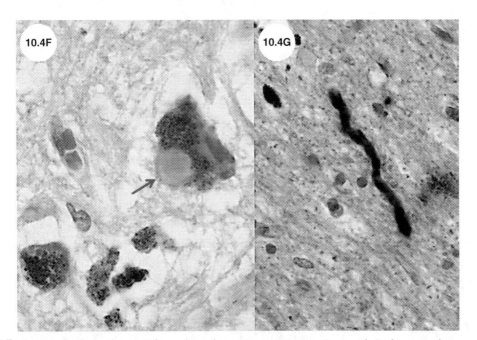

Image 10.4F: A Lewy body (red arrow) from the substantia nigra in a patient with Parkinson's disease.
Image 10.4G: Alpha-synuclein-positive Lewy neurite.

Source: Werner CJ, Heyny-von Haussen R, Mall G, Wolf S. Proteome analysis of human substantia nigra in Parkinson's disease. *Proteome Sci.* 2008;6, 8. doi:10.1186/1477-5956-6-8.

- Jerky action tremor
- Flexed neck
- Axial postural abnormalities (camptocormia, Pisa syndrome)
- Cold, dusky hands and feet
- Contractures of hands or feet
- Severe dysphonia, dysarthria, or dysphagia
- Emotional incontinence
- Wide-based gait

Treatment

- There is no treatment to alter the course of PD, though a wide range of symptomatic treatments exists. Medications should be introduced when the symptoms begin to interfere with a patient's life. These medications include:

1. Presynaptic dopamine replacement therapy with levodopa
2. Dopamine agonists that bind directly to the postsynaptic receptors
3. Catechol-*O*-methyltransferase (COMT) inhibitors that inhibit the enzymatic breakdown of dopamine at the presynaptic terminal

- The most common surgery for PD is currently deep brain stimulation (DBS). An electrode placed in the brain is connected to a generator that delivers electrical stimulation, which can be adjusted externally. The subthalamic nucleus is

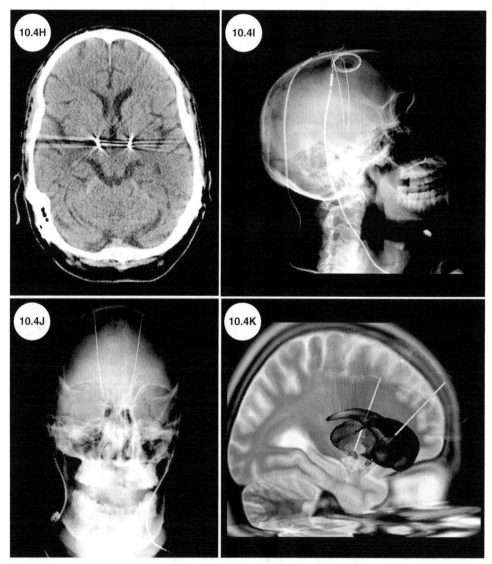

Images 10.4H–10.4J: Axial CT and lateral skull and anteroposterior radiographs demonstrate bilateral electrode placement terminating in the subthalamic nuclei. **Image 10.4K:** Illustration demonstrating electrode placement in the subthalamic nuclei (image credit Andreashorn; https://en.wikipedia.org/wiki/Deep_brain_stimulation#/media/File:Deep_brain_stimulation_electrode_placement_reconstruction.png).

the most common target, but the globus pallidus interna is also a target.

■ The best candidates for DBS are those who have a clear diagnosis of idiopathic PD and an obvious response to levodopa but have significant fluctuations in response to medications or drug-induced dyskinesias. These fluctuations and dyskinesias respond most dramatically to DBS, and as a rule, a patient's best response to medication preoperatively is what can be expected postoperatively. Patients with DBS are often able to lower their doses of medications. Symptoms such as postural instability, hypophonia, micrographia, and nonmotor symptoms will not be improved by DBS. Contraindications to DBS include significant cognitive impairment or psychiatric illness.

■ Nonmotor symptoms such as depression, constipation, and hypotension should be asked about at clinical visits and treated with available medications.

References

1. Beitz JM. Parkinson's disease: a review. *Front Biosci (Schol Ed)*. January 2014;6:65–74.
2. Klockgether T. Parkinson's disease: clinical aspects. *Cell Tissue Res*. October 2004;318(1):115–120.
3. Varrone A, Halldin C. New developments of dopaminergic imaging in Parkinson's disease. *Q J Nucl Med Mol Imaging*. February 2012;56(1):68–82.
4. Lyons KE, Pahwa R. Diagnosis and initiation of treatment in Parkinson's disease. *Int J Neurosci*. 2011;121(Suppl. 2):27–36.
5. Blausen gallery 2014. *Wikiversity Journal of Medicine*. 2014. doi:10.15347/wjm/2014.010. ISSN 20018762.
6. Werner CJ, Heyny-von Haussen R, Mall G, Wolf S. Proteome analysis of human substantia nigra in Parkinson's disease. *Proteome Sci*. 2008;6, 8. doi:10.1186/1477-5956-6-8.

10.5 Multiple System Atrophy

Case History

A 54-year-old male presented with falls, dizziness, lightheadedness, and increasing speech difficulties for the past 4 years. He had been wheelchair-bound for the past 6 months. On examination, he was found to have anterocollis, dysarthria, orthostatic hypotension, and ataxia. He was started on Sinemet without any clinical improvement.

Diagnosis: Multiple System Atrophy

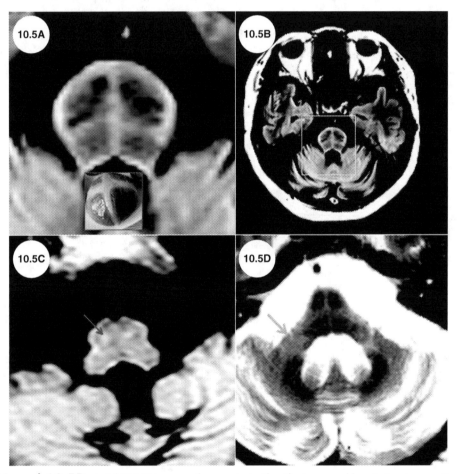

Images 10.5A and 10.5B: Axial FLAIR images demonstrate the "hot crossed bun" sign in a patient with MSA.
Image 10.5C: Axial FLAIR image demonstrates a hyperintense signal (red arrow) due to atrophy of the inferior olive.
Image 10.5D: Axial T2-weighted image demonstrates hyperintensity and atrophy of the middle cerebellar peduncles (blue arrow).

Introduction

- Multiple system atrophy (MSA) is a sporadic, neurodegenerative synucleinopathy. It is a rare disorder with a prevalence of 2 to 4 per 100,000 population.

- Patients typically present between the ages of 50 and 60, and it is more common in males than females.

- A number of structures are degraded in patients with MSA. These include:

- Basal ganglia (striatum)
- Substantia nigra
- Locus coeruleus
- Pontine nuclei
- Dorsal vagal nuclei
- Purkinje cells of the cerebellum
- Inferior olives

■ In PD there is dopamine depletion, but dopamine receptors remain the same; in MSA, there is depletion of both dopamine and dopamine receptors.

Clinical Presentation

■ MSA can be characterized by parkinsonism as well as cerebellar dysfunction, autonomic dysfunction, and corticospinal tract dysfunction. Patients present with certain features more than others, leading to the division of MSA into cerebellar type (MSA-C) and parkinsonian type (MSA-P), depending on which feature predominates initially. This distinction fades as the disease progresses and patients develop features of all types (**Table 10.5.1**).

Table 10.5.1 Clinical Characteristics of Various Subtypes of MSA

MSA	Clinical Features
MSA-P	Muscle rigidity, shuffling gait, akinesia, resting tremors
MSA-C	Wide-based gait, intention tremors, ataxia, nystagmus, scanning speech
MSA-P and C	Orthostatic hypotension, supine hypertension, reduced ability to sweat, bladder dysfunction, erectile dysfunction, impotence, constipation

■ Other MSA symptoms are anterocollis, dysarthria or dysarthrophonia, laryngeal stridor, sleep apnea or REM *sleep* behavior disorder, rigidity, and bradykinesia. In contrast to PD in which tremor often predominates, in MSA, rigidity and bradykinesia are more prominent than tremor. Other distinguishing features between PD and MSA are listed in **Table 10.5.2**.

Radiographic Appearance and Diagnosis

■ A characteristic radiographic feature of MSA-C is the "hot crossed bun" sign seen in the pons

Table 10.5.2 Characteristics of PD and MSA

Characteristics	PD	MSA
Axial rigidity	++	++
Limb dystonia	+	+
Postural instability	++	++
Rest tremors	++	--
Symmetry of deficits	+	+++
Vertical gaze palsy	+	++
Dysautonomia	+	++
Frontal behavior	+	+

on T2-weighted images. This sign is due to a selective loss of myelinated transverse pontocerebellar fibers and neurons in the pontine raphe with preservation of the pontine tegmentum and corticospinal tracts. Hyperintensity on T2-weighted images is often seen in the inferior olives and middle cerebellar peduncles. These areas are atrophied as well. A linear rim of hyperintensity surrounding the putamen on T2-weighted images, the "putaminal rim" sign, is common in MSA-P, signifying atrophy of the putamen.

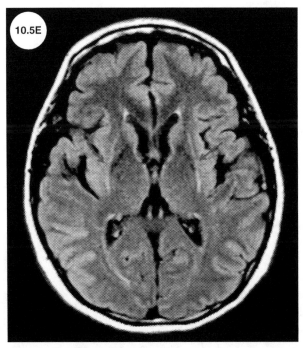

Image 10.5E: Axial FLAIR image demonstrates the "putaminal rim" sign (red arrow) in a patient with MSA.

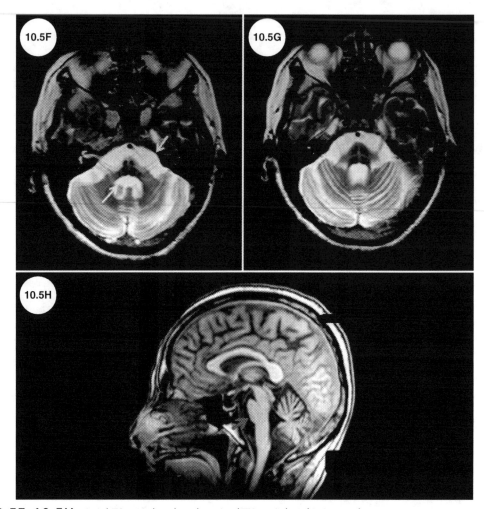

Images 10.5F–10.5H: Axial T2-weighted and sagittal T1-weighted images demonstrate severe atrophy of the pons (red arrow) and cerebellum, with a widened fourth ventricle (yellow arrow), and an enlarged cerebellopontine angle (green arrow) in a patient with MSA-C.

- In MSA-C, imaging may be normal early in the disease; there will eventually be diffuse atrophy of the brainstem and cerebellum. The pons is typically flattened, and the fourth ventricle and cerebellopontine angle are enlarged.

- Pathologically, there is altered function and accumulation of p25α within oligodendroglia and reduction of myelin basic protein (MBP) and deposition of degraded MBP in the affected cell body. The histological core feature of MSA are glial cytoplasmic inclusions (GCIs, Papp-Lantos bodies) in all types of oligodendroglia that contain aggregates of misfolded α-Synuclein (α-Syn).

Treatment

- There is no specific treatment for MSA. Supportive treatments are listed in **Table 10.5.3**.

Table 10.5.3 Supportive Treatment for Various Subtypes of MSA

MSA	Treatment
MSA-P	Levodopa, Comtan, amantadine, physical and occupational therapy, speech therapy
MSA-C	Physical and occupational therapy
MSA-A	Fluid intake, sodium, pressure stockings, midodrine, fludrocortisone, oxybutynin, tolterodine, sildenafil (Viagra), vardenafil (Levitra), tadalafil (Cialis), avanafil (Stendra)

References

1. Matsusue E, Fujii S, Kanasaki Y, Sugihara S, Miyata H, Ohama E, Ogawa T. Putaminal lesion in multiple system atrophy: postmortem MR-pathological correlations. *Neuroradiology.* July 2008;50(7):559–567.

2. Wenning GK, Colosimo C, Geser F, Poewe W. Multiple system atrophy. *Lancet Neurol*. February 2004;3(2):93–103.

3. Köllensperger M, Geser F, Ndayisaba JP, et al. Presentation, diagnosis, and management of multiple system atrophy in Europe: final analysis of the European multiple system atrophy registry. *Mov Disord*. November 2010;25(15): 2604–2612.

4. Deguchi K, Ikeda K, Kume K, et al. Significance of the hot-cross bun sign on T2*-weighted MRI for the diagnosis of multiple system atrophy. *J Neurol*. June 2015;262(6):1433–1439.

5. Gilman S, Wenning GK, Low PA, Brooks DJ, Mathias CJ, Trojanowski JQ. Second consensus statement on the diagnosis of multiple system atrophy. *Neurology*. August 2008;71(9): 670–676.

6. Geser F, Wenning GK, Seppi K. Progression of multiple system atrophy (MSA): a prospective natural history study by the European MSA Study Group (EMSA SG). *Mov Disord*. February 2006;21(2):179–186.

7. Robertson D, Biaggioni I, Burnstock G, Low PA, Paton JFR. *Primer on the Autonomic Nervous System*. San Diego, CA: Elsevier; 2012:1–702.

8. Ubhi K, Low P, Masliah E. Multiple system atrophy: a clinical and neuropathological perspective. *Trends Neurosci*. November 2011;34(11):581–590.

10.6 | Progressive Supranuclear Palsy

Case History

A 67-year-old man developed rigidity and impaired vertical eye movements. His wife reported that he had suffered several significant falls in the past few months.

Diagnosis: Progressive Supranuclear Palsy

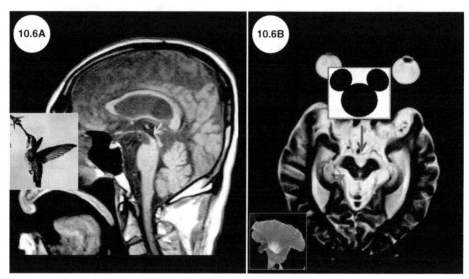

Image 10.6A: Postcontrast sagittal T1-weighted image demonstrates atrophy of the midbrain (yellow arrow), creating the "hummingbird" sign. **Image 10.6B:** Axial T2-weighted image demonstrates an increased space between the cerebral peduncles (red arrow), creating the "Mickey Mouse" sign, as well as a concavity of the lateral margins of the tegmentum (pink arrow) known as the "morning glory" sign.

Introduction

■ Progressive supranuclear palsy (PSP) is an idiopathic, sporadic, neurodegenerative disorder of the brainstem and basal ganglia that affects patients between the ages of 50 and 70 years. It is one of the most common causes of idiopathic parkinsonism, aside from PD itself. There is significant neuronal loss in the subthalamic nucleus, substantia nigra, globus pallidus, nucleus basalis of Meynert, superior colliculi, and locus coeruleus.

Clinical Presentation

■ The hallmarks of the disease are:

1. **Supranuclear vertical gaze palsy:** Damage to the vertical gaze centers in the midbrain impairs vertical eye movements. The palsy can be overcome by the Doll's eye maneuver in the vertical direction.

2. **Imbalance:** Backward falls are common and are often the presenting symptom of the disease.

3. **Parkinsonism:** Early in the course of the disease, it can be mistaken for PD due to the rigidity and bradykinesia. However, the symmetrical onset of symptoms, lack of tremor, vertical gaze palsy, and very minimal response to dopaminergic agents help distinguish PSP from PD.

4. **Behavioral changes:** Patients often suffer from dementia, depression, apathy, pseudobulbar palsy, and personality changes.

5. **Additional features:** Patients have a wide-eyed stare, referred to as a "reptilian stare" due to impaired control of eyelid movements. Patients often have eyebrow/forehead wrinkling, known as the "procerus sign." The "applause sign" is so named as patients instructed to clap three times will often be unable to stop clapping and will clap several times more. Patients often have hypophonia and dysphagia.

Radiographic Appearance and Diagnosis

■ The diagnosis is a clinical one as there are no specific diagnostic tests. On MRI, there is atrophy of the midbrain tegmentum with general sparing of the tectum and cerebral peduncles. This leads to an increased angle between the two cerebral peduncles in patients with PSP and is called the "Mickey Mouse" sign on axial MRI. On sagittal MRI, the ratio of the midbrain to pons area is significantly reduced and this measurement is the most sensitive imaging measure of PSP. The appearance of the atrophied midbrain on sagittal MRI is called the "hummingbird" sign. It is seen in about 75% of patients. Concavity of the lateral margins of the tegmentum of the midbrain is termed the "morning glory" sign due to its resemblance to this flower.

Treatment

■ There is no direct treatment; however, there may be a small and temporary response to dopaminergic treatment. The life expectancy is 5 to 7 years after diagnosis.

References

1. Massey LA, Jäger HR, Paviour DC, et al. The midbrain to pons ratio: a simple and specific MRI sign of progressive supranuclear palsy. *Neurology.* May 2013;80(20):1856–1861.
2. Adachi M, Kawanami T, Ohshima H, Sugai Y, Hosoya T. Morning glory sign: a particular MR finding in progressive supranuclear palsy. *Magn Reson Med Sci.* December 2004;3(3):125–132.
3. Lubarsky M, Juncos JL. Progressive supranuclear palsy: a current review. *Neurologist.* March 2008;14(2):79–88.
4. Oba H, Yagishita A, Terada H, et al. New and reliable MRI diagnosis for progressive supranuclear palsy. *Neurology.* June 2005;64(12):2050–2055.

10.7 | Corticobasal Degeneration

Case History

A 59-year-old woman presented with several falls. On examination, she had asymmetric rigidity with a shuffling gait. She also developed uncontrolled movements of her left arm.

Diagnosis: Corticobasal Degeneration

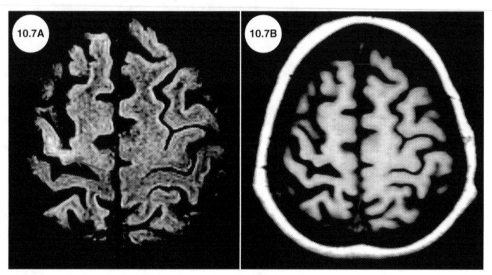

Images 10.7A and 10.7B: Axial FLAIR and T1-weighted images demonstrate hyperintensity (red arrow) and atrophy of the precentral gyrus and superior parietal lobule on the right.

Introduction

- Corticobasal degeneration (CBD) is a rare, sporadic, neurodegenerative disease characterized by progressive degeneration of the cerebral cortex and the basal ganglia. It is a tauopathy that presents around the age of 60.

Clinical Presentation

- Affected individuals develop parkinsonism (rigidity, bradykinesia, postural instability, and dysphagia). Classically, one limb is dystonic and myoclonic. Cortical sensory loss and apraxia of that limb are common findings as well. A relatively unique feature of this illness is that up to 60% of patients may develop alien limb phenomenon. Cognitive impairment and aphasia are commonly seen in the later stages of the disease.

- The corticobasal syndrome can be found under autopsy to actually be AD, PSP, or FTD. Statistically, it is probably more likely for the corticobasal syndrome to be one of these other conditions as CBD is rare under autopsy. In general, there is a tremendous amount of clinical overlap among all these conditions, highlighting the clinical overlap of the tauopathies as a group.

Radiographic Appearance and Diagnosis

- There is no specific diagnostic test. The MRI in patients with CBD typically shows asymmetric posterior parietal and frontal cortical atrophy. The superior parietal lobule is most commonly affected, and there is commonly hyperintensity on T2-weighted images of the affected areas. Atrophy of the midbrain, basal ganglia, and corpus callosum is also seen.

Treatment

- There is no specific treatment for CBD, and treatment is based on symptoms. Patients do not benefit from dopamine replacement therapy. Behavioral disturbances may respond to medication and behavioral therapies. Death usually occurs within 6 to 8 years.

References

1. Marsili L, Suppa A, Berardelli A, Colosimo C. Therapeutic interventions in parkinsonism: Corticobasal degeneration. *Parkinsonism Relat Disord.* September 2015;22:S96–S100. pii: S1353-8020(15)00398-3.

2. Armstrong MJ. Diagnosis and treatment of corticobasal degeneration. *Curr Treat Options Neurol.* March 2014;16(3):282.

3. Armstrong MJ, Litvan I, Lang AE, et al. Criteria for the diagnosis of corticobasal degeneration. *Neurology.* February 2013;80(5):496–503.

4. Alexander SK, Rittman T, Xuereb JH, et al. Validation of the new consensus criteria for the diagnosis of corticobasal degeneration. *J Neurol Neurosurg Psychiatry.* August 2014;85(8):925–929.

10.8 Amyotrophic Lateral Sclerosis

Case History

A 56-year-old man presented with progressive weakness in his legs and hands and slurred speech over the past few months. On examination, the patient had dysarthria, and fasciculations were seen in deltoid muscles on both sides and tongue. There was preferential wasting of the thenar and first dorsal interosseous muscles with relative sparing of hypothenar muscles ("split hand"). There was mild atrophy of the tongue. Muscle strength was 3/5 in distal leg muscles and 2/5 in distal hand muscles. There were no sensory deficits. He had diffuse hyperreflexia, bilateral ankle clonus, jaw jerk, and positive Hoffmann's reflex in both hands.

Diagnosis: Amyotrophic Lateral Sclerosis

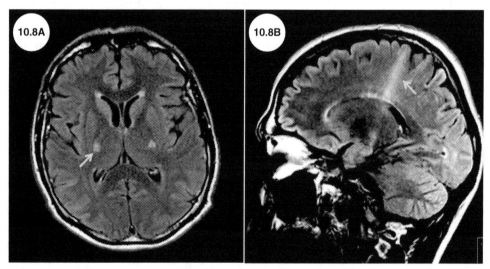

Images 10.8A and 10.8B: Axial and sagittal FLAIR images demonstrate hyperintensity throughout the corticospinal tract (yellow arrows). The corticospinal tract is seen in the posterior limb of the internal capsule on the axial image.

Introduction

■ Amyotrophic lateral sclerosis (ALS) is an adult-onset, progressive disorder characterized by degeneration of upper and lower motor neurons.

■ It has an annual incidence of 1 to 3:100,000. Most cases are sporadic, with about 5% to 10% being familial. About 20% of familial ALS (FALS) are associated with mutations in the gene that codes for the protein Cu/Zn superoxide dismutase 1 (SOD 1) located on chromosome 21. About

two-thirds of familial cases can be attributed to genetic mutations in C9ORF72, SOD1, TARDBP, or FUS.

■ Males are affected more frequently than females.

■ Juvenile ALS is more frequently familial in nature than the adult-onset forms. Mutations in the alsin (ALS2), senataxin (SETX), and spatacsin (SPG11) have been associated with FALS with juvenile onset and slow progression. However, SOD1 and FUS mutations can lead to juvenile-onset malignant forms of ALS and should be screened in

ALS patients with an earlier age of onset and an aggressive progression, even if there is no apparent family history.

Clinical Presentation

■ Most patients present with asymmetric weakness in the distal extremities. About 20% present with bulbar symptoms—dysarthria, dysphonia, dysphagia, or difficulty breathing.

■ Later symptoms include constipation, early satiety, bloating with delayed gastric emptying, urinary urgency without incontinence, and weight loss. Patients may also display executive dysfunction, subjective sensory symptoms (ie, tingling), or parkinsonism. Pseudobulbar palsy, a condition of "emotional incontinence" in which patients laugh or cry without experiencing the underlying emotion, is a common symptom.

■ On exam, patients have both upper motor neuron (UMN) signs (hyperreflexia, spasticity) and lower motor neuron (LMN) signs (muscle atrophy and fasciculations). There are no differences between familial and sporadic ALS on neurological exam except for occasional sensory loss in patients with FALS (**Table 10.8.1**).

Table 10.8.1 Types of Motor Neuron Disease

Typical	Atypical
UMN and LMN: ALS	Mills hemiplegic variant
UMN only: Primary lateral sclerosis	Scapulohumeral form
LMN only: Spinal muscular atrophy	Monomelic form (Hirayama's disease)
Bulbar only: Progressive bulbar palsy	Wasted-leg syndrome
Familial ALS	Flail arm syndrome
Juvenile ALS	Unilateral leg hypertrophy

ALS, amyotrophic lateral sclerosis; LMN, lower motor neuron; UMN, upper motor neuron.

Radiographic Appearance and Diagnosis

■ Hyperintensity of the corticospinal tract may be seen on T2-weighted images throughout its course in the brain, brainstem, and spinal cord. The appearance of the corticospinal tract in the spinal cord is called the "snake-eye" sign due to its resemblance to a pair of dice, each rolled to one.

■ Cortical iron deposition may be seen on susceptibility-weighted imaging.

■ PET studies have shown diffuse gliosis in white matter tracts due to loss of inhibitory cortical interneurons in the motor cortex.

■ The diagnosis can be confirmed with an electromyography (EMG), which shows fibrillation and fasciculation potentials. The motor units may be polyphasic with increased amplitude and long duration. With chronic denervation there are large motor unit potentials.

■ **The El Escorial criteria (EEC)** for the diagnosis of ALS requires:

A criteria:
A1: evidence of LMN degeneration by clinical, electrophysiological, or neuropathological examination
A2: evidence of UMN degeneration by clinical examination
A3: progressive dissemination beyond typical nerve supply areas
B criteria:
B1: electrophysiological and pathological evidence of other disease processes that might explain the signs of LMN and/or UMN degeneration, and
B2: neuroimaging evidence of other disease processes that may explain the clinical symptoms

The EEC defines four body regions to be evaluated:

1. Brainstem (bulbar)
2. Cervical (neck and upper extremities)
3. Thoracic (trunk, abdominal wall)
4. Lumbosacral (lumbar spine and lower extremities)

■ **Diagnostic categories**

  ▪ **Clinically definite ALS** is defined on clinical evidence alone by the presence of UMN, as well as LMN signs, in three regions.

  ▪ **Clinically probable ALS** is defined on clinical evidence alone by UMN and LMN signs in at least two regions with some UMN signs necessarily rostral to (above) the LMN signs.

  ▪ **Clinically probable–laboratory-supported ALS** is defined when clinical signs of UMN and LMN dysfunction are in only one region, or when UMN signs alone are present in one region, and LMN signs defined by EMG

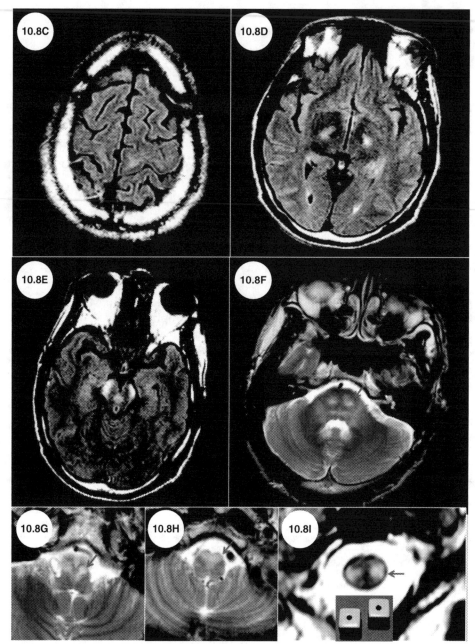

Image 10.8C: Axial FLAIR images demonstrate hyperintensity in the corticospinal tracts in the primary motor cortex of the frontal lobe can be seen as a subtle hyperintensity. **Image 10.8D:** Axial FLAIR image demonstrates the corticospinal tract in the posterior limb of the internal capsule. **Image 10.8E:** Axial FLAIR image demonstrates the corticospinal tract in the cerebral peduncle. **Image 10.8F:** Axial T2-weighted image demonstrates the corticospinal tract in the pons. **Image 10.8G:** Axial T2-weighted image demonstrates the corticospinal tract in the upper medulla. **Image 10.8H:** Axial T2-weighted image demonstrates corticospinal tract in the lower medulla, at the level of the pyramids where the corticospinal tract decussates. **Image 10.8I:** Axial T2-weighted image demonstrates now crossed corticospinal tract in the upper cervical cord. The appearance there is known as the "snake-eye" sign. In all images the red arrow points to the corticospinal tract.

criteria are present in at least two limbs, with proper application of neuroimaging and clinical laboratory protocols to exclude other causes.

Clinically possible ALS is defined when clinical signs of UMN and LMN dysfunction are found together in only one region or UMN signs are found alone in two or more

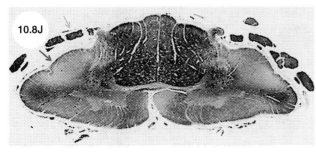

Image 10.8J: Wallerian degeneration of lateral fasciculi (red arrow) of spinal cord in a patient with ALS-FTD-complex. The dorsal, sensory nerve root (blue arrow) is preserved, while the anterior, motor nerve root is significantly atrophied.

Source: Luty AA, Kwok JB, Thompson EM, et al. Pedigree with frontotemporal lobar degeneration—motor neuron disease and Tar DNA binding protein-43 positive neuropathology: genetic linkage to chromosome 9. *BMC Neurol.* 2008;8:32.

regions; or LMN signs are found rostral to UMN signs and the diagnosis of clinically probable–laboratory-supported ALS cannot be proven by evidence on clinical grounds in conjunction with electrodiagnostic, neurophysiologic, neuroimaging, or clinical laboratory studies. Other diagnoses must have been excluded to accept a diagnosis of clinically possible ALS.

Treatment

■ Riluzole, a glutamate antagonist, is the only Food and Drug Administration (FDA) approved drug for the treatment of ALS. It prolongs survival by 3 to 6 months. Physical and occupational therapy is essential to maintain the patient's mobility and daily function for as long as possible.

■ ALS is a progressive disease. The median survival from the time of diagnosis is 3 to 5 years, and neuromuscular respiratory failure is the most common cause of death. However, approximately 10% of ALS patients can live for 10 years or more after diagnosis.

■ **Table 10.8.2** enlists different drug and nondrug therapies for patients with ALS.

Table 10.8.2 Pharmacological and Nonpharmacological Therapies for Patients With ALS

Disease-Modifying Treatment	Riluzole
Multidisciplinary clinic care	Speech therapy, physiotherapy, occupational therapy, orthotics, psychology, nutrition
Respiratory support	Noninvasive ventilation (NIV), Bi-PAP
Spasticity	Baclofen, Flexeril, tizanidine, dantrolene, diazepam, Botox injection, physical therapy, hydrotherapy
Sialorrhea	Amitriptyline, scopolamine patch, Botox injection, atropine, benztropine, radiation therapy to parotid glands, glycopyrrolate (Robinul)
Miscellaneous supportive treatment	For constipation, depression, anxiety, fatigue, cramps; nutrition—percutaneous endoscopic gastrostomy (PEG) tube may be necessary in some patients for nutritional support
Pseudobulbar affect	Dextromethorphan and quinidine (Nuedexta)
Bronchial secretions	Guaifenesin, portable suction devices, cricopharyngeal myotomy; high frequency chest wall oscillation device (VEST)

References

1. Kiernan MC, Vucic S, Cheah BC, et al. Amyotrophic lateral sclerosis. *Lancet.* March 2011;377(9769):942–955.
2. Chiò A, Pagani M, Agosta F, Calvo A, Cistaro A, Filippi M. Neuroimaging in amyotrophic lateral sclerosis: insights into structural and functional changes. *Lancet Neurol.* December 2014;13(12):1228–1240.
3. Miller RG, Jackson CE, Kasarskis EJ, et al. Practice parameter update: the care of the patient with amyotrophic lateral sclerosis: multidisciplinary care, symptom management, and cognitive/behavioral impairment (an evidence-based review): report of the Quality Standards Subcommittee of the American Academy of Neurology. *Neurology.* 2009;73:1227–1233.
4. Luty AA, Kwok JB, Thompson EM, et al. Pedigree with frontotemporal lobar degeneration—motor neuron disease and Tar DNA binding protein-43 positive neuropathology: genetic linkage to chromosome 9. *BMC Neurol.* 2008;8:32.

10.9 | Wilson's Disease

Case History

A 29-year-old female presented with psychosis, abnormal movements, and jaundice.

Diagnosis: Wilson's Disease

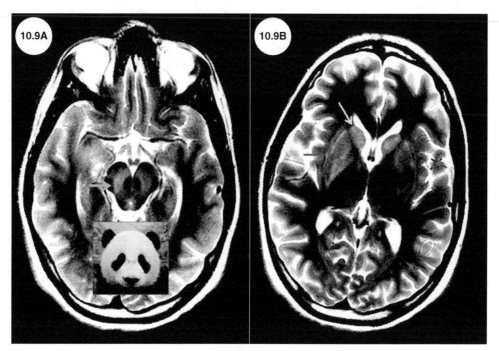

Images 10.9A and 10.9B: Axial T2-weighted images demonstrate hyperintensities of the substantia nigra (blue arrow), caudate nucleus (yellow arrow), and putamen (red arrow) in a patient with Wilson's disease. The appearance of the midbrain is known as the "face of the giant panda" sign.

Introduction

■ Wilson's disease (WD), also known as hepatolenticular degeneration, is an autosomal-recessive disorder in which there is a deficiency of the copper-carrying protein, ceruloplasmin. This leads to an accumulation of copper in multiple parts of the body, mainly the liver, cornea, and the basal ganglia.

Clinical Presentation

■ The primary manifestation is liver disease, appearing in late childhood or early adolescence as acute or chronic hepatitis or cirrhosis.

■ For those with a neurological presentation, the first symptom can be essentially any movement

disorder or ataxia. The classic presentation is a "wing beating tremor." Dysphagia and dysarthria are common as well. About half of patients will have psychiatric symptoms, which range from mood disturbances to psychosis.

■ The characteristic ocular finding is the Kayser–Fleischer ring, which is caused by deposition of copper around the periphery of the cornea's Descemet's membrane.

Radiographic Appearance and Diagnosis

■ The characteristic finding on T2-weighted images is the "face of the giant panda" sign. This is seen in the midbrain and is created by areas

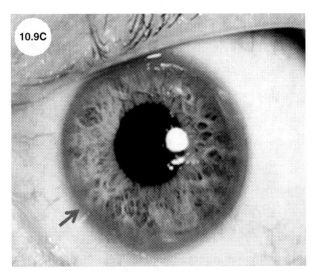

Image 10.9C: A Kayser–Fleischer ring (red arrow) (image credit Dr. Herbert L. Fred).

of hyperintensity adjacent to the substantia nigra and red nucleus. Additionally, hyperintensity on T2-weighted images can be seen in the caudate, putamen, globus pallidus, and thalamus.

■ Decreased serum ceruloplasmin supports the diagnosis. Copper levels are elevated in the urine and can be elevated, normal, or decreased in the serum. The gold standard for diagnosis is an elevated copper concentration on liver biopsy.

Treatment

■ Treatment includes avoiding foods with high copper (chocolate, nuts, shellfish), zinc salts to block copper absorption, and chelation therapy with D-penicillamine and trientine to increase urinary excretion of copper. In severe disease liver transplantation can be curative.

References

1. Bandmann O, Weiss KH, Kaler SG. Wilson's disease and other neurological copper disorders. *Lancet Neurol.* January 2015;14(1):103–113.
2. Lorincz MT. Neurologic Wilson's disease. *Ann N Y Acad Sci.* January 2010;1184:173–187.
3. Lorincz MT. Recognition and treatment of neurologic Wilson's disease. *Semin Neurol.* November 2012;32(5):538–543.

10.10 Normal Pressure Hydrocephalus

Case History

A 69-year-old female presented with cognitive impairment and an unsteady gait.

Diagnosis: Normal Pressure Hydrocephalus

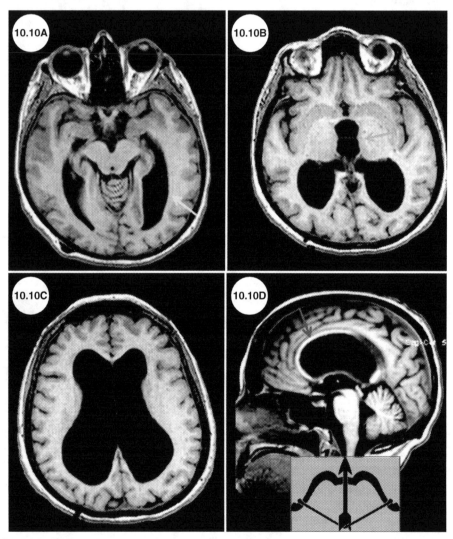

Images 10.10A–10.10D: Axial and sagittal T1-weighted images demonstrate massively enlarged ventricles in a patient with NPH. There is enlargement of the temporal horns (yellow arrow) as well as the third ventricle (blue arrow). The corpus callosum is thinned and "bowed" (red arrow).

Introduction

■ Cerebrospinal fluid (CSF) is formed in the choroid plexus, located in the lateral ventricles. It then flows from the lateral ventricles through the third and fourth ventricles, then into the subarachnoid space where it is absorbed into the systemic circulation through the arachnoid villi. The ventricular system contains approximately 150 ml of CSF and it is recycled several times daily (**Illustration 10.10.1**).

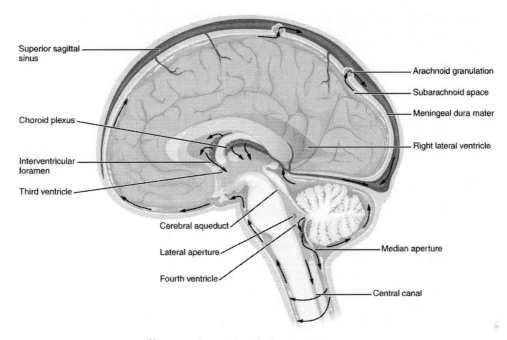

Illustration 10.10.1: The CSF system.

Source: Anatomy & Physiology. Connexions website. http://cnx.org/content/col11496/1.6.

■ Normal pressure hydrocephalus (NPH) is characterized by pathologically enlarged ventricles with normal opening pressure on lumbar puncture. NPH can arise either due to an overproduction of CSF or a failure in the absorption process, which is the suspected pathogenesis in secondary NPH. It can occur either as an idiopathic condition or secondary to another condition, such as subarachnoid hemorrhage or meningitis. The hydrocephalus is communicating in that there is no focal obstruction in the ventricular system, which impedes the outflow of CSF.

■ When idiopathic, the average age of onset is 60 years, and the incidence increases with advanced age. It can occur at any age if secondary to another condition.

Clinical Presentation

■ NPH classically presents with cognitive disturbance, gait abnormality, and urinary incontinence, presumably secondary to disruption of the periventricular white matter tracts. The gait associated with NPH is typically described as "magnetic," as patients shuffle their feet along the ground. The steps are small and the stance is wide-based. Gait disturbance is the earliest and most prominent symptom. It is considered a gait apraxia, as patients are able to mimic walking normally while sitting in a chair or lying down, but their feet seem glued to the floor when they actually try to walk.

■ The cognitive disturbances are psychomotor slowing, apathy, and decreased attention and concentration. It is considered a treatable form of dementia.

Diagnosis and Radiographic Appearance

■ The hallmark is ventricular enlargement out of proportion to normal age-related brain atrophy. There is enlargement of the temporal horns in particular, and the third ventricle is enlarged. Other imaging findings include transependymal flow of CSF.

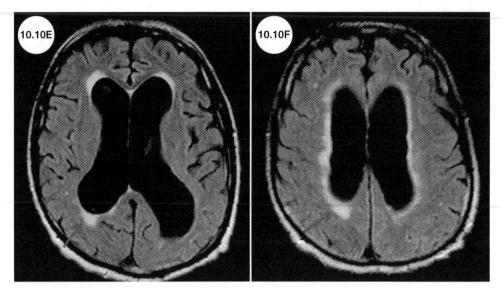

Images 10.10E and 10.10F: Axial FLAIR images demonstrate massively enlarged ventricles and transependymal flow of CSF (red arrows).

■ Often, a prominent flow void can be seen on T2-weighted images in the cerebral aqueduct due to increased CSF velocity.

■ In longstanding NPH, the corpus callosum becomes thin and elevated, taking on a "bowed" appearance. Often, the floor of the sella turcica is eroded as well.

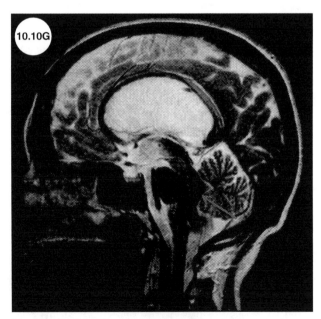

Image 10.10G: Sagittal T2-weighted image demonstrates a prominent flow void in the cerebral aqueduct and fourth ventricle (red arrow).

■ In patients with a suggestive presentation, the diagnosis is made by removing a large volume of CSF (20–30 mL). This will reveal a low to normal opening pressure and may result in improvement of the gait abnormality, which can further support the diagnosis. In certain institutions, a lumbar drain is left in place for several days to mimic the effect of a ventricular shunt.

Treatment

■ Treatment involves the placement of a ventriculoperitoneal shunt.

■ The ideal surgical candidate would show imaging evidence of ventriculomegaly and the following:

1. Presence of a clearly identified etiology of the hydrocephalus

2. Gait difficulties with mild cognitive impairment

3. Substantial improvement after removal of CSF

4. Lack of atrophy and white matter lesions on imaging

5. Presence of aqueductal flow void on T2-weighted image

■ In about 15% of patients with nonobstructive hydrocephalus, lesions may develop in the corpus callosum after placement of a shunt. The

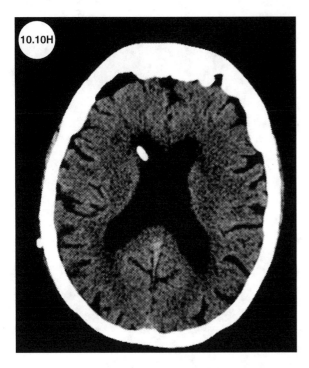

Image 10.10H: Axial CT image demonstrates placement of a ventricular shunt (red arrow) in a patient with NPH.

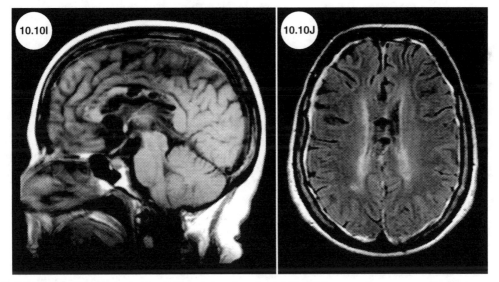

Images 10.10I and 10.10J: Sagittal T1-weighted and axial FLAIR images demonstrate extensive cystic lesions (red arrows) in the corpus callosum after the placement of a ventricular shunt.

exact mechanism of these lesions is not known, but may be due to ischemia in patients with long-standing hydrocephalus followed by rapid ventricular decompression. The clinical significance of these lesions is also not known.

References

1. Shprecher D, Schwalb J, Kurlan R. Normal pressure hydrocephalus: diagnosis and treatment. *Curr Neurol Neurosci Rep.* September 2008;8(5):371–376.

2. Ghosh S, Lippa C. Diagnosis and prognosis in idiopathic normal pressure hydrocephalus. *Am J Alzheimers Dis Other Demen.* November 2014;29(7):583–589.

3. Torsnes L, Blåfjelldal V, Poulsen FR. Treatment and clinical outcome in patients with idiopathic normal pressure hydrocephalus--a systematic review. *Dan Med J.* October 2014;61(10):A4911.

4. Toma AK, Papadopoulos MC, Stapleton S, Kitchen ND, Watkins LD. Systematic review of the outcome of shunt surgery in idiopathic normal-pressure hydrocephalus. *Acta Neurochir (Wien).* October 2013;155(10):1977–1980.

5. Anatomy & Physiology. Connexions website. http://cnx.org/content/col11496/1.6. Accessed June 19, 2013.

CHAPTER 11

TOXIC/METABOLIC DISORDERS

11.1 | Central Pontine Myelinolysis

Case History

A 56-year-old alcoholic was found obtunded in the street. He was found to have a serum sodium of 114 mEq/L, which was aggressively corrected by the emergency department (ED) to a value of 144 mEq/L in the next few hours.

Diagnosis: Central Pontine Myelinolysis

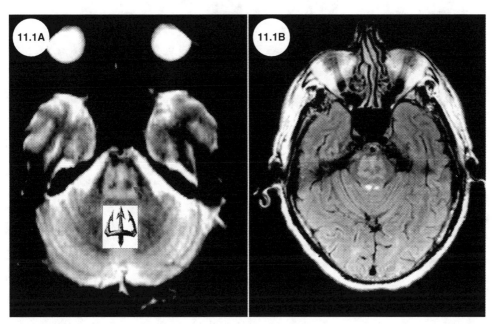

Images 11.1A and 11.1B: Axial T2-weighted and fluid-attenuated inversion recovery (FLAIR) images demonstrate hyperintensity in the center of the pons with sparing of corticospinal tracts (red arrow), the "trident" sign.

Introduction

■ Central pontine myelinolysis (CPM) is a demyelinating disorder that occurs when there is rapid correction of hyponatremia leading to changes in cell osmolarities and shifts of free water. Patients typically have had severe hyponatremia (less than 120 mEq/L) for at least 48 hours.

Clinical Presentation

■ CPM occurs most commonly in alcoholics or chronically malnourished, medically ill patients. It presents with parkinsonism, quadriparesis, locked-in syndrome, bulbar dysfunction, and coma. Symptoms appear 48 to 72 hours after the correction of hyponatremia.

Radiographic Appearance and Diagnosis

■ On T2-weighted images, there is hyperintensity in the central pons with sparing of the corticospinal tracts, creating the "trident" sign. Extrapontine myelinolysis occurs in about 10% of patients, most commonly in the caudate and putamen. Other affected locations include the ventrolateral thalami, the external and extreme capsules, and the gray–white matter junction.

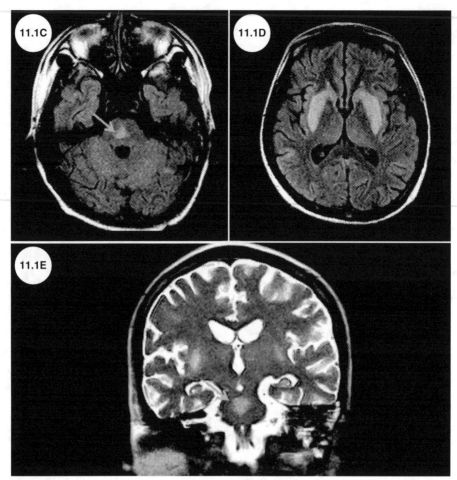

Images 11.1C–11.1E: Axial FLAIR and coronal T2-weighted images demonstrate hyperintensity in the central pons (blue arrows) and striatum (red arrows) in a patient with CPM.

Treatment

■ Treatment of CPM is supportive. It can be fatal in up to 25% of cases, and many survivors are left with permanent neuropsychiatric dysfunction.

■ To avoid CPM, patients with severe hyponatremia should have their sodium corrected at a rate of no more than 12 to 20 mmol/L daily.

References

1. Singh TD, Fugate JE, Rabinstein AA. Central pontine and extrapontine myelinolysis: a systematic review. *Eur J Neurol*. December 2014;21(12):1443–1450.
2. Huq S, Wong M, Chan H, Crimmins D. Osmotic demyelination syndromes: central and extrapontine myelinolysis. *J Clin Neurosci*. July 2007;14(7):684–688. Epub 2007 April 25.
3. Brown WD. Osmotic demyelination disorders: central pontine and extrapontine myelinolysis. *Curr Opin Neurol*. December 2000;13(6):691–697.

11.2 | Familial Cerebrovascular Ferrocalcinosis

Case History

A 43-year-old man presented with dystonia and choreoathetoid movements, and was paranoid that his neighbors were spying on him.

Diagnosis: Familial Cerebrovascular Ferrocalcinosis

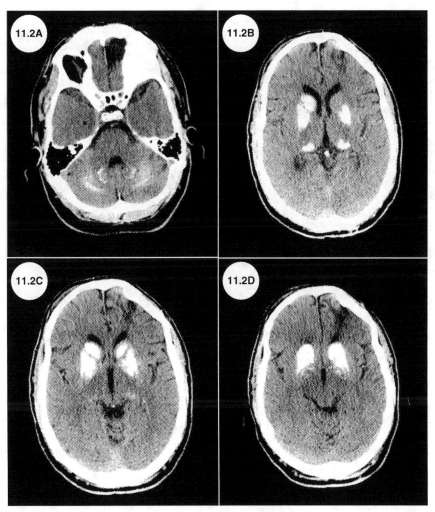

Images 11.2A–11.2D: Axial CT images demonstrate dense bilateral calcification of the dentate nuclei of the cerebellum, basal ganglia, and pulvinar nucleus of thalamus.

Introduction

■ Familial cerebrovascular ferrocalcinosis (Fahr's disease) is a rare, autosomal-dominant disease characterized by abnormal calcium deposition in the brain.

Clinical Presentation

■ It presents with a variety of movement disorders, including parkinsonism, dystonia, chorea, as well as neuropsychiatric impairment. Symptoms typically start in the fourth or the fifth decade, though some patients present younger.

Radiographic Appearance and Diagnosis

■ It is characterized by bilateral, symmetric calcifications of the basal ganglia, thalamus, dentate nucleus of the cerebellum, and occasionally the subcortical white matter. These are best seen on CT.

■ There is a variable appearance on MRI, but often calcium crystals will appear hyperintense on unenhanced T1-weighted images.

■ Calcification of the basal ganglia may be associated with hypoparathyroidism and abnormalities

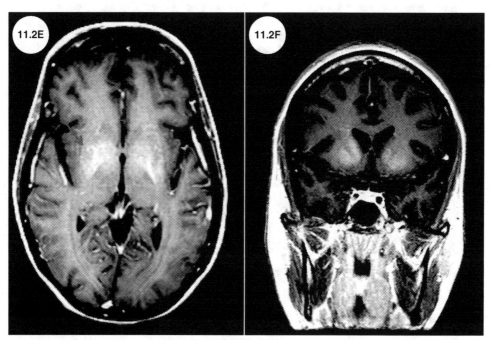

Images 11.2E and 11.2F: Axial and coronal T1-weighed images demonstrate basal ganglia hyperintensities (red arrows) in a patient with familial cerebrovascular ferrocalcinosis.

of phosphate and calcium. Serum calcium, phosphorus, magnesium, alkaline phosphatase, calcitonin, and parathyroid hormone should also be measured to rule out metabolic causes. It may also occur after neurocysticercosis or tuberculosis. Often no cause is found.

Treatment

■ There is no specific treatment for the disease beyond trying to alleviate the symptoms.

References

1. Wider C, Dickson DW, Schweitzer KJ, Broderick DF, Wszolek ZK. Familial idiopathic basal ganglia calcification: a challenging clinical-pathological correlation. *J Neurol.* May 2009;256(5):839–842.
2. Rosenberg DR, Neylan TC, el-Alwar M, Peters J, Van Kammen DP. Neuropsychiatric symptoms associated with idiopathic calcification of the basal ganglia. *J Nerv Ment Dis.* January 1991;179(1):48–49.
3. Saleem S, Aslam HM, Anwar M, et al. Fahr's syndrome: literature review of current evidence. *Orphanet J Rare Dis.* October 2013;8:156.

Case History

A 65-year-old alcoholic man presented with several days of confusion and jaundice. On exam, he did not know the date, location, or his age. He had ascites and asterixis.

Diagnosis: Hepatic Encephalopathy

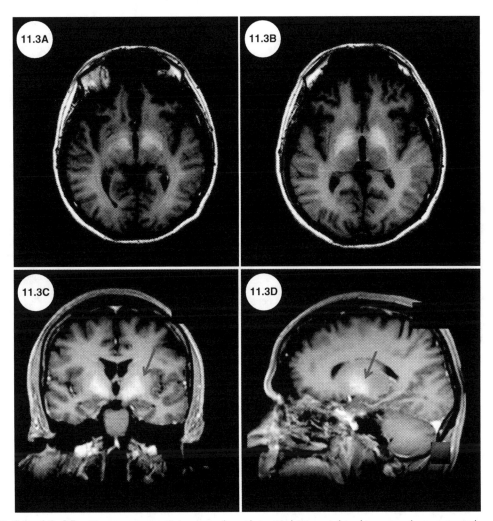

Images 11.3A–11.3D: Noncontrast axial, coronal, and sagittal T1-weighted images demonstrate hyperintensity (red arrows) of the globus pallidus descending into the cerebral peduncles without mass effect in a patient with hepatic encephalopathy.

Introduction

■ Hepatic encephalopathy occurs in cirrhotic patients when there is diversion of portal venous blood into the systemic circulation.

■ It can be caused by a variety of pathologies (see **Table 11.3.1**).

Clinical Presentation

■ Patients present with neuropsychiatric dysfunction, which may range from mild confusion to coma. Movement disorders, such as asterixis and parkinsonism, are common. It can present acutely, especially if there is a precipitating

Table 11.3.1 Causes of Hepatic Encephalopathy

Category	Causes
Excessive nitrogen	Gastrointestinal bleeding, renal failure, constipation, high protein diet
Electrolyte or metabolic disturbance	Hyponatremia, hypokalemia (often from diuretic therapy), hypoxia, hypoglycemia, alkalosis
Toxic	Benzodiazepines, opiates, antidepressants, antipsychotics, alcohol, valproic acid
Infection	Pneumonia, urinary tract infection, bacterial peritonitis
Focal hepatic pathology	Hepatocellular carcinoma, hepatic vein or portal vein thrombosis

infection. Such cases may be fatal. The degree of impairment is categorized by the West Haven criteria (see **Table 11.3.2**).

Radiographic Appearance and Diagnosis

■ Noncontrast T1-weighted images demonstrate bilateral, symmetric hyperintense lesions in the basal ganglia, most commonly the globus pallidus. These are believed to be due to impaired metabolism of metals, manganese in particular, but are not specific for hepatic encephalopathy. On T2-weighted and diffusion-weighted images, there may be swelling and hyperintensity of the cortex, as well as the thalami, and posterior limbs of the internal capsules. These findings are more common with acute cases and are reversible.

■ In addition to elevated hepatic function tests, ammonia levels are commonly elevated, though the level does not correlate with functional impairment.

■ An electroencephalogram (EEG) will classically reveal triphasic waves.

Table 11.3.2 West Haven Criteria

Stage	Consciousness	Cognition and Behavior	Neurological Exam
0	Normal	Normal	Normal examination; or mild psychomotor slowing
1	Mild confusion	Decreased attention span	Impaired addition or subtraction; mild asterixis or tremor
2	Lethargy	Disoriented; inappropriate behavior	Asterixis; dysarthria
3	Somnolent but arousable	Gross disorientation; disorganized behavior	Rigidity, diffuse clonus and hyperreflexia
4	Coma	Coma	Decerebrate posturing

Treatment

■ Specific treatment depends on addressing the underlying cause. General treatment includes lactulose, which decreases ammonia production and absorption, and antibiotics (such as rifaximin) to decrease ammonia-producing bacteria in the gut. L-ornithine and L-aspartate (LOLA) can be used to remove ammonia by converting it into urea. Supplementation of branched-chain amino acids and the use of probiotics have shown benefit. Restriction of dietary protein is no longer recommended as many patients are chronically malnourished.

■ Liver transplantation is curative in appropriate patients.

References

1. Rovira A, Alonso J, Córdoba J. MR imaging findings in hepatic encephalopathy. *AJNR Am J Neuroradiol.* October 2008;29(9):1612–1621.
2. Ellul MA, Gholkar SA, Cross TJ. Hepatic encephalopathy due to liver cirrhosis. *MJ.* August 2015;351:h4187.
3. Wright G, Jalan R. Management of hepatic encephalopathy in patients with cirrhosis. *Best Pract Res Clin Gastroenterol.* 2007;21(1):95–110.
4. Córdoba J, Mínguez B. Hepatic encephalopathy. *Semin Liver Dis.* February 2008;28(1):70–80.

11.4 Cerebellar Atrophy

Case History

A 34-year-old man with history of seizures since childhood presented with chronic gait ataxia.

Diagnosis: Cerebellar Atrophy

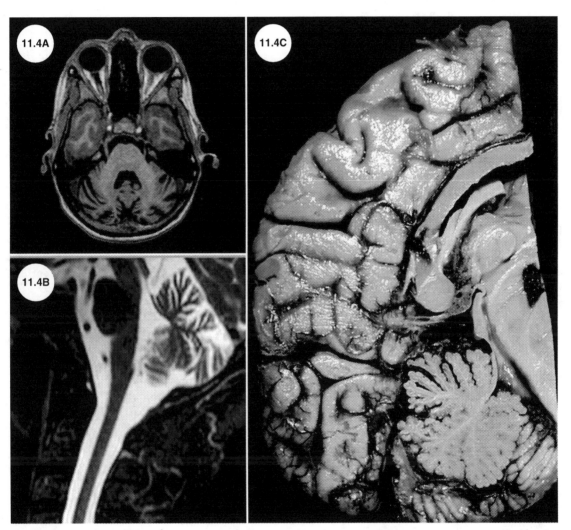

Images 11.4A and 11.4B: Axial T1-weighted and sagittal T2-weighted images demonstrate atrophy of cerebellum due to chronic antiepileptic therapy. **Image 11.4C:** Gross pathology demonstrates cerebellar atrophy.

Introduction

■ A number of toxins, namely older antiepileptic medications such as phenytoin and alcohol, can result in atrophy of the cerebellum with chronic use.

■ Patients with neurodegenerative diseases, such as olivopontocerebellar atrophy and the spinocerebellar ataxias, have a similar clinical and radiographic presentation.

■ Paraneoplastic cerebellar degeneration (PCD) can occur with a number of malignancies due to production of antineuronal antibodies that target Purkinje cells throughout the cerebellar cortex. Gynecologic cancers are most commonly implicated, though the condition is rare overall, occurring in less than 1% of cancers. Ovarian and breast cancers are associated with anti-Yo and anti-Ri antibodies, lung cancer is associated with anti-Hu antibodies, and Hodgkin's lymphoma is associated with (anti-Tr and anti-mGluR1) antibodies.

Clinical Presentation

■ Patients develop a wide-based, ataxic gait, slurred, scanning speech, and nystagmus. The arms are relatively spared with toxic cerebellar degeneration.

■ With PCD, symptoms can develop rapidly over the course of several months. Patients then stabilize, but are often debilitated by their symptoms.

Radiographic Appearance and Diagnosis

■ The superior vermis is affected earliest and the cerebellar hemispheres are affected only in the most severe cases. Skull thickening can also be seen with long-term use of phenytoin.

Treatment

■ There is no treatment beyond stopping the offending medication or alcohol use. PCD responds poorly to immunotherapy. With non-gynecologic cancers, the condition may improve with treatment of the underlying neoplasm.

References

1. Ney GC, Lantos G, Barr WB, Schaul N. Cerebellar atrophy in patients with long-term phenytoin exposure and epilepsy. *Arch Neurol.* August 1994;51(8):767–771.
2. Shams'ili S, Grefkens J, de Leeuw B, et al. Paraneoplastic cerebellar degeneration associated with antineuronal antibodies: analysis of 50 patients. *Brain.* June 2003;126(Pt. 6):1409–1418.

11.5 | Cyclosporin Toxicity

Case History

A 56-year-old kidney transplant patient developed confusion and headache after being started on a medication.

Diagnosis: Cyclosporine

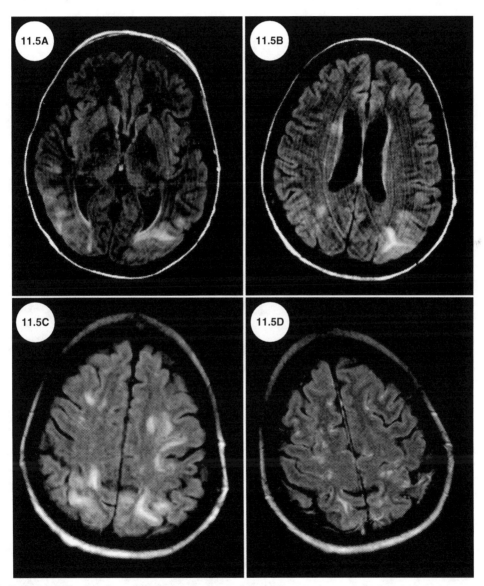

Images 11.5A–11.5D: Axial FLAIR images demonstrate confluent white matter hyperintensities, primarily in the posterior temporal and occipital lobes in a patient treated with cyclosporine.

Introduction

■ Cyclosporine is an immunosuppressant medication used to prevent organ rejection in transplantation. Neurotoxicity occurs in up to 25% of patients, especially when high doses are used. Breakdown of the blood brain barrier is the likely mechanism.

Clinical Presentation

■ Patients present with seizures, cortical blindness, headaches, psychosis, and encephalopathy. Electrolyte abnormalities are a risk factor.

Radiographic Appearance

■ White matter hyperintensities are seen on T2-weighted images primarily in the parietal and occipital lobes. They may be seen more diffusely throughout the brain in severe cases. Microhemorrhages may be seen as well.

Treatment

■ In the vast majority of patients, symptoms resolve with lowering the dose or drug cessation.

References

1. Magnasco A, Rossi A, Catarsi P, et al. Cyclosporin and organ specific toxicity: clinical aspects, pharmacogenetics and perspectives. *Curr Clin Pharmacol*. September 2008;3(3):166–173.
2. Shah AK. Cyclosporine A neurotoxicity among bone marrow transplant recipients. *Clin Neuropharmacol*. March–April 1999;22(2):67–73.
3. Edwards LL, Wszolek ZK, Normand MM. Neurophysiologic evaluation of cyclosporine toxicity associated with bone marrow transplantation. *Acta Neurol Scand*. November 1996;94(5):358–364.

11.6 | Heroin Leukoencephalopathy

Case History

A 45-year-old heroin addict was found sleeping on the street. He was lethargic and disoriented in the ED. Over the next few weeks, he developed diffuse weakness, hyperreflexia, and tremors.

Diagnosis: Heroin Leukoencephalopathy

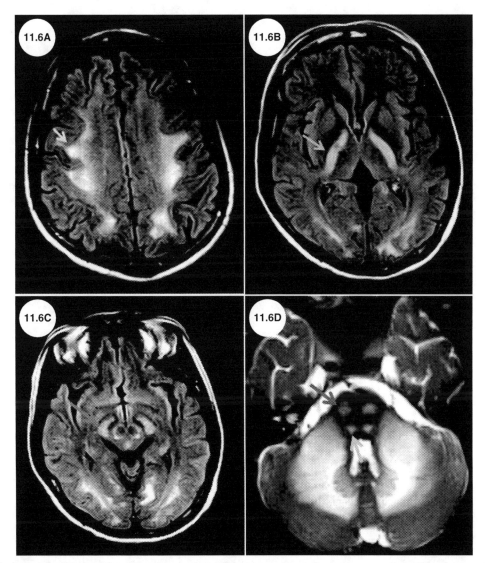

Images 11.6A–11.6D: Axial FLAIR images demonstrate symmetric hyperintensities in the subcortical white matter (yellow arrow), posterior limb of the internal capsule (blue arrow), cerebral peduncles (pink arrow), corticospinal tract (red arrow) and medial lemniscus (green arrow) in the pons, and cerebellum in a patient who smoked heroin.

Introduction

■ "Chasing the dragon" is a method of smoking heroin that involves placing a powder on an aluminum foil, which is then heated underneath. The vapor is then inhaled. It is known to produce a spongiform leukoencephalopathy.

Clinical Presentation

■ The syndrome progresses over several stages.

1. **Initial symptoms include:**
   - Soft speech
   - Ataxia
   - Restlessness
   - Cognitive changes, most commonly apathy

2. **After 2 to 4 weeks, 50% of patients develop worsening cerebellar symptoms and additional features:**
   - Spastic weakness and hyperreflexia
   - Tremor and myoclonus
   - Chorea and athetosis

3. **Several weeks after this, 25% of patients enter the terminal stage, which is characterized by:**
   - Hypotonic paresis and areflexia
   - Akinetic mutism
   - Central pyrexia
   - Spasms
   - Death in certain cases

Radiographic Appearance and Diagnosis

■ On MRI the pattern is typical for a toxic leukoencephalopathy. It is characterized by symmetric, hyperintensity on T2-weighted images of the subcortical white matter, posterior limb of the internal capsule, the corticospinal tract, and the cerebellum. The gray matter and subcortical u-fibers are typically uninvolved.

Treatment

■ Treatment is supportive.

References

1. Kass-Hout T, Kass-Hout O, Darkhabani MZ, Mokin M, Mehta B, Radovic V. "Chasing the dragon"—heroin-associated spongiform leukoencephalopathy. *J Med Toxicol.* September 2011;7(3):240–242.
2. Hagel J, Andrews G, Vertinsky T, Heran MK, Keogh C. "Chasing the dragon"—imaging of heroin inhalation leukoencephalopathy. *Can Assoc Radiol J.* October 2005;56(4):199–203.
3. Bach AG, Jordan B, Wegener NA, et al. Heroin spongiform leukoencephalopathy (HSLE). *Clin Neuroradiol.* December 2012;22(4):345–349.

11.7 | Marchiafava–Bignami Disease

Case History

A 61-year-old man with alcoholism presented with rapid-onset dementia.

Diagnosis: Marchiafava–Bignami Disease

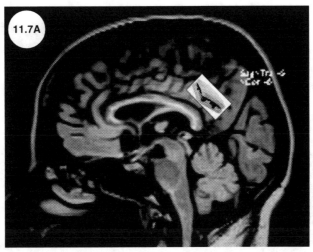

Image 11.7A: Sagittal FLAIR image demonstrates hyperintensity in the central layers of the corpus callosum in a patient with Marchiafava–Bignami disease, the "sandwich" sign.

Introduction

- Marchiafava–Bignami disease is a rare disorder characterized by symmetrical areas of demyelination and necrosis, primarily of the corpus callosum (CC).

Clinical Presentation

- It occurs most commonly in middle-aged, male alcoholics, but may occur in any chronically malnourished patient. It presents with a rapid-onset dementia and is thought to be due to a deficiency of vitamin B complex.

Radiographic Appearance and Diagnosis

- Imaging abnormalities characteristically start in the body of the CC and later involves the genu and then splenium. It preferentially involves the central layers with sparing of peripheral dorsal and ventral layers, a finding known as the "sandwich sign" on sagittal MRI imaging.

Treatment

- Replacement of B vitamins may result in improvement in some patients.

Reference

1. Hillbom M, Saloheimo P, Fujioka S, Wszolek ZK, Juvela S, Leone MA. Diagnosis and management of Marchiafava-Bignami disease: a review of CT/MRI confirmed cases. *J Neurol Neurosurg Psychiatry.* February 2014;85(2):168–173.

11.8 | B12 Deficiency

Case History

A 36-year-old man presented with severe burning and tingling in his feet, legs, and hands for several months. He had recently attended several music festivals where he abused nitrous oxide. On examination, he was weak in his legs with an unsteady gait. He was unable to feel a tuning fork on his legs and had profoundly impaired joint-position sense.

Diagnosis: Subacute Combined Degeneration

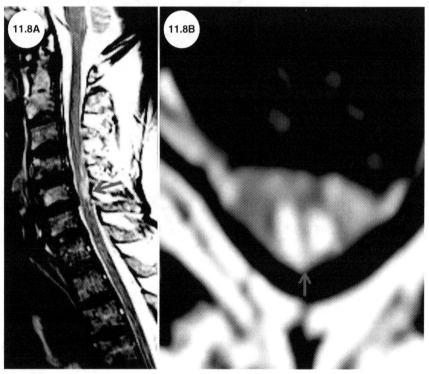

Images 11.8A and 11.8B: Sagittal and axial T2-weighted images of the cervical spine demonstrate hyperintensities in the dorsal columns (red arrows).

Introduction

- B12 (cyanocobalamin) is involved in fatty acid and amino acid metabolism, as well as DNA synthesis and regulation. It cannot be produced endogenously, and is obtained entirely through dietary sources.

- Deficiencies may occur in strict vegetarians, patients with inflammatory bowel disease, post-gastric bypass patients, patients with impaired absorption of B12 (pernicious anemia), or in patients who abuse nitrous oxide. Certain medications, namely proton pump inhibitors and histamine 2 receptor antagonists, can also decrease B12 absorption. Overall, pernicious anemia is the most common cause. Gastric parietal cells are destroyed in an autoimmune process, leading to atrophic gastritis and a deficiency of intrinsic factor, a protein necessary for B12 absorption in the ileum. It usually presents in older adults.

Clinical Presentation

- Deficiency causes accumulation of methylmalonic acid and neurological dysfunction in the peripheral nerves, optic nerves, dorsal and lateral columns of the spinal cord, and the brain. It is the combined degeneration of the dorsal and lateral columns that led to the term subacute combined degeneration.

■ Patients can experience a wide range of symptoms, including neuropathy, myelopathy, or neuropsychiatric manifestations. Typically, patients develop a cold sensation, numbness, or tingling that starts in the toes and then ascends up the legs, eventually involving the fingertips and hands. Some patients may experience excruciating lancinating pains. Limb weakness and gait ataxia can be seen in advanced cases. Patients may develop neuropsychiatric manifestations including depression and psychosis. Cognitive dysfunction is common and may be severe enough to cause frank dementia.

■ Neurological examination initially reveals impaired vibration and joint-position sense, which progresses over time to loss of light touch, pain, and temperature. The feet and legs are affected before arms. The ankle jerks are absent,

with relative hyperreflexia at the knees. The bait is wide-based and Romberg sign is usually positive.

■ Systemic signs and symptoms include shortness of breath, tachycardia, weight loss, nausea, and pallor. Patients may have a smooth, beefy red tongue and impaired taste, and sores at the corner of the mouth (angular cheilitis).

■ Hematological findings include hypersegmented neutrophils and a macrocytic anemia. When combined with the neuropsychiatric dysfunction, B12 deficiency is called "megaloblastic madness."

Radiographic Appearance and Diagnosis

■ As seen in **Images 11.8A and 11.8B**, in patients with myelopathy, spine MRI may reveal hyperintensities in the dorsal columns on T2-weighted images. In exceptional cases, there may be enhancement of the dorsal columns. This produces the "inverted-V" sign.

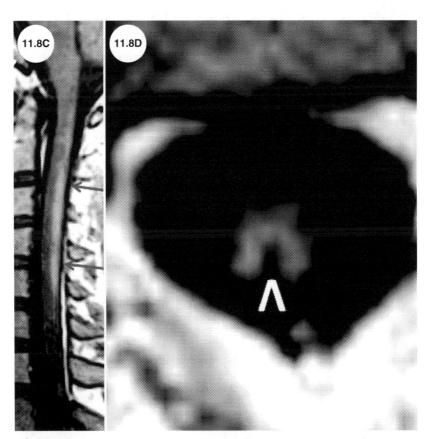

Images 11.8C and 11.8D: Postcontrast sagittal and axial T1-weighted images of the cervical spine demonstrate hyperintensities in the dorsal columns (red arrows) and the "inverted-V" sign.

11.8E

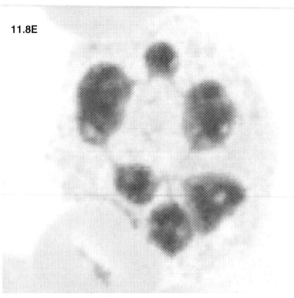

Image 11.8E: A hypersegmented neutrophil (image credit courtesy of and copyright by Gabriel Caponetti [2014]; from https://commons.wikimedia.org/wiki/File:Hypersegmented_neutrophil_-_by_Gabriel_Caponetti,MD.jpg).

- Spinal cord atrophy can be seen in chronic cases. A similar clinical and radiographic pattern can occur in patients with HIV-associated myelopathy.

- Serum studies may reveal a macrocytic anemia, and hypersegmented neutrophils are seen on peripheral smear.

- Importantly, patients can experience neurological symptoms with low–normal B12 values. Elevated levels of homocysteine and methylmalonic acid are the most sensitive markers of B12 deficiency.

- Patients with an unclear etiology for their deficiency should be evaluated for pernicious anemia by testing for antiparietal cell and intrinsic factor antibodies.

Treatment

- Treatment is with replacement of B12. Though injections are often needed initially, high doses of oral B12 are sufficient in most patients, even those with pernicious anemia. Neurological symptoms will stabilize, but not improve with treatment, however.

Reference

1. Sen A, Chandrasekhar K. Spinal MR imaging in Vitamin B12 deficiency: Case series; differential diagnosis of symmetrical posterior spinal cord lesions. *Ann Indian Acad Neurol*. April–June 2013;16(2):255–258.

11.9 | Copper Deficiency Myelopathy

Case History

A 56-year-old woman presented with an unsteady gait and pain in her feet several years after undergoing gastric bypass surgery.

Diagnosis: Copper Deficiency Myelopathy

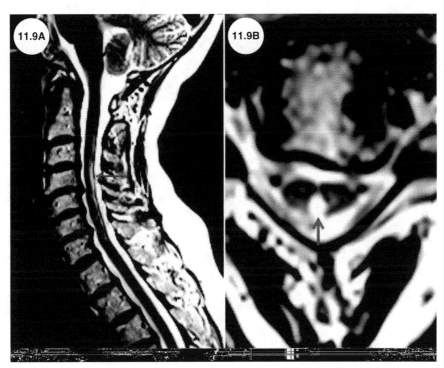

Images 11.9A and 11.9B: Sagittal and axial T2-weighted images of the cervical spine demonstrate a long segment hyperintensity in the dorsal columns (red arrows).

Introduction

■ Copper deficiency myelopathy (CDM) is an acquired, noncompressive myelopathy, which closely mimics subacute combined degeneration due to vitamin B12 deficiency.

■ Etiologies for impaired copper absorption in the upper gastrointestinal tract include prior gastric surgery, zinc overload, and various malabsorption syndromes. In some cases, no cause is found.

■ CDM is most common in patients in their 40s and 50s, and women are more commonly affected than men.

Clinical Presentation

■ Patients present with a slowly progressive gait ataxia and paresthesias in the hands and feet. Polyneuropathy is a near universal finding.

■ Neurological examination will reveal:

　▪ Wide-based ataxic and spastic gait and spastic paraparesis

　▪ Sensory ataxia and impaired vibration and joint-position sense

　▪ Sensory loss in a stocking–glove distribution and/or a sensory level

　▪ Positive Romberg sign

Radiographic Appearance and Diagnosis

- MRI is the imaging modality of choice, though it may be normal in half of the patients. Spinal MRI demonstrates long segment hyperintensities on T2-weighted images in the posterior columns of the cervical and/or thoracic spinal cord.

- The diagnosis can be confirmed by detecting low serum copper and ceruloplasmin levels. Copper levels are usually decreased in the urine, in contrast to Wilson's disease. Elevated zinc levels are common. Anemia and neutropenia are common findings as well.

Treatment

- CDM is treated with copper supplementation, which can stabilize symptoms, though many patients do not improve. The radiographic abnormalities may improve with treatment as well.

References

1. Jaiser SR, Winston GP. Copper deficiency myelopathy. *J Neurol.* June 2010;257(6):869–881. doi:10.1007/s00415-010-5511-x. Epub March 16, 2010.
2. Kumar N, Gross JB Jr, Ahlskog JE. Copper deficiency myelopathy produces a clinical picture like subacute combined degeneration. *Neurology.* July 2004;63(1):33–39.
3. Kumar N, Ahlskog JE, Klein CJ, Port JD. Imaging features of copper deficiency myelopathy: a study of 25 cases. *Neuroradiology.* February 2006;48(2):78–83. Epub October 28, 2005.

11.10 Wernicke's Encephalopathy

Case History

A 64-year-old alcoholic man presented with confusion and ataxia. On exam, he was delirious, not knowing the date or location. He was unable to adduct either eye.

Diagnosis: Wernicke's Encephalopathy

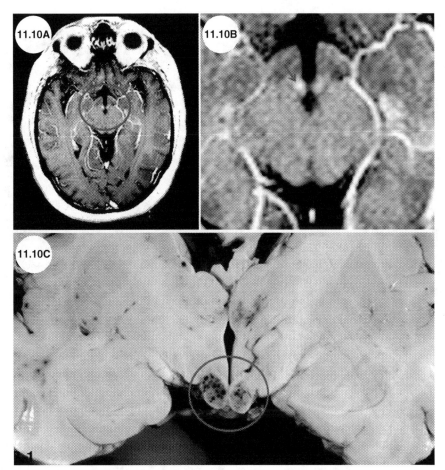

Images 11.10A and 11.10B: Postcontrast axial T1-weighted images demonstrate enhancement of the mammillary bodies (red circles and arrow). **Image 11.10C:** Gross pathology demonstrates petechiae in the mammillary bodies.

Introduction

- Wernicke–Korsakoff encephalopathy is due to a deficiency of thiamine (vitamin B1). It most commonly occurs in patients with chronic alcoholism, but can also occur in patients with poor nutritional intake due to eating disorders or prolonged vomiting, patients on chronic parenteral

---

nutrition, or as a complication of bariatric surgery or gastric malignancies.

Clinical Presentation

■ Wernicke's encephalopathy is characterized by the triad of delirium, ataxia, and ophthalmologic abnormalities, including nystagmus, ophthalmoparesis, and impaired pupillary reaction. Few patients present with this complete triad, and the most common symptoms are confusion and memory impairment. Most individuals have a 4- to 6-week store of thiamine; however, acute deficiency states can be triggered by glucose loading in patients with already low thiamine levels.

■ Korsakoff's psychosis is a more advanced form of the illness characterized by anterograde and retrograde amnesia, confabulation, and psychosis. It often follows Wernicke's encephalopathy in alcoholics, but is less common in other etiologies.

Radiographic Appearance and Diagnosis

■ T2-weighted image MRI reveals symmetrical hyperintensity in the mammillary bodies, medial

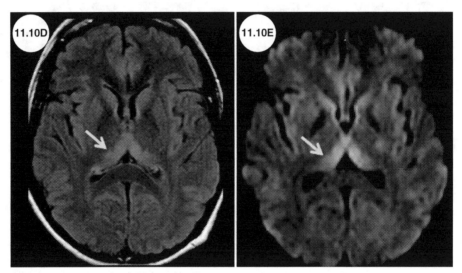

Images 11.10D and 11.10E: Axial FLAIR and diffusion-weighted images demonstrate hyperintensity and restricted diffusion of the posterior thalamus (yellow arrows).

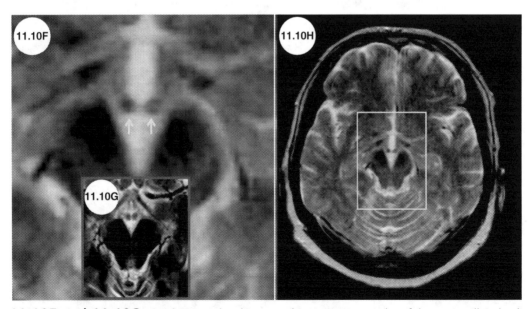

Images 11.10F and 11.10G: Axial T2-weighted images demonstrate atrophy of the mammillary bodies (yellow arrows). **Image 11.10H:** A normal MRI is shown for comparison.

thalami, quadrigeminal plate, and periaqueductal area.

- As seen in **Images 11.10A and 11.10B,** enhancement on postcontrast imaging is frequently seen, especially in alcoholics. Atrophy of the mammillary bodies is seen in chronic cases.

Treatment

- Treatment is with thiamine replacement.

References

1. Manzo G, De Gennaro A, Cozzolino A, Serino A, Fenza G, Manto A. MR imaging findings in alcoholic and nonalcoholic acute Wernicke's encephalopathy: a review. *Biomed Res Int.* 2014;2014:503596.
2. Sechi G, Serra A. Wernicke's encephalopathy: new clinical settings and recent advances in diagnosis and management. *Lancet Neurol.* May 2007;6(5):442–455.
3. Zuccoli G, Pipitone N. Neuroimaging findings in acute Wernicke's encephalopathy: review of the literature. *AJR Am J Roentgenol.* February 2009;192(2):501–508.

11.11 | Radiation Necrosis

Case History

A 39-year-old man presented with seizures and a right homonymous hemianopsia several years after being treated with radiation for an arteriovenous malformation (AVM).

Diagnosis: Radiation Necrosis

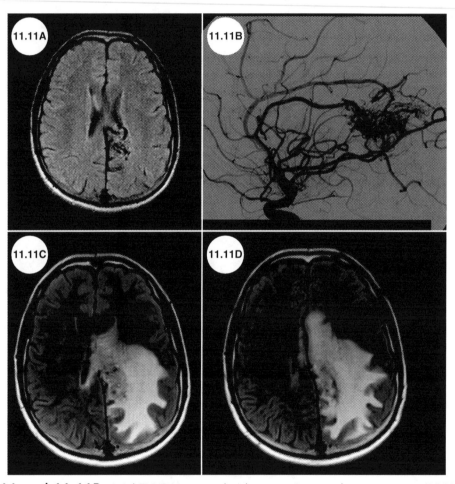

Images 11.11A and 11.11B: Axial FLAIR image and catheter angiogram demonstrate an AVM in the left occipital lobe due to an AVM. **Images 11.11C and 11.11D:** Axial FLAIR images demonstrate hyperintensity of the lesion and reactive edema after radiation.

Introduction

- Therapeutic radiation is used to treat cerebral malignancies and AVMs.

- Radiation necrosis refers to postradiation brain necrosis. Blood vessels are acutely vulnerable to radiation, leading to vasogenic edema. Oligodendrocytes are also vulnerable to radiation, leading to demyelination.

Clinical Presentation

- There are three stages of radiation-induced central nervous system (CNS) injury:

  1. **Acute encephalopathy** is due to disruption of the blood–brain barrier and occurs in the first month.

  2. **Early delayed complications** occur after 1 to 4 months and are characterized by vasogenic

edema and demyelination. Patients may present with encephalopathy or a return of their original tumor symptoms.

3. **Radiation necrosis** occurs after months to years. Patients present with seizures, recurrence of the initial tumor symptoms, or signs of increased intracranial pressure (ICP) if there is enough edema and mass effect.

Radiographic Appearance

■ There are a variety of radiographic appearances. On T2-weighted images, there is typically edema in the white matter with mass effect. With the addition of contrast, there may be cystic enhancement.

■ It may be difficult to distinguish radiation-induced changes from tumor recurrence. MR perfusion studies may be helpful in this setting,

as tumors show increased relative cerebral blood volume, while radiation necrosis does not.

■ Over time, there is atrophy of the necrotic area.

Treatment

■ Treatment is indicated in patients with symptoms due to mass effect and increased ICP. Steroids can be used, and are most effective in the acute and early delayed stages.

References

1. Miyatake S, Nonoguchi N, Furuse M, et al. Pathophysiology, diagnosis, and treatment of radiation necrosis in the brain. *Neurol Med Chir (Tokyo)*. 2015;55(Suppl. 1):50–59.
2. Na A, Haghigi N, Drummond KJ. Cerebral radiation necrosis. *Asia Pac J Clin Oncol*. March 2014;10(1):11–21.
3. Parvez K, Parvez A, Zadeh G. The diagnosis and treatment of pseudoprogression, radiation necrosis and brain tumor recurrence. *Int J Mol Sci*. July 2014;15(7):11832–11846.

11.12 | Carbon Monoxide

Case History

A 45-year-old man was found unconscious, his wife dead beside him.

Diagnosis: Carbon Monoxide Poisoning

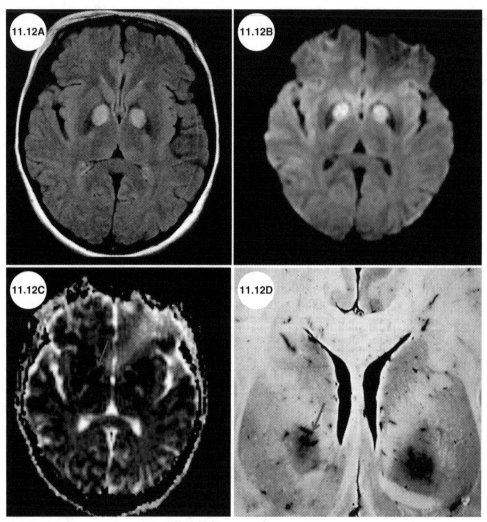

Images 11.12A–11.12C: Axial FLAIR, diffusion-weighted, and apparent diffusion coefficient map images demonstrate symmetric hyperintensity and restricted diffusion (red arrow) in the globus pallidus.
Image 11.12D: Gross pathology demonstrates multiple punctate hemorrhages in the globus pallidus.

Introduction

- Carbon monoxide (CO) is a colorless, odorless, tasteless, gas. CO combines with hemoglobin to form carboxyhemoglobin, which in turn prevents oxygen from binding to hemoglobin.

Clinical Presentation

- With mild cases, patients develop nonspecific symptoms such as nausea, headache, and fatigue. In more severe cases, patients develop apathy, rigidity, bradykinesia, and dystonia. In severe cases it is fatal. Patients may experience a delayed deterioration several weeks after the initial insult, manifested by depression, memory loss, and psychosis.

Radiographic Appearance and Diagnosis

■ On T2-weighted images, there is hyperintensity and restricted diffusion in the globus pallidus. Other characteristic findings are hippocampal and cerebellar injury and diffuse cerebral edema. Carboxyhemoglobin in the serum confirms the diagnosis.

Treatment

■ Acute treatment involves administering 100% oxygen or hyperbaric oxygen therapy, which hastens the removal of CO from hemoglobin.

References

1. Roderique JD, Josef CS, Feldman MJ, Spiess BD. A modern literature review of carbon monoxide poisoning theories, therapies, and potential targets for therapy advancement. *Toxicology*. August 2015;334:45–58.
2. Dubrey SW, Chehab O, Ghonim S. Carbon monoxide poisoning: an ancient and frequent cause of accidental death. *Br J Hosp Med (Lond)*. March 2015;76(3):159–162.
3. Weaver LK. Clinical practice. Carbon monoxide poisoning. *N Engl J Med*. March 2009;360(12):1217–1225.

11.13 Transient Signal Alterations in Splenium of Corpus Callosum

Case History

A 61-year-old man with epilepsy presented with several seizures in one day.

Diagnosis: Transient Hyperintensity of the Splenium of Corpus Callosum

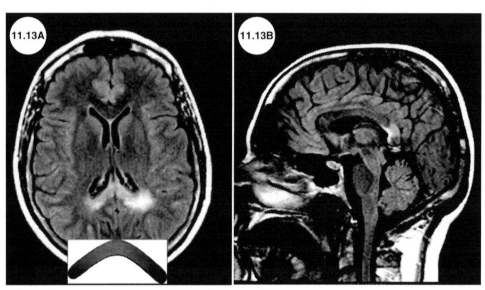

Images 11.13A and 11.13B: Axial and sagittal FLAIR images demonstrate hyperintensity within the splenium of the corpus callosum, the boomerang sign.

Introduction

■ The corpus callosum (CC) is the largest white matter tract connecting the two cerebral hemispheres. It is divided into three parts. From anterior to posterior these are the genu, body, and splenium.

■ Transient signal alterations in splenium of the CC are most commonly seen in patients suffering from focal status epilepticus or in patients who abruptly stop antiepileptic medications. A wide variety of other pathologies can cause this finding including infections, hypoglycemia, trauma, hyponatremia/hypernatremia, infections, posterior reversible encephalopathy syndrome, thiamine deficiency in alcoholics, hemolytic–uremic syndrome with encephalopathy, and hemicrania continua.

Clinical Presentation

■ Confusion and delirium are the most common presentations. Patients do not typically suffer from disconnection syndromes, such as alexia without agraphia, seen in other lesions of the splenium of the CC.

Radiographic Appearance and Diagnosis

■ There is hyperintensity on T2-weighted images involving the splenium of the CC. The radiographic appearance is known as the "boomerang" sign. The lesions are transient and improve or entirely resolve on subsequent imaging.

Treatment

■ Treatment is directed at the underlying cause. There is generally a good prognosis.

References

1. Hirsch KG, Hoesch RE. Boomerang sign on MRI. *Neurocrit Care*. 2012 Jun;16(3):450–451.
2. Malhotra HS, Garg RK, Vidhate MR, Sharma PK. Boomerang sign: Clinical significance of transient lesion in splenium of corpus callosum. *Ann Indian Acad Neurol*. April–June 2012;15(2):151–157.
3. Doherty MJ, Jayadev S, Watson NF, Konchada RS, Hallam DK. Clinical implications of splenium magnetic resonance imaging signal changes. *Arch Neurol*. March 2005;62(3):433–437.

CHAPTER 12

PEDIATRICS

12.1 Acute Cerebellar Ataxia

Case History

A 4-year-old boy presented with gait unsteadiness and increased falls several days after recovering from a flu-like illness.

Diagnosis: Acute Cerebellar Ataxia

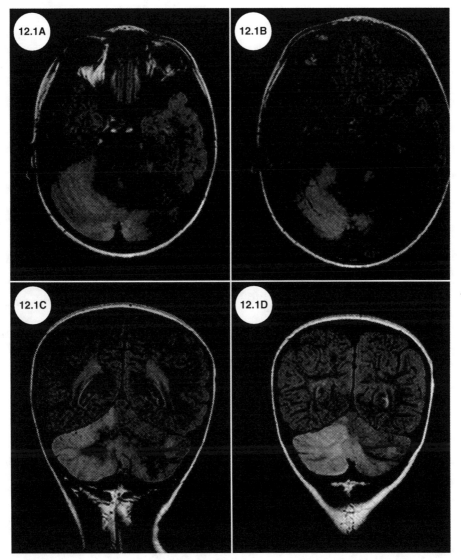

Images 12.1A–12.1D: Axial and coronal fluid-attenuated inversion recovery (FLAIR) images demonstrate hyperintensity of the cerebellum, the right more than the left, in a patient with acute cerebellar ataxia.

Introduction

■ Ataxia is a disturbance in the smooth, accurate coordination of the limbs, eyes, and gait, usually resulting from cerebellar dysfunction. Acute ataxia is defined as unsteadiness of walking or of fine motor movement, of less than 72 hours duration, in a previously well child.

■ Causes include infection, postinfectious inflammatory conditions, toxins, tumors, trauma, and vascular disorders. Most are benign and self-limiting, though some conditions are potentially life-threatening.

Clinical Presentation

■ Acute cerebellar ataxia is the most common cause of acute ataxia, representing 30% to 50% of cases. It affects children aged 2 to 5 years, with boys more affected than girls. It is a postinfectious condition, often seen after infection with the varicella or Epstein–Barr virus. It may also be seen after vaccination, though less commonly than with vaccine-preventable diseases.

■ It presents with an unsteady gait, ranging from a wide-based gait to the complete inability to walk. Examination reveals a wide-based, unsteady gait, characterized by lurching and staggering. Symptoms develop over hours to days.

■ Other signs of cerebellar dysfunction include dysarthria, abnormal truncal tone with titubation or sporadic jerking movements of the trunk, arm ataxia, nausea and vomiting, and nystagmus. On general examination, patients may exhibit evidence of viral exanthema.

Radiographic Appearance and Diagnosis

■ In acute cerebellar ataxia, the characteristic finding is hyperintensity of the cerebellum on T2-weighted images (T2WIs), which is often asymmetric. There may be restricted diffusion and mild cortical and meningeal enhancement with the addition of contrast. CT scans are less sensitive, but are appropriate to rule out life-threatening conditions, such as hydrocephalus, trauma, hemorrhage, and mass lesions.

■ There is no specific test to diagnose acute cerebellar ataxia. Though it is the most common cause of acute ataxia in children, life-threatening etiologies must be ruled out first. Accidental toxic ingestion is a common cause of acute ataxia in children, and should be investigated with a toxicology screen. Basic metabolic panel is important to evaluate for hypoglycemia. In select cases where there is concern for an underlying metabolic disorder, appropriate labs should be ordered.

■ Cerebrospinal fluid (CSF) analysis may reveal a mild protein elevation or a mild lymphocytic pleocytosis.

Treatment

■ Acute cerebellar ataxia is generally a self-limiting process, with most patients returning to normal after several weeks. Less than 10% of patients are left with permanent symptoms. In rare cases, cerebellar edema may lead to occlusion of the fourth ventricle and ventricular drainage may be lifesaving.

■ Some children have recurrent attacks, typically preceded by illness. Such patients are sometimes managed with immunotherapies prophylactically to shorten courses of symptoms.

References

1. Nussinovitch M, Prais D, Volovitz B, Shapiro R, Amir J. Post-infectious acute cerebellar ataxia in children. *Clin Pediatr (Phila)*. September 2003;42(7):581–584.
2. De Bruecker Y, Claus F, Demaerel P, Ballaux F, Sciot R, Lagae L, Buyse G, Wilms G. MRI findings in acute cerebellitis. *Eur Radiol*. August 2004;14(8):1478–1483.
3. Desai J, Mitchell WG. Acute cerebellar ataxia, acute cerebellitis, and opsoclonus-myoclonus syndrome. *J Child Neurol*. November 2012;27(11):1482–1488.

12.2 | Germinal Matrix Hemorrhage

Case History

A premature child had a routine head ultrasound.

Diagnosis: Germinal Matrix Hemorrhage

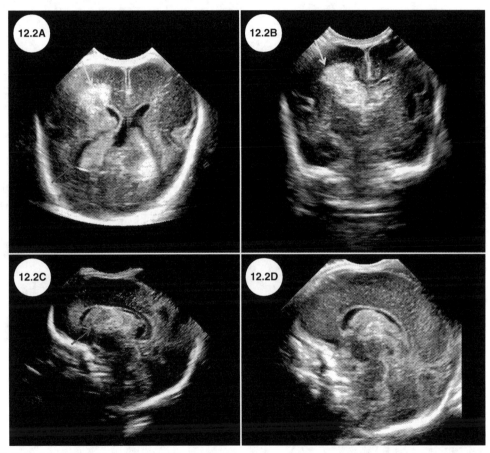

Images 12.2A–12.2D: Ultrasound showing blood throughout the ventricles (red arrows) and brain parenchyma (yellow arrows).

Introduction

■ The germinal matrix is a thick layer of immature neuronal and glial cells under the ependymal lining of the ventricles where glial and neuronal differentiation occurs during embryogenesis. Cells migrate peripherally from there using radial glia to form the cerebral cortex. It is densely vascular,

though the walls of the blood vessels are weak and vulnerable to ischemia with subsequent hemorrhage in premature infants. The risk of hemorrhage is directly related to the gestational age. Nearly 80% of infants born before 24 weeks have such hemorrhages, with the risk declining every week thereafter. Other risk factors include prolonged labor and low birthweight. By 35 to 36 weeks gestation the germinal matrix has disappeared and there is no risk of hemorrhage.

- Most hemorrhages are thought to occur during delivery or in the first few hours after birth. The bleeding occurs initially between the caudate nucleus and the thalamus, at the floor of the lateral ventricle near the foramen of Monro, an area known as the caudothalamic groove. Larger bleeds may expand into the lateral ventricles leading to an intraventricular hemorrhage (IVH).

Clinical Presentation

- The clinical outcome is directly related to the grade of the bleed. Grade I and II hemorrhages have a favorable outcome. There is a 20% to 25% mortality in grade III hemorrhages, and over 90% mortality with grade IV hemorrhages. Survivors are at high risk for cerebral palsy and mental retardation. Over 90% are found within 4 days of birth, and nearly half within 5 hours.

Radiographic Appearance and Diagnosis

- Suspected cases are best investigated with ultrasounds. As seen in **Images 12.2A–12.2C**, germinal

matrix hemorrhages are echogenic regions. The choroid plexus is normally located there, but any hemorrhage located anterior to this groove is pathological.

- Hemorrhages are graded on a four-point scale:

  1. **Grade I:** The bleed remains in the subependymal region.
  2. **Grade II:** The bleed extends into the ventricles, but fills less than half of the volume.
  3. **Grade III:** The blood fills and dilates the ventricles.
  4. **Grade IV:** The blood extends into the brain parenchyma. Examples are shown in **Images 12.2A–12.2C**.

- In **Images 12.2A–12.2D**, a grade IV IVH is shown on the right, and a grade III IVH is shown on the left.

- Complications of survivors include hydrocephalus.

- Another complication is periventricular white matter infarction, which is thought to be a venous infarct of the white matter adjacent to the hemorrhage. Other patients may develop porencephalic cysts.

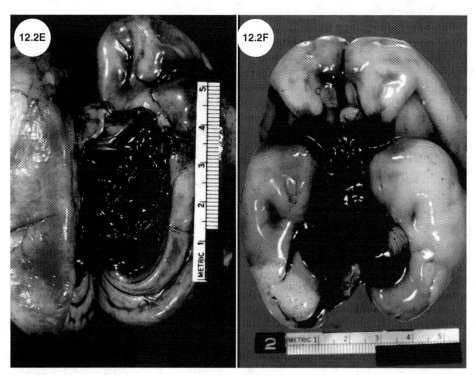

Images 12.2E and 12.2F: Gross pathology of grade 4 IVHs (image credit www.wikidoc.org via Professor Peter Anderson, DVM, PhD, and published with permission © PEIR, University of Alabama at Birmingham, Department of Pathology).

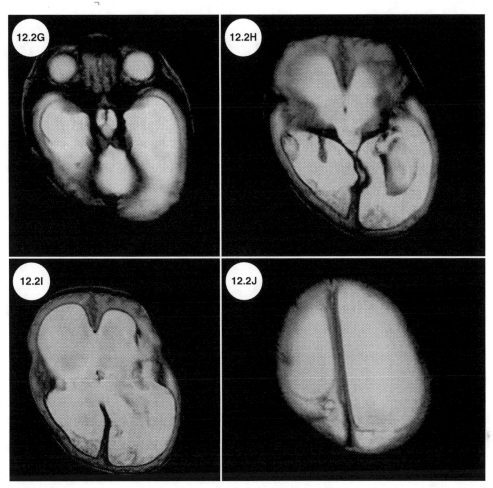

Images 12.2G–12.2J: Axial T2-weighted images demonstrate massive hydrocephalus in an infant who suffered a grade IV IVH.

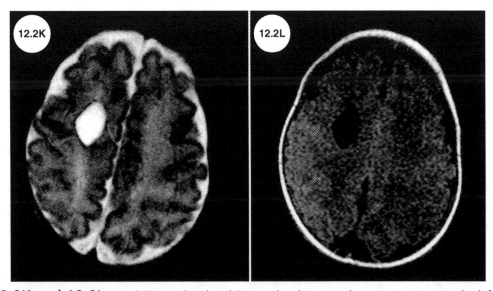

Images 12.2K and 12.2L: Axial T2-weighted and T1-weighted images demonstrate a cyst in the left frontal lobe. This is the same patient whose ultrasound is shown in Images 12.2A–12.2D.

Treatment

■ In grade III and IV hemorrhages, CSF drainage may be attempted to relieve hydrocephalus. Postnatal administration of phenobarbital was found to increase the need for mechanical ventilation.

References

1. Fukui K, Morioka T, Nishio S, et al. Fetal germinal matrix and intraventricular haemorrhage diagnosed by MRI. *Neuroradiology*. January 2001;43(1):68–72.

2. Woodward LJ, Andeson PJ, Austin NC, Howard K, Inder TE. Neonatal MRI to predict neurodevelopmental outcomes in preterm infants. *N Engl J Med*. 2006;355:685–694.

3. Ballabh P. Intraventricular hemorrhage in premature infants: mechanism of disease. *Pediatr Res*. 2010;67:1–8.

4. Meneguel JF, Guinsburg R, Miyoshi MH, et al. Antenatal treatment with corticosteroids for preterm neonates: impact on the incidence of respiratory distress syndrome and intra-hospital mortality. *Sao Paulo Med J*. March 2003;121(2): 45–52.

5. McCrea HJ, Ment LR. The diagnosis, management, and post-natal prevention of intraventricular hemorrhage in the preterm neonate. *Clin Perinatol*. December 2008;35(4):777–792.

12.3 | Hypoxic-Ischemic Encephalopathy

Case History

A newborn infant was found to have low Apgar scores and was unable to breathe independently after labor was complicated by placental abruption.

Diagnosis: Hypoxic-Ischemic Encephalopathy

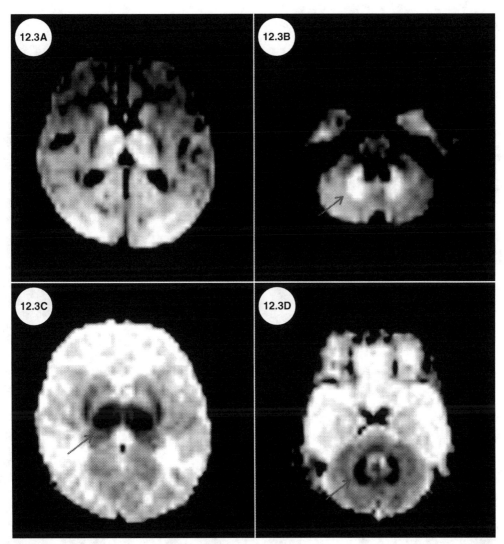

Images 12.3A–12.3D: Diffusion-weighted images and apparent diffusion coefficient (ADC) map demonstrate restricted diffusion of the thalami (red arrows).

Introduction

■ Hypoxic-ischemic encephalopathy (HIE) occurs in a newborn when there is global hypoxic-ischemic brain injury.

Clinical Presentation

■ Severely affected newborns have low Apgar scores at birth. Within 24 hours, they develop seizures and apnea. Patients with mild injury may make a full recovery, but survivors suffer from a spectrum of cerebral palsy and seizures. It accounts for approximately 25% of neonatal deaths. The prognosis for preterm infants is worse. Mildly affected infants may have no immediate symptoms, but are at risk of spastic weakness, cognitive delay, and vision and hearing impairments.

Radiographic Appearance and Diagnosis

■ MRI is the modality of choice to image neonates with suspected HIE. There is a variable appearance depending on whether the ischemia is total or partial, whether the infant is preterm or term, and the timing of the imaging after the injury. Though there is some overlap, several main patterns are recognized in HIE. In order of descending frequency, they are:

1. **Watershed Injury.** The white matter and cortex of the vascular watershed areas are vulnerable to injury. The changes can be unilateral or bilateral and are first visible on diffusion-weighted images.

■ Necrosis of the periventricular white matter is seen and is referred to as periventricular

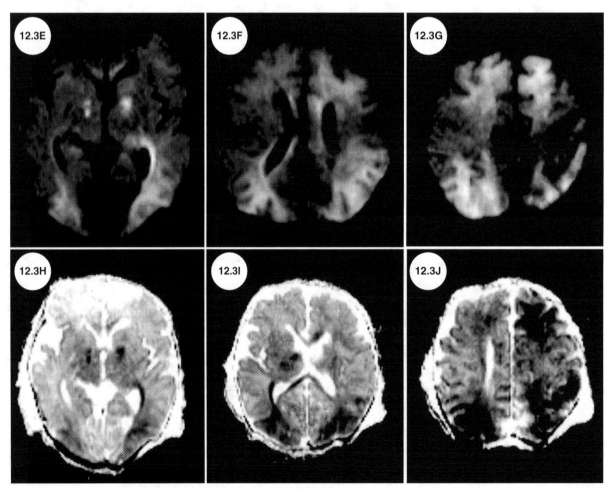

Images 12.3E–12.3J: Diffusion-weighted images and ADC map demonstrate acute infarctions of the bilateral frontal and occipital lobes and deep gray matter in a newborn with HIE.

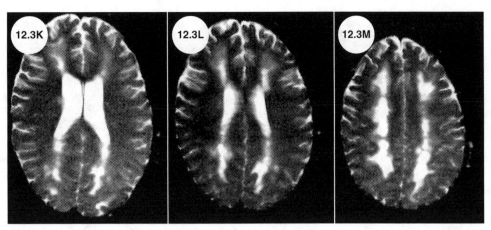

Images 12.3K–12.3M: Axial T2-weighted images demonstrate extensive periventricular white matter hyperintensities due to periventricular leukomalacia.

leukomalacia. This is followed by cyst formation and eventually parenchymal loss and hydro-cephalus ex vacuo.

2. **Basal Ganglia and Thalamic Lesions.** This occurs after acute and severe hypoxia in term birth. Mechanisms include a ruptured uterus, placental abruption, or cord prolapse. The earliest and most sensitive finding is restricted diffusion in the thalami, posterior limb of the internal capsule, and/or basal ganglia, as seen in **Images 12.3A and 12.3B**. Other characteristic findings include hyperintensity on unenhanced T1-weighted images (T1WIs) in the thalami and basal ganglia. The brainstem can also be involved in severe cases.

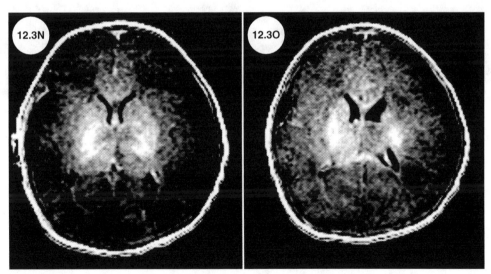

Images 12.3N and 12.3O: Axial T1-weighted images demonstrate hyperintensity of the basal ganglia, thalamus, and brainstem in an infant with HIE.

■ In normal, full-term newborns, the posterior limb of the internal capsule is hyperintense on T1WI and hypointense on T2WI. In infants with severe, acute HIE, absence of normal hyperintensity on T1WI is characteristic, and is known as the "absent posterior limb sign."

3. **Multicystic Encephalopathy.** Multicystic encephalopathy occurs after infants experience mild signs of hypoxia ischemia, followed by an unexpectedly severe encephalopathy, most commonly after term birth. The presumed mechanism is a protracted, difficult

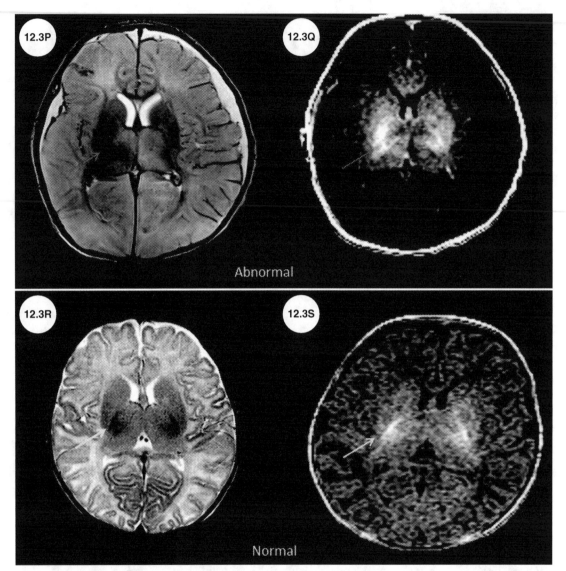

Images 12.3P and 12.3Q: Axial T2-weighted and T1-weighted images demonstrate hyperintensity of the brainstem, basal ganglia, and thalami. There is hypointensity of the posterior limb of the internal capsule (red arrows).
Images 12.3R and 12.3S: Axial T2-weighted and T1-weighted images demonstrate normal hypointensity and hyperintensity of the posterior limb of the internal capsule (yellow arrows).

delivery. It presents radiographically with multiple cysts of the white matter and cerebral cortex. The cystic cavities are traversed by a web of delicate glial strands and contain fluid, debris, and macrophages. Ulegyria refers to shrunken deep cortical gyri, usually in the parasagittal region. It is one of the leading causes of epilepsy arising from the posterior cortex.

▨ Over time, severe cases of multicystic encephalopathy may cause necrosis such that the brain

essentially vanishes, leaving only the meninges remaining.

Treatment

▨ A number of randomized controlled trials have shown that therapeutic hypothermia is beneficial in term and late preterm newborns with HIE in both reducing mortality and improving neurodevelopment outcomes in both term and preterm infants if started before 6 hours of age.

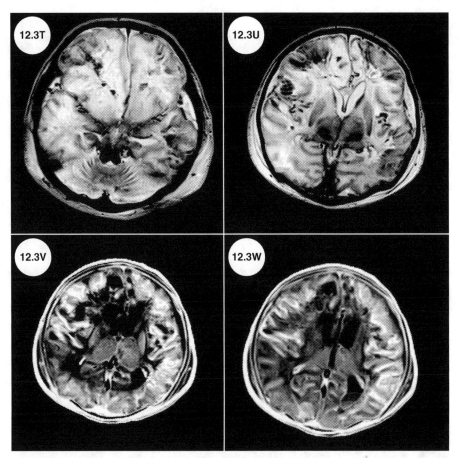

Images 12.3T–12.3W: Axial T2-weighted and T1-weighted images demonstrate diffuse cortical signal abnormality in a patient and cystic changes in the white matter in a patient with multicystic encephalopathy.

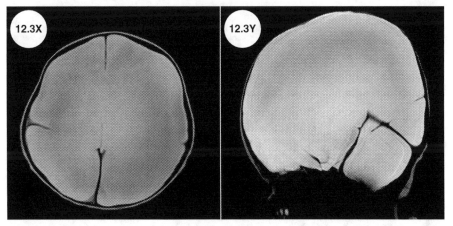

Images 12.3X and 12.3Y: Axial and sagittal T2-weighted images demonstrate complete loss of the brain in a child with severe HIE.

References

1. Heinz ER, Provenzale JM. Imaging findings in neonatal hypoxia: a practical review. *AJR Am J Roentgenol.* January 2009;192(1):41–47.
2. Cabaj A, Bekiesińska-Figatowska M, Mądzik J. MRI patterns of hypoxic-ischemic brain injury in preterm and full term infants—classical and less common MR findings. *Pol J Radiol.* July–September 2012;77(3):71–76.
3. Jacobs SE, Berg M, Hunt R, Tarnow-Mordi WO, Inder TE, Davis PG. Cooling for newborns with hypoxic ischaemic encephalopathy. *Cochrane Database Syst Rev.* January 2013:1.
4. de Vries LS, Groenendaal F. Patterns of neonatal hypoxic–ischaemic brain injury. *Neuroradiology.* June 2010;52(6): 555–566.
5. Douglas-Escobar M, Weiss MD. Hypoxic-ischemic encephalopathy: a review for the clinician. *JAMA Pediatr.* April 2015;169(4):397–403.

12.4 | Mitochondrial Encephalomyopathy, Lactic Acidosis, and Stroke-Like Episodes (MELAS)

Case History

A 10-year-old boy presented with acute visual loss and headaches. A similar episode happened two years ago. He was found to have a right homonymous hemianopsia on examination.

Diagnosis: Mitochondrial Encephalomyopathy, Lactic Acidosis, and Stroke-Like Episodes (MELAS)

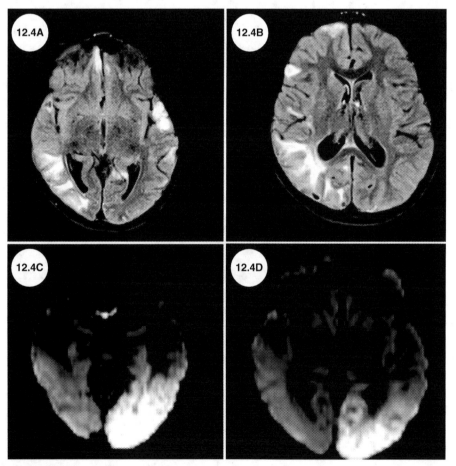

Images 12.4A–12.4D: Axial FLAIR and diffusion-weighted images demonstrate acute infarction in the left temporal and occipital lobes and older lesions in the right occipital and frontal and bilateral temporal lobes in a patient with MELAS.

Introduction

■ MELAS is a rare mitochondrial disorder that results from mutations in multiple different genes. As it is a mitochondrial disorder, the condition is inherited only from mothers, though both sexes are equally affected.

Clinical Presentation

■ It presents in patients under 40 with weakness, myalgias, headaches, loss of appetite, vomiting, and seizures. Patients have "stroke-like" events, which are so named because they often do not conform to specific vascular territories. Clinically, the episodes present with hemiparesis, encephalopathy, deafness, visual field defects, aphasia, and headaches. Though they may be temporary initially, there is permanent damage over time. Generalized and partial seizures can occur. Dementia is common at the end stage of the illness.

■ Lactic acidosis can lead to muscle pain, weakness, spasms, and fatigue as well as gastrointestinal (GI) disturbances (vomiting, incontinence, and abdominal pain), and dyspnea.

■ Non-neurological symptoms include endocrinopathies, short stature, renal impairment, and cardiac dysfunction.

Radiographic Appearance and Diagnosis

■ MRI shows infarctions, primarily in the parietal, occipital, or posterior temporal lobes. They may be symmetric or asymmetric, and acute infarctions will show restricted diffusion.

■ Basal ganglia calcifications are common in older patients and are best seen on CT.

■ **MR spectroscopy** may demonstrate elevated lactate level, even in normal-appearing brain and CSF.

■ Ragged red fibers are a characteristic finding on muscle biopsy.

■ Elevated lactic acid can be found in the serum.

Treatment

■ The disease is progressive and eventually fatal. Though controlled trials are lacking, a number of supplements and antioxidants have shown benefits including CoQ10, L-carnitine,

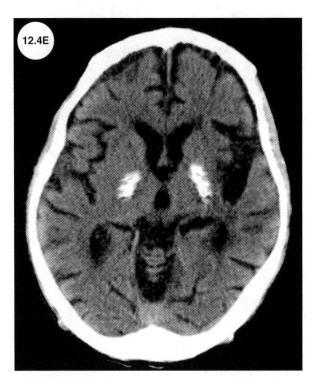

Image 12.4E: Axial CT image demonstrates bilateral basal ganglia calcifications.

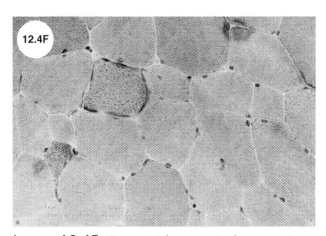

Image 12.4F: Gomori trichrome stain demonstrating ragged red fibers in a patient with MELAS (photo credit Nephron).

citrulline, arginine, and vitamins K-3 and K-1. MELAS patients have a decreased nitrous oxide dependent vasodilation, and this may represent a future therapeutic target. Management of seizures and other symptoms is paramount.

References

1. Santa KM. Treatment options for mitochondrial myopathy, encephalopathy, lactic acidosis, and stroke-like episodes (MELAS) syndrome. *Pharmacotherapy.* November 2010;30(11):1179–1196.

2. El-Hattab AW, Emrick LT, Chanprasert S, Craigen WJ, Scaglia F. Mitochondria: role of citrulline and arginine supplementation in MELAS syndrome. *Int J Biochem Cell Biol*. March 2014;48:85–91.

3. El-Hattab AW, Adesina AM, Jones J, Scaglia F. MELAS syndrome: Clinical manifestations, pathogenesis, and treatment options. *Mol Genet Metab*. September–October 2015;116(1–2):4–12.

4. Koga Y, Povalko N, Nishioka J, Katayama K, Yatsuga S, Matsuishi T. Molecular pathology of MELAS and L-arginine effects. *Biochim Biophys Acta*. May 2012;1820(5):608–614.

5. El-Hattab AW, Emrick LT, Craigen WJ, Scaglia F. Citrulline and arginine utility in treating nitric oxide deficiency in mitochondrial disorders. *Mol Genet Metab*. November 2012;107(3): 247–252.

12.5 | Septo-Optic Dysplasia

Case History

A 2-year-old child presented with short stature. He had nystagmus as an infant.

Diagnosis: Septo-Optic Dysplasia

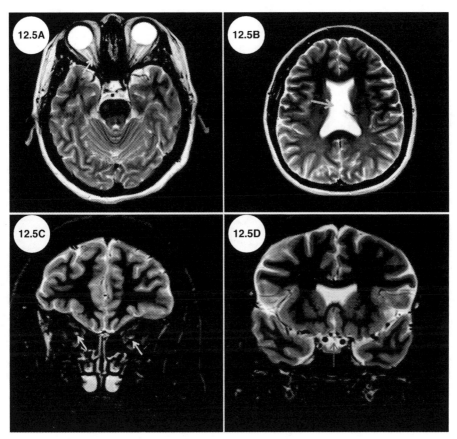

Images 12.5A–12.5D: Axial and coronal T2-weighted images demonstrate atrophy of the optic nerves (yellow arrows) and chiasm (red arrow) as well as absence of the septum pellucidum (blue arrow).

Introduction

■ Septo-optic dysplasia (SOD) is a congenital disorder characterized by:

  ▩ Absence of septum pellucidum

  ▩ Hypoplasia of the optic nerves

  ▩ Hypoplasia of the pituitary gland

■ Two of these three features are needed for diagnosis, and only one-third of patients have all three.

■ It is rare, affecting about 1:10,000 newborns.

■ There is no single cause, but it has been linked to young maternal age, maternal diabetes, substance use during pregnancy, and certain medications. It is sporadic in most cases, but in some families, a genetic cause has been discovered.

Clinical Presentation

■ There is a highly variable clinical presentation. Patients present with visual dysfunction, which ranges from a mild decrease in visual acuity to total blindness. Nystagmus is common in infants. Similarly, there is a wide range of dysfunction of the pituitary–hypothalamic axis. Deficiency of growth hormone is the most common symptom. Severe cases cause panhypopituitarism, and newborns suffer from neonatal jaundice and hypoglycemia. Some patients suffer seizures, and while most patients have cognitive dysfunction, some have normal intellectual functioning.

Radiographic Appearance and Diagnosis

■ The findings of SOD are best visualized on MRI. It will show absence of the septum pellucidum as well as hypoplasia of the pituitary stalk and optic nerves/chiasm.

■ It is associated with schizencephaly in 50% of cases as well as holoprosencephaly and cortical malformations, such as polymicrogyria (PMG) and cortical dysplasia.

Treatment

■ Replacement of pituitary hormones is the mainstay of treatment along with antiepileptic medications.

References

1. Maurya VK, Ravikumar R, Bhatia M, Rai R. Septo-optic dysplasia: Magnetic Resonance Imaging findings. *Med J Armed Forces India.* July 2015;71(3):287–289.
2. Shammas NW, Brown JD, Foreman BW, Marutani DR, Maddela D, Tonner D. Septo-optic dysplasia associated with polyendocrine dysfunction. *J Med.* 1993;24(1):67–74.
3. Campbell CL. Septo-optic dysplasia: a literature review. *Optometry.* July 2003;74(7):417–426.

12.6 | Aicardi Syndrome

Case History

A 4-month-old infant presented with infantile spasms.

Diagnosis: Aicardi Syndrome

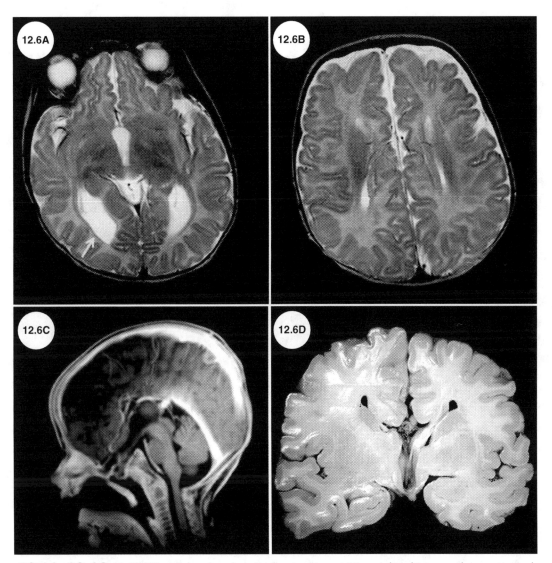

Images 12.6A–12.6C: Axial T2-weighted and sagittal postcontrast T1-weighted images demonstrate absence of the corpus callosum (red arrows), dilatation of the occipital horns of the lateral ventricles (yellow arrow), and mild cerebellar hypoplasia. **Image 12.6D:** Gross pathology demonstrates absence of the corpus callosum.

Introduction

■ **Aicardi syndrome** is a rare X-linked genetic developmental disorder. Mostly females are affected as this disorder can be fatal in males except those with 47XXY karyotype (Klinefelter syndrome). All cases are sporadic.

■ It affects less than 1 in 100,000 newborns.

Clinical Presentation

■ It presents due to pathology of the eye, brain, and spine. There is a wide spectrum of severity.

■ Infantile spasms are the common presenting feature and start around 5 months of age. Seizures are often progressive and refractory to medications. Intellectual disability and microcephaly are common.

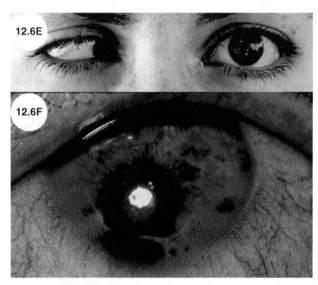

Image 12.6E: Microphthalmia of the right eye (image credit Etan J. Tal). **Image 12.6F:** Coloboma (image credit National Eye Institute).

■ Chorioretinal lacunes are holes in the pigmented layer of the retina adjacent to the optic disc and are consistently found in aqueductal stenosis. Other ocular abnormalities include microphthalmia (small or poorly developed eyes) and a coloboma (a gap or hole in the optic nerve). Blindness is common.

■ In the spine, scoliosis and spina bifida are common as are dysmorphic facial features.

■ Many patients have GI disturbances including reflux, constipation, and poor feeding.

Radiographic Appearance and Diagnosis

■ Agenesis or malformation of the corpus callosum is a characteristic feature. Cerebellar hypoplasia is seen in over 90% of cases. Other findings include microcephaly, polymicrogyria porencephalic cysts, and colpocephaly (enlargement of the occipital horns of the lateral ventricle).

Treatment

■ There is no direct treatment. Treatment involves controlling of seizures and therapy for developmental delay. Porencephalic cysts may require surgical drainage, and hydrocephalus may require shunting.

References

1. Crow YJ. Aicardi-Goutières syndrome. *Handb Clin Neurol.* 2013;113:1629–1635.
2. Crow YJ, Livingston JH. Aicardi-Goutières syndrome: an important Mendelian mimic of congenital infection. *Dev Med Child Neurol.* June 2008;50(6):410–416.
3. Hopkins B, Sutton VR, Lewis RA, Van den Veyver I, Clark G. Neuroimaging aspects of Aicardi syndrome. *Am J Med Genet A.* November 2008;146A(22):2871–2878.

12.7 Joubert's Syndrome

Case History

A 2-year-old child presented with developmental delay and macrocephaly. The child was hypotonic, but with brisk reflexes on exam.

Diagnosis: Joubert's Syndrome

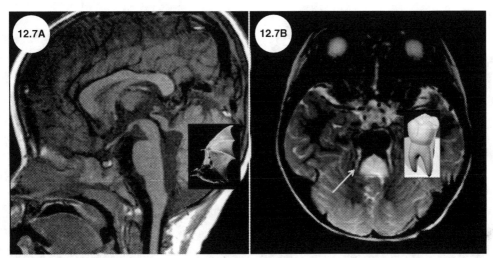

Images 12.7A and 12.7B: Sagittal T1-weighted and axial T2-weighted images demonstrate atrophy of the cerebellar vermis, creating the "bat-wing" appearance of the fourth ventricle (red arrow) and "molar tooth" sign. The dentate nuclei of the cerebellum are dysplastic (yellow arrow).

Introduction

- Joubert's syndrome is a ciliopathy, a genetic disorder of the cellular cilia, that causes abnormal development of the brainstem and atrophy of the cerebellar vermis.

- It affects 1 in 80,000 and 1 in 100,000 newborns. It has an autosomal-recessive pattern of inheritance and at least 20 different genes have been discovered.

Clinical Presentation

- Infants present with hypotonia, which evolves into ataxia in early childhood. Additional features include episodes of tachypnea or bradypnea, nystagmus, and poor smooth pursuit.

- Distinctive facial features include a broad forehead, arched eyebrows, ptosis, widely spaced eyes, low-set ears, cleft lip or palate, and a triangle-shaped mouth. Some patients have polydactyly and renal or hepatic dysfunction. Nearly half of the cases have retinal dysplasia. Intellectual disability is common and ranges from moderate to severe.

Radiographic Appearance

- Atrophy of the cerebellar vermis leads to enlargement of the fourth ventricle, which takes on a "bat-wing" appearance on sagittal images. On axial images, the shape of the brainstem takes on a "molar tooth" appearance. There is often dysplasia or heterotopia of cerebellar and inferior olivary nuclei.

Treatment

- There is no direct treatment, and physical, occupational, and speech therapy are the main treatment modalities.

References

1. Kumandas S, Akcakus M, Coskun A, Gumus H. Joubert syndrome: review and report of seven new cases. *Eur J Neurol.* August 2004;11(8):505–510.
2. Brancati F, Dallapiccola B, Valente EM. Joubert Syndrome and related disorders. *Orphanet J Rare Dis.* July 2010;5:20.

12.8 | Fabry's Disease

Case History

A 9-year-old boy presented with pain in his legs when playing soccer and pain when eating.

Diagnosis: Fabry's Disease

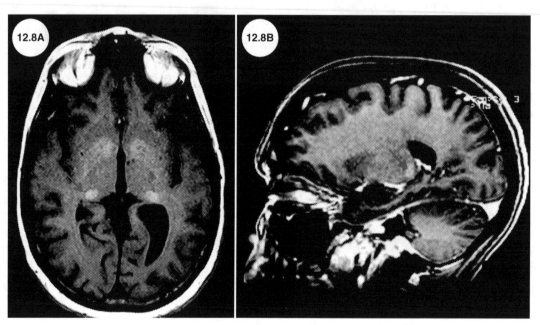

Images 12.8A and 12.8B: Axial and sagittal T1-weighted images demonstrate round hyperintensities in the pulvinar nuclei of the thalamus (red arrows).

Introduction

■ Fabry's disease is due to a deficiency of the enzyme *alpha-galactosidase-A (GLA)*, which degrades a lipid called globotriaosylceramide. Inadequate breakdown results in harmful lipid accumulation in the blood vessels of the heart, eyes, kidneys, and nervous system.

■ It is the only X-linked lipid storage disease, affecting 1 in 40,000 to 60,000 males. However, it is unique in that it may cause significant morbidity in females who inherit a single altered copy of the *GLA* gene, though symptoms are typically milder and begin at a later age.

Clinical Presentation

■ It manifests in childhood or adolescence. Symptoms include:

  ▪ **Acroparesthesias:** a painful, burning sensation in the extremities that may be exacerbated by heat and exercise

  ▪ **Gastrointestinal pain:** lipid accumulation in the microvasculature of the GI tract can obstruct blood flow and cause pain

  ▪ **Renal insufficiency**

  ▪ **Cardiomyopathy**

  ▪ **Anhidrosis:** decreased or absent sweating

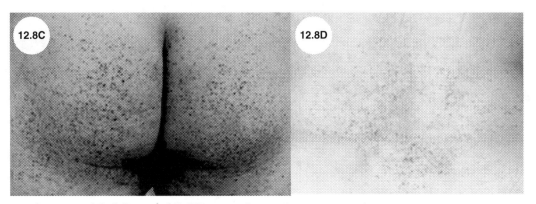

Images 12.8C and 12.8D: Angiokeratomas (image credit Dominique P. Germain).

- **Hearing loss and tinnitus**
- **Autonomic dysfunction:** Patients have decreased sweating.
- **Angiokeratomas:** Small, dark red or purple papules found on the abdomen, buttocks, thighs, and groin.
- **Ocular involvement:** Clouding of the corneas and corneal verticillata, which are whorl-like golden brown or gray deposits in the inferior interpalpebral portion of the cornea.

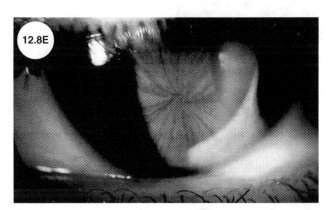

Image 12.8E: Cornea verticillata (image credit Alessandro P Burlina, Katherine B Sims, Juan M Politei, Gary J Bennett, Ralf Baron, Claudia Sommer, Anette Torvin Møller, and Max J Hilz: Early diagnosis of peripheral nervous system involvement in Fabry disease and treatment of neuropathic pain: the report of an expert panel. In: BMC Neurology 2011, 11:61).

Radiographic Appearance and Diagnosis

- Unenhanced T1-weighted images show hyperintensity of the pulvinar nucleus of the thalamus. This is known as the "pulvinar" sign, and may also be seen in other diseases, such as Creutzfeldt–Jakob disease.

- The diagnosis is made by measuring the level of alpha-galactosidase activity in leukocytes.

Treatment

- Enzyme replacement therapy with hydroxylase alpha-galactosidase is the mainstay of treatment. Many patients require dialysis or kidney transplants. Life expectancy is decreased by several decades due to strokes, heart attacks, and renal failure.

References

1. Mehta A, Beck M, Eyskens F, et al. Fabry disease: a review of current management strategies. *QJM*. September 2010;103(9):641–659.
2. Laney DA, Peck DS, Atherton AM, et al. Fabry disease in infancy and early childhood: a systematic literature review. *Genet Med*. May 2015;17(5):323–330.
3. Schaefer RM, Tylki-Szymańska A, Hilz MJ. Enzyme replacement therapy for Fabry disease: a systematic review of available evidence. *Drugs*. November 2009;69(16): 2179–2205.

12.9 Pantothenate Kinase-Associated Neurodegeneration

Case History

A 7-year-old child presented with trouble walking due to leg stiffness.

Diagnosis: Pantothenate Kinase-Associated Neurodegeneration

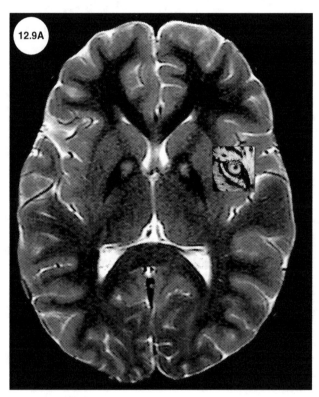

Image 12.9A: Axial T2-weighted image demonstrates hypointensity in bilateral globus pallidus with a central hyperintensity, the "eye of the tiger" sign.

Introduction

- Pantothenate kinase-associated neurodegeneration (formerly Hallervorden–Spatz syndrome) is a rare autosomal-recessive disorder caused by a mutation in the pantothenate kinase gene (*PANK2*), located on chromosome 20. It is essential to form coenzyme A, and is active in mitochondria.

- Deficiency of this enzyme leads to accumulation of N-pantothenoyl-cysteine and pantetheine. This in turn leads to accumulation of iron chelates in the brain, specifically in the globus pallidus and the substantia nigra. It is the most common disease in a family of diseases collectively known as **neurodegeneration with brain iron accumulation**.

- It is a rare disease, affecting 1 to 3 per million people.

Clinical Presentation

■ The illness begins in childhood, usually before 6 years. Gait disturbances are the usual presenting symptom. Patients develop dystonia and a variety of parkinsonian symptoms (rigidity, tremors), dysphagia, dysarthria, as well as progressive cognitive defects. Retinitis pigmentosa causes nyctalopia (night blindness) in most patients, which eventually progresses to complete blindness. Physical examination often reveals spasticity and upgoing toes.

■ About 25% of patients have an "atypical form." They present after 10 years, sometimes as late as 40 years, with speech deficits and psychiatric disturbances. Retinal dysfunction is rare in these patients. Disease progression is slower in these patients.

Radiographic Appearance and Diagnosis

■ T2WIs demonstrate hypointensity of the globus pallidus and pars reticulata of the substantia nigra. A central hyperintensity within the medial globus pallidus creates the "eye of the tiger" sign. In advanced cases, there may be atrophy of the head of the caudate.

■ Fundoscopy will reveal optic nerve pallor, pigment deposits in the retina, and thin retinal vessels characteristic of retinitis pigmentosa.

■ Genetic tests can confirm the diagnosis.

Treatment

■ There is no direct treatment, and the goal is alleviating symptoms with physical and occupational therapy. Oral dystonia may lead to tongue trauma,

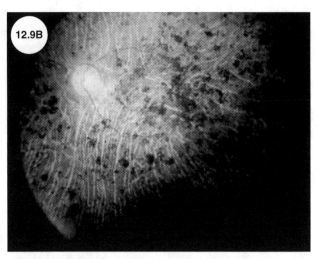

Image 12.9B: Fundoscopy reveals the characteristic findings of retinitis pigmentosa (image credit Christian Hamel).

severe enough to require dental extraction. It is fatal in early adulthood, usually due to secondary infections.

References

1. Hayflick SJ. Unraveling the Hallervorden-Spatz syndrome: pantothenate kinase-associated neurodegeneration is the name. *Curr Opin Pediatr.* December 2003;15(6):572–577.
2. Hayflick SJ, Hartman M, Coryell J, Gitschier J, Rowley H. Brain MRI in neurodegeneration with brain iron accumulation with and without PANK2 mutations. *AJNR Am J Neuroradiol.* June–July 2006;27(6):1230–1233.
3. Thomas M, Hayflick SJ, Jankovic J. Clinical heterogeneity of neurodegeneration with brain iron accumulation (Hallervorden-Spatz syndrome) and pantothenate kinase-associated neurodegeneration. *Mov Disord.* January 2004;19(1): 36–42.
4. Gregory A, Hayflick SJ. Pantothenate Kinase-Associated Neurodegeneration. *Gene Reviews.* http://www.ncbi.nlm.nih.gov/books/NBK1490.

12.10 Polymicrogyria

Case History

A 4-year-old child presented with developmental delay and partial seizures.

Diagnosis: Polymicrogyria

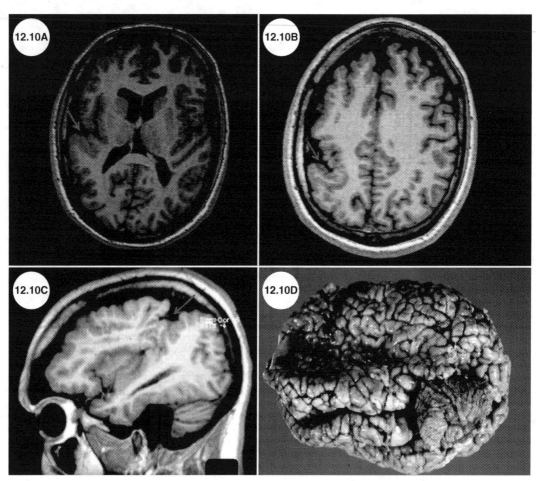

Images 12.10A–12.10C: Axial and sagittal T1-weighted images demonstrate polymicrogyria on the right, around the Sylvian fissure (red arrows). **Image 12.10D:** Gross image of polymicrogyria.

Source: www.wikidoc.org/index.php/File:Arnold-Chiari_Malformation_0003.jpg

Introduction

■ Polymicrogyria (PMG) is a disorder of cortical neuronal organization and is thought to be due to a postmigrational disorder that occurs after the 20th week of gestation. In PMG, there are multiple small gyri separated by shallow sulci. The cortex has an irregular, serrated, or pebble-like appearance. It can affect small or large areas and can be unilateral or bilateral. In the most severe cases, the entire brain is affected.

■ Classic or idiopathic PMG is typically located in the peri-Sylvian fissures, likely because this area

All pathological images in this chapter are courtesy of Roberta J Seidman, MD, Associate Professor, Stony Brook School of Medicine, Department of Pathology, unless otherwise noted.

is more susceptible to intrauterine ischemic injuries. It is bilateral in 50% of patients, though often asymmetric. Secondary PMG is typically the result of cytomegalovirus (CMV) infection. It can be mild or severe, in which case it is associated with schizencephaly and microcephaly.

- It has also been described in association with several genetic syndromes including 22q11.2 deletion syndrome, Aicardi syndrome, oculocerebrocutaneous syndrome, Adams–Oliver syndrome, Joubert's syndrome, Galloway–Mowat syndrome, and Zellweger syndrome. In these cases, it is typically bilateral and symmetric. A severe form called bilateral frontoparietal PMG is due to a mutation in a gene known as *GPR56*, which is inherited in an autosomal-recessive pattern.

Clinical Presentation

- The clinical presentation varies depending on the degree and location of cortical involvement. The most severe cases can have encephalopathy, spastic paresis, cerebellar dysfunction, dysphagia, dysconjugate gaze, mental retardation, and medication-refractory epilepsy.

- In milder cases of unilateral focal PMG, there may be only a slight language delay or patients can be entirely normal.

Radiographic Appearance and Diagnosis

- On MRI, the cortex is serrated or thickened, though of normal signal intensity. There is reduced white matter volume and decreased interdigitation between the gray and white matter. White matter hyperintensity on T2-weighted images reflects undermyelination. Additional imaging findings include thin cortical ribbon, aberrant sulcation, shallow or deep sulci, decreased white matter volume, ventriculomegaly, thin interhemispheric commissures, hypoplasia of cerebral peduncles/pons/medullary pyramids, patterns of delayed myelination, and dysplastic vessels.

- Significant white matter hyperintensity on T2-weighted images, particularly in subcortical and periventricular regions, is highly suggestive of CMV infection. Calcifications are frequently seen in patients with congenital CMV.

- 45% of patients have an abnormal electroencephalogram (EEG), with the abnormality localized primarily to the frontal and temporal lobes. The severity of the EEG abnormality correlates with the extent of the abnormal cortex. PMG can be associated with electrical status epilepticus of sleep even when seizures are not a predominant feature of the patient's condition.

Treatment

- Treatment is symptomatic and primarily is aimed at controlling seizures, though many patients have medication-refractory epilepsy.

References

1. Teixeira KC, Montenegro MA, Cendes F, et al. Clinical and electroencephalographic features of patients with polymicrogyria. *J Clin Neurophysiol.* June 2007;24(3):244–251.
2. Stutterd CA, Leventer RJ. Polymicrogyria: a common and heterogeneous malformation of cortical development. *Am J Med Genet C Semin Med Genet.* June 2014;166C(2):227–239.
3. Guerrini R. Polymicrogyria and epilepsy. *Epilepsia.* February 2010;51(Suppl. 1):10–12.

12.11 Rhombencephalosynapsis

Case History

A 3-year-old child presented with cognitive dysfunction and dysmorphic facial features.

Diagnosis: Rhombencephalosynapsis

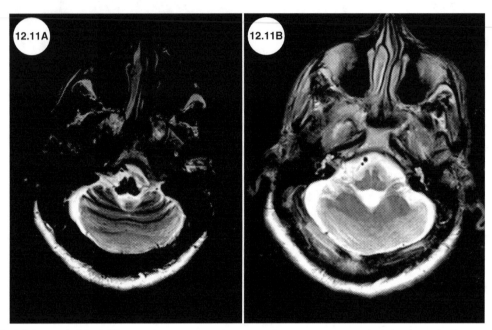

Images 12.11A and 12.11B: Axial T2-weighted images demonstrate a single-lobed cerebellum and with horizontal folia and the absence of a vermis.

Introduction

■ **Rhombencephalosynapsis** is a congenital abnormality characterized by absence of the cerebellar vermis and fusion of the cerebellar hemispheres, cerebellar nuclei, and superior cerebellar peduncles.

Clinical Presentation

■ It may occur in conjunction with two syndromes. VACTERL consists of *V*ertebral anomalies, *A*nal atresia, *C*ardiac defects, *T*racheoesophageal fistula and/or *E*sophageal atresia, *R*enal & *R*adial anomalies and *L*imb defects. It also occurs as part of the Gomez–Lopez–Hernandez syndrome, which includes parietal alopecia, numbness in the distribution of the trigeminal nerve, cognitive impairment, short stature, craniosynostosis, and dysmorphic facial features. It may also occur in isolation, and patients present with dysmorphic cranial features, such as a towering skull and hydrocephalus.

Radiographic Appearance and Diagnosis

■ There is a spectrum of severity ranging from mild hypoplasia of nodulus and vermis to complete absence of these structures. MRI reveals a single-lobed cerebellum with horizontal folia. The cerebellar vermis is hypoplastic or absent, and the fourth ventricle is enlarged and misshapen.

■ Additional features may include ventriculomegaly, hypoplasia or absence of the corpus callosum, anterior commissure, septum pellucidum, olfactory bulbs, posterior pituitary gland, and optic nerves/chiasm. In some cases, it is associated with holoprosencephaly.

Treatment

■ There is no specific treatment, and while most patients die in childhood, others survive into adulthood.

References

1. Ishak GE, Dempsey JC, Shaw DW, et al. Rhombencephalosynapsis: a hindbrain malformation associated with incomplete separation of midbrain and forebrain, hydrocephalus and a broad spectrum of severity. *Brain*. May 2012;135(Pt. 5):1370–1386.

2. Toelle SP, Yalcinkaya C, Kocer N, et al. Rhombencephalosynapsis: clinical findings and neuroimaging in 9 children. *Neuropediatrics*. August 2002;33(4):209–214.

3. Tan TY, McGillivray G, Goergen SK, White SM. Prenatal magnetic resonance imaging in Gomez-Lopez-Hernandez syndrome and review of the literature. *Am J Med Genet A*. November 2005;138(4):369–373.

4. Barth PG. Rhombencephalosynapsis: new findings in a larger study. *Brain*. May 2012;135(Pt. 5):1346–1347.

12.12   Schizencephaly

Case History

A 1-year-old infant presented with seizures and developmental delay. Her head circumference was in the second percentile.

Diagnosis: Schizencephaly

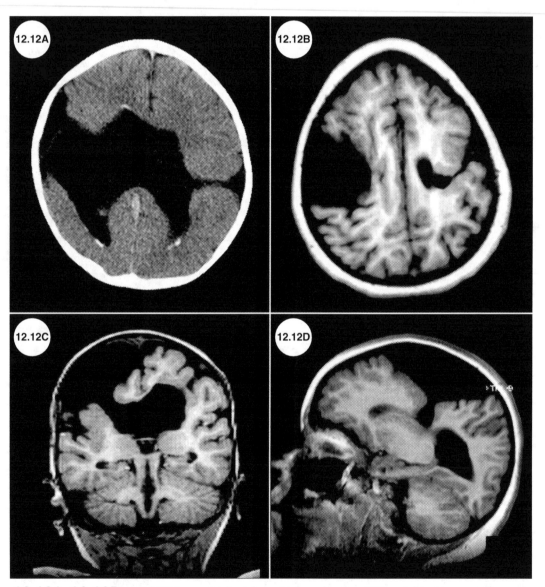

Images 12.12A–12.12D: Axial CT image and axial, sagittal, and coronal T1-weighted images demonstrate bilateral schizencephaly.

Introduction

■ Schizencephaly is a rare congenital malformation of cortical development that results in a cleft in the brain. The etiology is felt to be due to an in utero insult of the germinal matrix that prevents proper neuronal migration and differentiation. Damage to the radial glia prevents neurons from migrating to the cortex. The exact cause is not known, but it is thought to be secondary to fetal cerebral infarction, infection, or in utero toxic exposure. Mutations in the *COL4A1* gene occur in some patients.

Clinical Presentation

■ About 20% of infants are born prematurely and present with hydrocephalus. Later symptoms include seizures, hypotonia, and spastic hemiparesis or quadriparesis. Seizures can be the presenting symptom and can be intractable with seizure focus lying near the schizencephalic clefts. There is a range of overall severity, with 30% to 50% of patients severely affected, 35% moderately affected, and 17% to 25% mildly affected.

■ Bilateral schizencephaly is associated with severe mental retardation and spastic cerebral palsy. These patients are often microcephalic with epilepsy. In contrast, patients with unilateral clefts may have near normal intelligence with contralateral hemiparesis.

Radiographic Appearance

■ Neuroimaging will show clefts that extend from the ventricles to the subarachnoid space of the brain. They can be bilateral or unilateral, symmetric or asymmetric. They involve the posterior frontal or parietal lobes 75% of the time.

■ In **open lip** schizencephaly, the cleft walls are separated by a wide CSF connection between the subarachnoid space and ventricles. In **closed-lip** schizencephaly, the walls are in contact with one another, with a thin thread of CSF connecting the subarachnoid space and ventricles between them. They are lined by dysplastic gray matter, which distinguishes schizencephaly from a destructive process such as porencephaly.

■ Cortical malformations such as lissencephaly or pachygyria are common as well.

Treatment

■ Treatment is supportive, generally focusing on anticonvulsant therapy and physical/occupational therapy. Up to one-third of patients, typically infants, will have hydrocephalus requiring shunting.

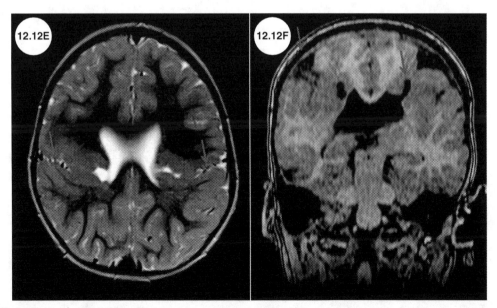

Images 12.12E and 12.12F: Axial T2-weighted and coronal T1-weighted images demonstrate bilateral closed-lip schizencephaly (red arrows) with associated cortical dysplasia.

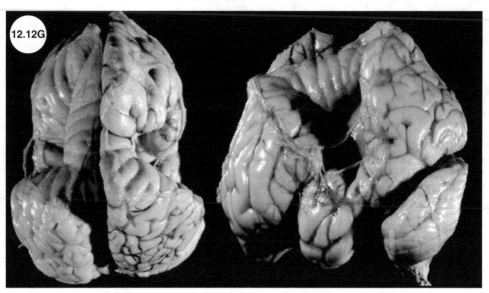

Image 12.12G: Gross pathology of bilateral schizencephaly.

References

1. Yoneda Y, Haginoya K, Kato M, et al. Phenotypic spectrum of COL4A1 mutations: porencephaly to schizencephaly. *Ann Neurol.* January 2013;73(1):48–57.
2. Abdel Razek AA, Kandell AY, Elsorogy LG, Elmongy A, Basett AA. Disorders of cortical formation: MR imaging features. *AJNR Am J Neuroradiol.* January 2009;30(1): 4–11.
3. Spalice A, Parisi P, Nicita F, Pizzardi G, Del Balzo F, Iannetti P. Neuronal migration disorders: clinical, neuroradiologic and genetics aspects. *Acta Paediatr.* March 2009;98(3): 421–433.

12.13 | Porencephaly

Case History

An 12-month-old presented with seizures, cognitive delay, and weakness and spasticity of her left side.

Diagnosis: Porencephaly

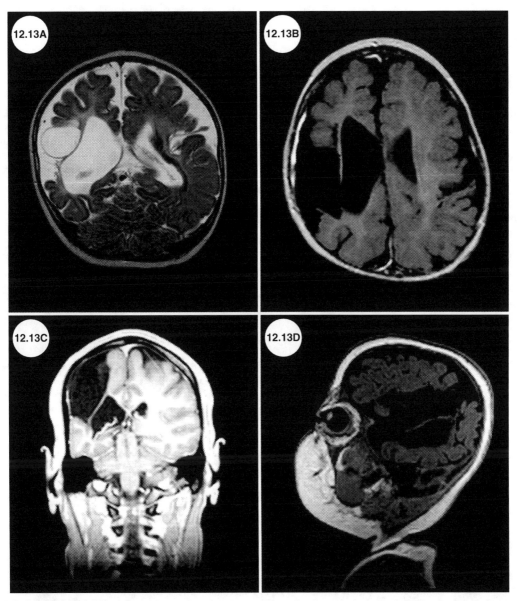

Images 12.13A–12.13D: Axial T2-weighted image and axial, coronal, and sagittal T1-weighted images demonstrate a porencephalic cyst on the right, in the territory of the MCA.

Introduction

■ Porencephaly refers to a rare, congenital, CSF-filled cyst within a cerebral hemisphere. Though different definitions exist, most radiologists use the term to refer to cysts that are in communication with both the ventricles and subarachnoid space.

■ They are mostly due to in utero infarctions in the middle cerebral artery (MCA) territory, though they can also be due to prenatal infection, trauma, or hemorrhage.

■ It is associated with mutations in the *COL4A1* gene, which expresses collagen and is crucial for the structural stability of vascular basement membranes. Mutations in this gene lead to fragile blood vessels and cerebral hemorrhages.

Clinical Presentation

■ There is a wide range of clinical symptoms and severity in patients with porencephalic cysts. Spasticity and seizures are often the presenting symptom and are evident during the first year of life. As patients age, language impairment, cognitive dysfunction, and motor deficits (most commonly, spastic hemiplegia or hypotonia) are also frequently encountered.

■ Head circumference is variable. It may be normal or small, or alternatively there may be progressive enlargement of the cyst, resulting in hydrocephalus and macrocephaly.

Radiographic Appearance and Diagnosis

■ The appearance of the cyst is isointense to CSF signal on all imaging modalities. It is most often located in the territory of the MCA and communicates with the ventricles and subarachnoid space. A thin membrane may separate the cavity from the lateral ventricle or the subarachnoid space. Porencephalic cysts are lined mostly by white matter, whereas the cavities of schizencephaly are lined by heterotopic gray matter.

Treatment

■ Treatment is primarily symptomatic, with antiepileptic therapy and physical and occupational therapies being the mainstays of therapy. Shunting of the ventricular system may be needed if there is hydrocephalus. Surgical fenestration of the cyst has also been used in patients with medication-refractory epilepsy.

References

1. Yoneda Y, Haginoya K, Kato M, et al. Phenotypic spectrum of COL4A1 mutations: porencephaly to schizencephaly. *Ann Neurol.* January 2013;73(1):48–57.
2. Verbeek E, Meuwissen ME, Verheijen FW, et al. COL4A2 mutation associated with familial porencephaly and small-vessel disease. *Eur J Hum Genet.* August 2012;20(8):844–851.

12.14 Colpocephaly

Case History

A 3-year-old child presented with seizures. His language development was delayed and his head circumference was in the second percentile.

Diagnosis: Colpocephaly

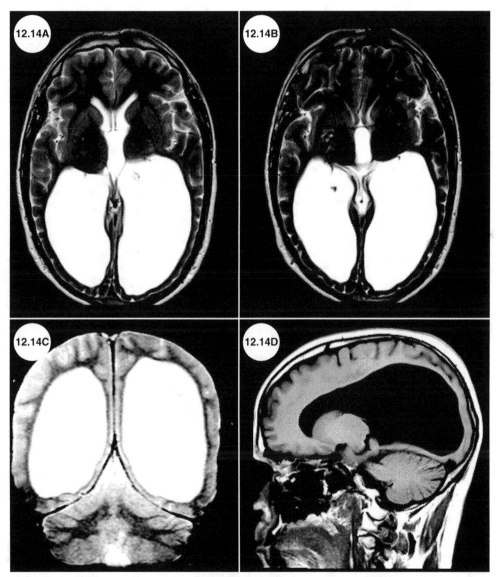

Images 12.14A–12.14D: Axial and coronal T2-weighted and sagittal T1-weighted images demonstrate enlargement of the occipital horns with normal caliber frontal horns.

Introduction

■ Colpocephaly is a congenital condition marked by dilatation of the occipital horns, but with normal caliber frontal horns. This dilatation is the result of white matter loss, not from increased intraventricular pressure.

■ It is primarily seen in two conditions:

1. Primary malformation from poorly laminated striate cortex, subcortical heterotopia, or defective ependymal lining of the occipital horns.

2. In association with agenesis of the corpus callosum due to absence of splenium and hypoplasia of white matter. This cluster of findings often occurs as part of **Aicardi syndrome**.

■ Acquired from periventricular leukomalacia, with loss of periventricular white matter, particularly in premature infants. The acquired form is most common and colpocephaly is associated with several syndromes and systemic disorders such as Zellweger (**cerebrohepatorenal**) syndrome, hemimegalencephaly, and several chromosomal disorders.

■ It can occur in association with agenesis of the posterior fibers of the corpus callosum and thus dilatation of the occipital horns, as a primary developmental malformation, or as a result of intrauterine infection or periventricular leukomalacia.

Clinical Presentation

■ The clinical picture is nonspecific, with varying degrees of mental retardation, seizures, spastic diplegia, and visual loss. Hypertelorism can be present, but is not indicative of visual function. Microcephaly is common.

Radiographic Appearance and Diagnosis

■ Neuroimaging demonstrates disproportionately dilated occipital horns with normal caliber frontal horns.

■ EEG findings range from normal to pseudo-hypsarrhythmia in those with myoclonic epilepsy, commonly with bilateral posterior slowing of low voltage occipital spikes.

Treatment

■ Treatment is with supportive management of symptoms. In contrast to congenital hydrocephalus, there is no role for surgical intervention.

References

1. Noorani PA, Bodensteiner JB, Barnes PD. Colpocephaly: frequency and associated findings. *J Child Neurol.* April 1988;3(2):100–104.
2. Landman J, Weitz R, Dulitzki F, et al. Radiological colpocephaly: a congenital malformation or the result of intrauterine and perinatal brain damage. *Brain Dev.* 1989;11(5):313–316.

12.15 | Holoprosencephaly

Case History

An infant with severe facial abnormalities died in the first week of life.

Diagnosis: Holoprosencephaly

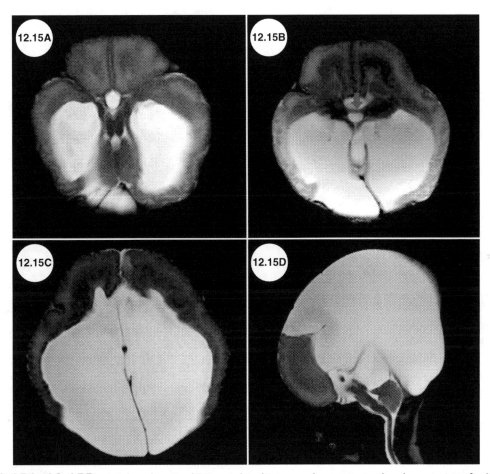

Images 12.15A–12.15D: Axial and sagittal T2-weighted images demonstrate the characteristic findings of lobar holoprosencephaly. The thalami are fused (red arrow).

Introduction

■ Holoprosencephaly is incomplete separation of the cerebral hemispheres due to defective cleavage of the embryonic forebrain. It occurs in 1 per 10,000 to 20,000 term births.

■ There are three forms depending on the degree of cleavage:

1. **Alobar:** Complete failure of hemispheric cleavage results in a small brain with a small midline vesicle.

2. **Semilobar:** The brain's hemispheres have somewhat divided.

3. **Lobar:** There is considerable evidence of separate brain hemispheres and the brain may be nearly normal.

- Approximately two-thirds of patients have the alobar forms and one-fourth have the semilobar form. The remainder of patients have the lobar form.

- Almost 50% of patients have a chromosomal abnormality, though less than 25% have a recognizable syndrome. Abnormalities on chromosome 13 account for the majority of chromosomal abnormalities that cause holoprosencephaly. An autosomal-dominant form of holoprosencephaly with sacral agenesis maps to the chromosome 7p36.2 locus.

Clinical Presentation

- The degree of developmental delay and motor abnormalities correlates with the type of holoprosencephaly. Most severely affected children (alobar) are stillborn or die in the early neonatal period. Survivors have severe cognitive, motor, and sensory impairments. Microcephaly, seizures, hypotonia, mental retardation, spasticity, athetoid movements, endocrinological dysfunction (including diabetes insipidus), and apnea are common. This is particularly the case when holoprosencephaly is associated with a chromosomal defect.

- Midline craniofacial dysplasia is associated with holoprosencephaly in up to 80% of patients. Craniofacial abnormalities include cyclopia, ocular hypotelorism, flat nose, cleft lip, and cleft palate. The degree of craniofacial abnormalities' severity predicts brain malformation severity.

- Non-neurological abnormalities associated with holoprosencephaly include congenital heart defects, clubbing of hands or feet, polydactyly or syndactyly, hypoplasia of the genitourinary system, accessory spleen and liver, and intestinal malrotation. Holoprosencephaly should be suspected in an infant with midline facial deformities, especially when malformations of other organs are present.

- While severely affected infants are stillborn or may only live hours to days to months, mildly affected patients can survive into adolescents and less often, beyond. Alobar patients who are most severely affected develop minimal motor and language skills, while semilobar and lobar patients can have more variable and promising outcomes.

Radiographic Appearance and Diagnosis

- Incomplete fusion of the cerebral hemispheres in ventral patterning affects deep structures such as the thalamic nuclei, basal ganglia, mesencephalon, and hypothalamic nuclei.

- **Alobar holoprosencephaly:** As seen in **Images 12.15A–12.15D**, the thalami are fused and there is a single, large posteriorly located ventricle. Midline structures are absent, including the septum pellucidum, olfactory tracts, and corpus callosum. The optic nerves may be fused as well, but also may be normal or absent. The middle cerebral artery (MCA) and anterior cerebral artery (ACA) are malformed and often intertwined with the internal carotid artery (ICA) and posterior cerebral artery (PCA). The anterior cerebral artery is usually a single azygous vessel coursing below the inner table of the skull. The sagittal sinuses are deformed or replaced by a network of large, abnormal veins.

- **Semilobar holoprosencephaly:** The basic structure of the cerebral lobes is present, but the lobes are fused most commonly anteriorly and at the thalami, with agenesis or hypoplasia

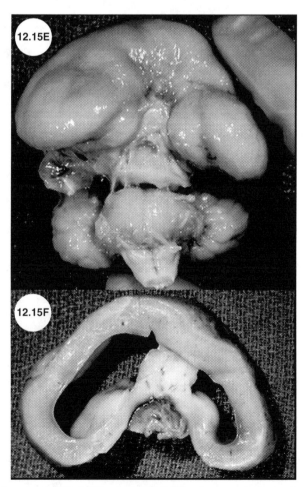

Images 12.15E and 12.15F: Gross pathology of holoprosencephaly.

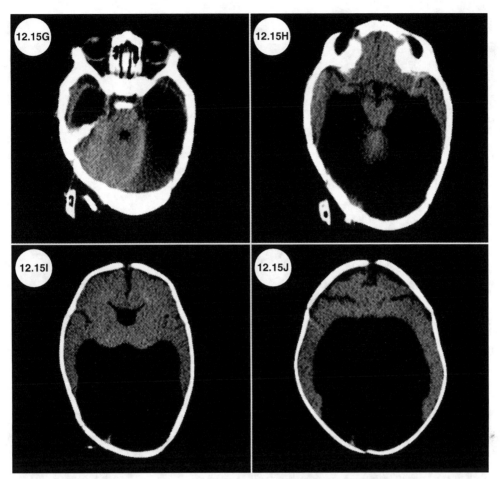

Images 12.15G–12.15J: Axial CT images demonstrate the characteristic findings of semilobar holoprosencephaly. The frontal lobes are fused anteriorly as are the thalami. There is a single, large ventricle.

of the corpus callosum. There is a single, massive ventricle posteriorly. The olfactory tracts are absent as is the septum pellucidum.

- **Lobar holoprosencephaly:** This is the least affected subtype. Images demonstrate more subtle areas of midline abnormalities such as fusion frontal horns of the lateral ventricle. The thalami may be fused, though incompletely. There may be hypoplasia of the body or complete absence of the corpus callosum. The lobes of the brain are well separated and the interhemispheric fissure and falx cerebri are normal.

- Molecular genetic testing is available.

- EEG will show multifocal spikes, which can evolve into a hypsarrhythmia pattern.

Treatment

- There is no specific treatment. If present, hydrocephalus may require a ventriculoperitoneal shunt. In patients with genetic abnormalities, only 2% survive to 1 year of age whereas 30% to 54% of patients without genetic abnormalities survive to 1 year.

References

1. Kauvar EF Muenke M. Holoprosencephaly: recommendations for diagnosis and management. *Curr Opin Pediatr.* 2010;22(6):687–695.
2. Dubourg C, Bendavid C, Pasquier L, Henry C, Odent S, David V. Holoprosencephaly. *Orphanet J Rare Dis.* 2007;2:8.

12.16   Lissencephaly

Case History

An 18-month-old girl presented with seizures and failure to reach developmental milestones. Her head circumference was in the first percentile.

Diagnosis: Lissencephaly

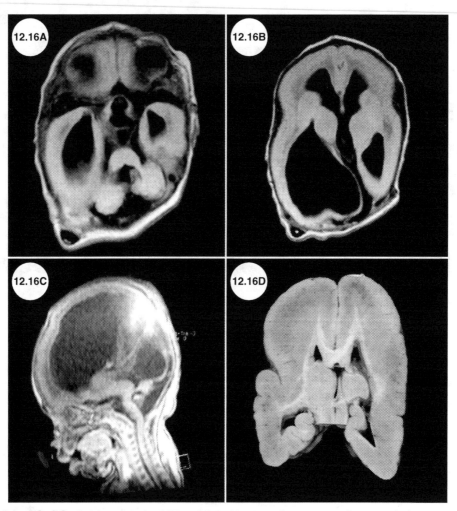

Images 12.16A–12.6C: Axial and sagittal T1-weighted images demonstrate lissencephaly.
Image 12.16D: Gross pathology of lissencephaly.

Introduction

■ Lissencephaly, meaning smooth brain, refers to the appearance of the cerebral cortex in disorders where incomplete neuronal migration in early brain development results in the absence of gyri causing a smooth cerebral surface. Lissencephaly is due to a migratory defect between 12 and 16 weeks gestation, preventing neurons from reaching their destinations.

■ The majority of patients have mutation of either the *LIS1* gene on chromosome 17p13.3 or the doublecortin gene (*DCX* or *XLIS* on the X chromosome). Doublecortin mutations result in anterior greater than posterior dysfunction while *LIS1* mutations result in posterior greater than anterior dysfunction.

■ Classic lissencephaly is likely due to a LIS1 mutation, while patients with subcortical band heterotopia are more likely to have mutations in the *DCX* gene.

Clinical Presentation

■ There is a variable clinical presentation with less severely affected patients having mild cognitive impairments and less severe epilepsy, while severely affected patients can have marked mental retardation, intractable epilepsy, and severe cerebral palsy. Fifty percent of patients have microcephaly.

Radiographic Appearance and Diagnosis

■ On imaging, there is a smooth cortical surface except for rudimentary sulci in the parietal, frontal, or whole brain. The Sylvian fissure is broadened and triangular, the interhemispheric fissure is widened, there are nests of gray matter within the white matter, the ventricles may be enlarged, and corpus callosum can be absent.

■ Several forms exist:

1. **Classic:** is associated with mutations in LIS1
2. **Cobblestone:** progressive hydrocephalus, muscular dystrophy, ocular anterior chamber abnormalities, retinal dysplasias, encephaloceles
3. **Miller–Dieker syndrome:** microcephaly, micrognathia, high forehead, short nose with anteverted nares, low-set ears, thin upper lip
4. **Lissencephaly with cerebellar hypoplasia:** microcephaly

■ It is associated with several other migratory defects such as gray matter heterotopia, macrogyria, PMG, and schizencephaly.

Treatment

■ While standard seizure treatments provide some benefit, seizures in these patients are usually intractable. Though long-term survival has been reported, death typically occurs during infancy, particularly in Miller–Dieker patients who tend to have more severe lissencephaly.

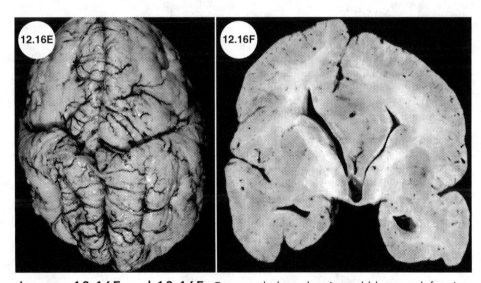

Images 12.16E and 12.16F: Gross pathology showing cobblestone deformity.

References

1. Ghai S, Fong KW, Toi A, Chitayat D, Pantazi S, Blaser S. Prenatal US and MR imaging findings of lissencephaly: review of fetal cerebral sulcal development. *Radiographics*. March–April 2006;26(2):389–405.
2. Hsieh DT, Jennesson MM, Thiele EA, Caruso PA, Masiakos PT, Duhaime AC. Brain and spinal manifestations of Miller-Dieker syndrome. *Neurol Clin Pract*. February 2013;3(1):82–83.
3. Lo Nigro C, Chong CS, Smith AC, Dobyns WB, Carrozzo R, Ledbetter DH. Point mutations and an intragenic deletion in LIS1, the lissencephaly causative gene in isolated lissencephaly sequence and Miller-Dieker syndrome. *Hum Mol Genet*. February 1997;6(2):157–164.

12.17 Hydranencephaly

Case History

A 3-week-old baby presented with seizures and failure to thrive. On exam, the child's head circumference was in the 99th percentile.

Diagnosis: Hydranencephaly

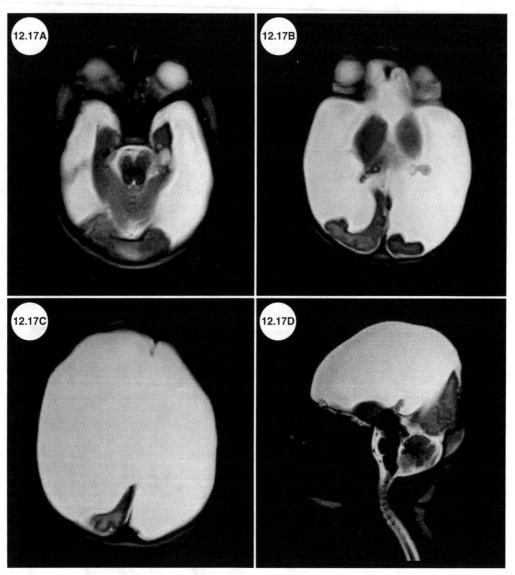

Images 12.17A–12.17D: Axial and sagittal T2-weighted images demonstrate preservation of the medial temporal lobes, occipital poles, cerebellum, thalami, and brainstem in an infant with hydranencephaly.

Introduction

- Hydranencephaly is a rare (less than 1:10,000) congenital condition in which the majority of the cerebral hemispheres and basal ganglia are replaced by glial tissue and CSF. The thalami, hypothalamus, and brainstem are unaffected, and primitive corticospinal and corticobulbar tracts exist.

- It is either a failure of normal brain development or a destructive intrauterine process. Potential intrauterine mechanisms include intrauterine infection, bilateral ICA infarction, fetal hypoxia, and defective embryogenesis causing schizencephaly and cortical agenesis. It has also been proposed that untreated, severe, progressive hydrocephalus may cause hydranencephaly as ventricular pressure destroys midline structures and cerebral parenchyma.

Clinical Presentation

- Babies have mild macrocephaly at birth, but appear healthy as primitive reflexes such as sucking, swallowing, crying, and moving the extremities are preserved. In the second or third postnatal week, head size quickly increases and neurological signs develop. These include hyperreflexia, hypertonia, quadriparesis, decerebration, irritability, infantile spasms, seizures, ocular impairments, failure to thrive, blindness, deafness, and eventually cognitive deficits.

- As the child ages, brainstem reflexes will remain intact, but higher cortical functions fail to develop. These patients are very unstable once the aforementioned conditions develop and have many medical emergencies such as seizures, pulmonary infections from aspiration and reflux, and autonomic instability.

Radiographic Appearance and Diagnosis

- Any imaging modality will reveal the diagnosis. The thalami and brainstem are intact. The cerebellum can be normal, hypoplastic, or dysplastic. While remnants of the occipital poles may remain, no other cortical tissue is present. Any vascular imaging will show absence of flow in the ICAs.

- Head ultrasound should be done on any infant with enlarged head or abnormal head circumference growth. Transillumination, simply shining a bright light at the skull, will reveal absence of the forebrain as the light passes through.

- The EEG can initially be normal but eventually evolves to abnormal patterns of diffuse slowing or isoelectricity. Visual-evoked potentials are absent, but brainstem audio-evoked potentials are present.

- Many cases are detected with prenatal ultrasound.

Treatment

- There is no specific treatment. It carries a very poor prognosis, with few infants surviving beyond 1 year.

References

1. Naidich TP, Griffiths PD, Rosenbloom L. Central nervous system injury in utero: selected entities. *Pediatr Radiol.* September 2015;45(Suppl. 3):454–462.
2. Cecchetto G, Milanese L, Giordano R, Viero A, Suma V, Manara R. Looking at the missing brain: hydranencephaly case series and literature review. *Pediatr Neurol.* February 2013;48(2):152–158.

12.18 | Aqueductal Stenosis

Case History

A 6-month-old girl presented with a head circumference in the 99th percentile.

Diagnosis: Aqueductal Stenosis

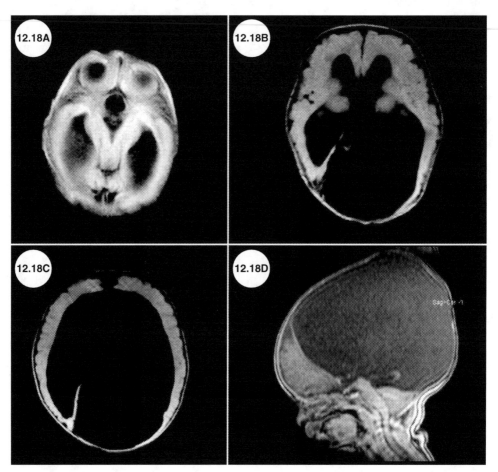

Images 12.18A–12.18D: Axial and sagittal T1-weighted images demonstrate massive dilation of the lateral and third ventricles in a patient with aqueductal stenosis. There is a thin rim of preserved neural tissue, which is not the case in hydranencephaly.

Introduction

■ The cerebral aqueduct connects the third and fourth ventricles and is lined by ependymal cells. At birth, it has a marked length to width discrepancy that makes the aqueduct vulnerable to a number of potential insults.

■ In aqueductal stenosis, the aqueduct is smaller in size but histologically normal without gliosis. Stenosis tends to occur at two places: beneath the midline of the superior quadrigeminal bodies and at the intercollicular sulcus.

- The incidence is 0.5 to 1 in 1,000 births, and AS is responsible for 20% of hydrocephalus cases.

- There are both genetic and acquired causes of acqueductal stenosis. Genetic causes include holoprosencephaly, Chiari II, X-linked hydrocephalus with aqueductal stenosis, and pachygyria, autosomal recessive hydrocephalus with aqueductal stenosis, mutation of dorsalizing gene in vertical axis of neural tube, primary defective ependymal, and choroid plexus epithelia.

- Acquired causes of acqueductal stenosis include IVH with a thrombus in the aqueduct, congenital infections (CMV, mumps), ependymitis/ventriculitis with gliosis around and within aqueduct, chronic arachnoiditis, aqueductal membrane across lumen, amnion rupture sequence, aneurysms/venous angiomas/vascular malformations, cystic dilatation of perivascular Virchow–Robin spaces in midbrain, tumors of aqueduct, and tumors compressing midbrain tectum from above. Alternatively, aqueductal gliosis is a postinfectious, noninflammatory process, usually from perinatal infection or hemorrhage, in which the aqueduct is slowly replaced by clusters of ependymal cells, and fibrillary gliosis resulting in progressive occlusion.

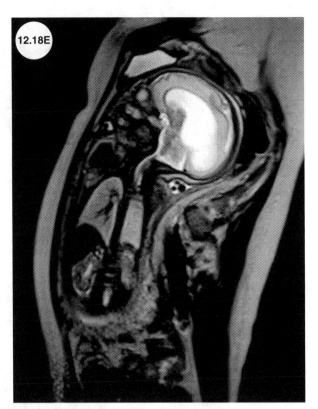

Image 12.18E: Sagittal T2-weighted image demonstrates hydrocephalus in a fetus.

Clinical Presentation

- In congenital acqueductal stenosis, findings include bossing of the forehead, dilated scalp veins, widened sutures, and tense, widened fontanelles. These are exaggerated with activities that raise intracranial pressure (ICP).

- The worsening of symptoms is gradual and can occur at any time in childhood or adulthood. In such instances, a downward deviation of the eyes resulting in sclera seen above iris (the sun-setting sign) and abducens nerve palsies can be appreciated.

- Other CNS malformations are seen in 75% of patients and include fusion of the quadrigeminal bodies, fusion of the oculomotor nuclei, and spina bifida cystica or occulta.

Radiographic Appearance and Diagnosis

- CT and MRI will show marked dilation of the lateral ventricles, third ventricle, and cephalic end of the cerebral aqueduct. The remainder of cerebral aqueduct and fourth ventricle will not be visualized. A thin band of remaining cortex is seen, helping to differentiate acqueductal stenosis from more destructive processes, such as hydranencephaly.

- The ventricles expand at 20 weeks gestation and prenatal diagnosis is common. When macrocephaly is present on an intrauterine ultrasound, alpha-fetoprotein levels should be drawn to detect neural tube defects. Prenatal ultrasound and MRI can show the malformation.

Treatment

- Hydrocephalus from congenital AS is severe, and the only option is ventriculoperitoneal shunt placement.

- With relief of the hydrocephalus, there is a possibility of normal development, and children tend to have better verbal than nonverbal skills. However, the associated anomalies may cause other neurological sequelae such as seizures and motor deficits. Often, prenatal diagnosis is made and elective termination is considered.

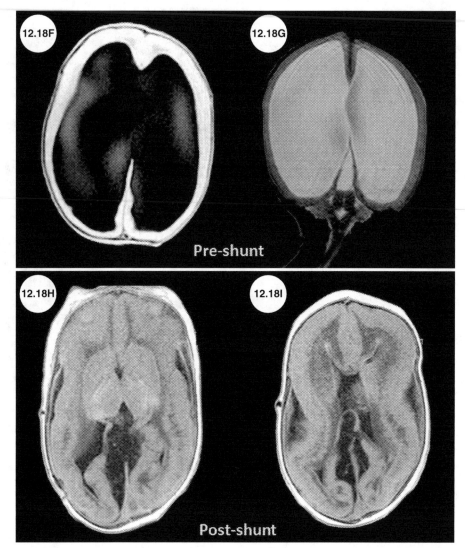

Images 12.18F and 12.18G: Axial T1-weighted and coronal T2-weighted images demonstrate aqueductal stenosis. **Images 12.18H and 12.18I:** Axial FLAIR images demonstrate expansion of the cortex after placement of a shunt.

References

1. Kahle KT, Kulkarni AV, Limbrick DD Jr, Warf BC. Hydrocephalus in children. *Lancet*. 2015;387:788–799. pii: S0140-6736(15)60694-8.

2. Cinalli G, Spennato P, Nastro A, et al. Hydrocephalus in aqueductal stenosis. *Childs Nerv Syst*. 2011;27(10):1621–1642.

3. Geng J, Wu D, Chen X, Zhang M, Xu B, Yu X. Aqueduct stent placement: indications, technique, and clinical experience. *World Neurosurg*. 2015;84:1347–1353. pii: S1878–8750(15)00779-2.

12.19 | Neurenteric Cyst

Case History

A 16-year-old boy presented with neck pain, weakness in his arms and legs, and bladder incontinence.

Diagnosis: Neurenteric Cyst

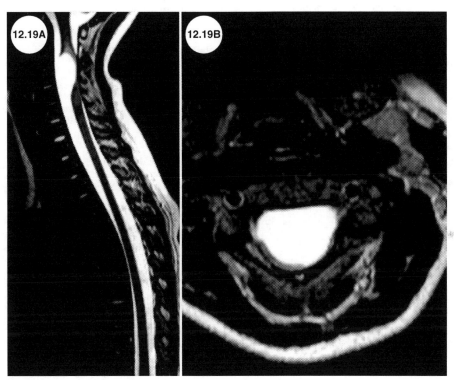

Images 12.19A and 12.19B: Sagittal and axial T2-weighted images demonstrate a large extraaxial cyst compressing the upper cervical spinal cord.

Introduction

■ A neurenteric cyst is an uncommon, congenital lesion of the spine thought to result from an abnormal connection between the primitive endoderm and ectoderm. They are composed of heterotopic endodermal tissue. During the third week of embryonic life, the neurenteric canal unites the yolk sac and amniotic cavity as it traverses the primitive notochordal plate. Persistence of the neurenteric canal prevents appropriate separation of endoderm and notochord. This anomalous union manifests as rare congenital cysts of the spine defined by the presence of mucus-secreting epithelium reminiscent of the GI tract.

■ Approximately 90% are located in the intradural/extramedullary compartment; the remaining 10% are divided between an extradural or intradural/intramedullary location. They are most common in the ventral, cervical cord. Rarely, they may be located intracranially, most commonly in the posterior fossa.

■ They are rare, accounting for about 1% of spinal tumors, and typically present in teenagers and young adults.

Clinical Presentation

■ Patients present with progressive focal pain at the level of spine lesion, radicular pain and paresthesias, weakness, and bladder and bowel dysfunction. In contrast to other spinal lesions, the symptoms may fluctuate as the size of the cyst changes due to hemodynamic and osmotic factors.

■ Neurological examination will reveal spastic paraparesis/quadriparesis and hyperreflexia with clonus and upgoing toes. A sensory level is usually present with loss of sensation below the level of lesion.

Radiographic Appearance and Diagnosis

■ On MRI, the cysts are isointense to CSF on both T1-weighted images and T2-weighted images. They do not enhance with the administration of contrast. CTs are better for detecting the bony malformations, such as scoliosis and spina bifida, which occur in nearly 50% of patients.

■ CT myelogram: positive meniscus sign (partial dye obstruction with intradural/extramedullary cysts and complete contrast obstruction with intradural/intramedullary cysts).

Treatment

■ They are treated surgically with the goal of gross total resection. Partial resections may lead to recurrence and arachnoiditis.

References

1. Savage JJ, Casey JN, McNeill IT, Sherman JH. Neurenteric cysts of the spine. *J Craniovertebr Junction Spine.* 2010;1(1):58–63.
2. Brooks BS, Duvall ER, el Gammal T, Garcia JH, Gupta KL, Kapila A. Neuroimaging features of neurenteric cysts: analysis of nine cases and review of the literature. *AJNR Am J Neuroradiol.* 1993;14(3):735–746.

12.20 | Diastematomyelia

Case History

A 10-year-old girl developed low back and trouble walking. On exam, she was weak in her legs.

Diagnosis: Diastematomyelia

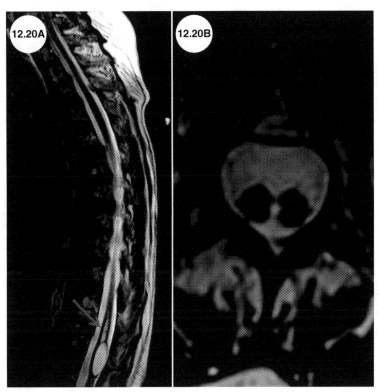

Images 12.20A and 12.20B: Sagittal and axial T2-weighted images demonstrate a longitudinal bifurcation of the spinal cord and hydromyelia (red arrow).

Introduction

- Diastematomyelia is a rare congenital malformation where a part of the spinal cord is split longitudinally. It usually occurs in the upper lumbar or lower thoracic cord. Females are affected more than males.

- Two types are recognized.

  1. **Type 1:** There is a duplicated dural sac. Hydromyelia (a fluid-filled dilatation of the central canal of the spinal cord) is present as is a midline bony or cartilaginous spur. Cutaneous and vertebral anomalies, such as spina bifida, butterfly or hemivertebrae, are common. This type is more symptomatic.

  2. **Type 2:** There is a single dural sac and the division of the cord may be incomplete. A hydromyelia and bony abnormalities are often absent and patients are less symptomatic.

Clinical Presentation

- It usually presents in children with low pain, urinary incontinence, paraparesis, and scoliosis. Cutaneous manifestations including a dimple, hairy patch, hemangioma, meningocele, or lipoma over the affected area are seen in 50% of the cases. Though rare, in adults it presents with slowly progressive paraparesis, sensory loss, and blower/bladder incontinence.

Radiographic Appearance and Diagnosis

■ MRI is the preferred imaging modality. On axial imaging the spinal cord will divide into two branches. A hydromyelia, if present, will appear as a cyst within the spinal cord, isodense to CSF on all sequences. CT scans are more sensitive for revealing bony abnormalities. The diagnosis is commonly made on prenatal ultrasound.

Treatment

■ Symptomatic patients may benefit from surgical decompression of neural elements and removal of any bony or fibrous spur. This also allows for repair of duplicated dural sacs.

References

1. Cheng B, Li FT, Lin L. Diastematomyelia: a retrospective review of 138 patients. *J Bone Joint Surg Br.* 2012;94(3): 365–372.
2. Huang SL, He XJ, Xiang L, Yuan GL, Ning N, Lan BS. CT and MRI features of patients with diastematomyelia. *Spinal Cord.* 2014;52(9):689–692.

12.21 | Chiari I Malformation

Case History

A 39-year-old woman presented with severe headaches whenever she sneezed. She noticed that her hands were weak for the past few months and they were atrophied on physical examination. She also had decreased sensation to pinprick over her upper back, shoulders, and upper arms.

Diagnosis: Chiari I Malformation

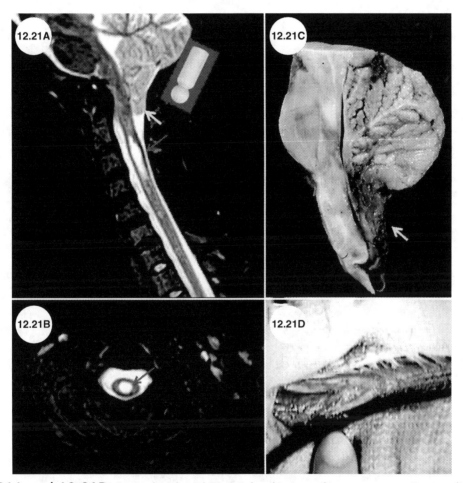

Images 12.21A and 12.21B: Sagittal and axial T2-weighted images demonstrate a syringomyelia in the upper cervical spine (red arrow) and "peg-like" tonsils, which herniate into the foramen magnum (yellow arrow).
Image 12.21C: Gross specimen demonstrates herniation of the cerebellar tonsils. **Image 12.21D:** Gross specimen demonstrates a syringomyelia.

Source: Images 12.21C and 12.21D, www.wikidoc.org.

Introduction

■ Chiari malformation type I (CMI) describes the displacement of otherwise normal cerebellar tonsils more than 5 mm below the plane of the foramen magnum, into the cervical canal. Most cases appear to occur spontaneously. CMI is due to a combination of a developmental skull malformation, cerebrovascular physiology, and low spinal CSF pressures. CSF pressure gradients or decreased cerebral compliance from cerebral venous hypertension can push the tonsils downward into the spinal canal.

■ CMI often occurs in conjunction with a syringomyelia, meaning "cavitation of the spinal cord." Syringomyelia is felt to result from CMI as downward displaced cerebellar tonsils cause pulsating pressure waves into the CSF in the spinal compartment. This pressure drives CSF into the spinal cord and dilates the perivascular spaces (Virchow–Robin spaces), leading to interstitial edema, microcysts, and syrinx. Syringomyelia can also be seen in association with myelomeningocele, trauma, arachnoiditis, and intrinsic spinal cord tumor. Syringobulbia is a cystic cavity in the brainstem, which can cause symptoms of lower cranial nerve dysfunction.

■ The prevalence of asymptomatic CMI in the general population is 1.1 per 1,000.

Clinical Presentation

■ CMI is generally asymptomatic in childhood with symptoms beginning in adolescence and adulthood. The average age of presentation is 41 years with slight female predominance, though symptoms have been reported as early as infancy. Symptoms result from both compression of the cerebellar tonsils and from a syringomyelia if present.

■ Symptoms from cerebellar tonsillar compression are headache (valsalva-induced), neck pain, inconsolable crying, torticollis, dysphagia with resultant failure to thrive, dysphonia, sleep-disordered breathing, downward beating nystagmus, scoliosis, gait disturbance, impairment of the limbs (especially hand movements), vertigo, ataxia, tinnitus, and hoarseness. Twenty percent of symptomatic patients have lower cranial nerve dysfunction.

■ Symptoms of syringomyelia are neck and back pain, paresthesias, numbness, and pain of the limbs or trunk, weakness and atrophy of the limbs (especially in the hands), gait disturbance, scoliosis, bladder incontinence, and sexual dysfunction. Children are more likely than adults to experience scoliosis.

■ Signs on physical exam are ataxia, spastic quadriparesis, downbeating nystagmus, decreased sensation in "cape-like" distribution, and wasting of intrinsic muscles of hands. This pattern is called central cord syndrome. The hand weakness and atrophy are due to involvement of the anterior horn cells that give motor innervation to the upper extremities, while the "cape-like" sensory loss is due to disruption of the fibers of the spinothalamic tract as it decussates in the center of the spinal cord.

■ Craniofacial dysostoses, skeletal dysplasias, hydrocephalus, pseudotumor cerebri, and spontaneous intracranial hypotension can all be related to CMI.

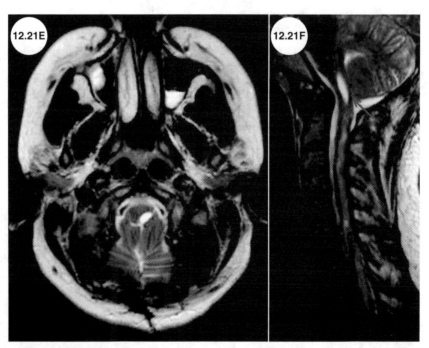

Images 12.21E and 12.21F: Axial and sagittal T2-weighted images demonstrate syringobulbia (red arrows).

Radiographic Appearance and Diagnosis

- MRI is the gold standard for diagnosis. It will show "peg-like" cerebellar tonsils, which lie 5 mm or more below the plane of the foramen magnum. As a syringomyelia is fluid-filled, it will be a cavity in the central spinal cord, isodense to CSF on all sequences. If the lesion extends into the brainstem (syringobulbia), there may be tongue atrophy and palatal weakness.

- Lack of CSF flow behind the cerebellum can also be useful in making the diagnosis.

Treatment

- Posterior fossa decompression is indicated for headaches resistant to pharmacological intervention, syringomyelia in association with neuropathic pain, scoliosis, or neurological dysfunction. The goal is alleviating the compression of brainstem and spinal cord and to restore CSF pulsation across the craniocervical junction. Craniocervical decompression has reduction or complete resolution of syringomyelia in 80% of the cases. Acute and subacute neurological symptoms have an 80% response rate, but chronic neurological symptoms will stabilize with surgery, not improve.

- Management of asymptomatic syringomyelia is less certain. Some surgeons will intervene only if there are symptoms or evidence of expansion of the cavity. Others believe that syringomyelia represents spinal tissue destruction and will inevitably result in neurological symptoms that may not be reversible once present, and thus intervene prospectively.

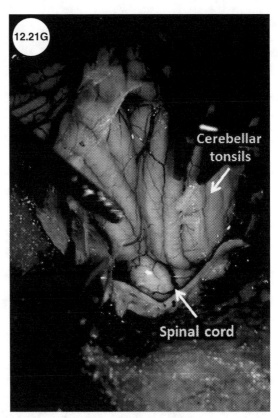

Image 12.21G: Intraoperative picture demonstrating decompression of a Chiari malformation.

References

1. Greitz D. Unraveling the riddle of syringomyelia. *Neurosurg Rev.* October 2006;29(4):251–263.
2. Koyanagi I, Houkin K. Pathogenesis of syringomyelia associated with Chiari type 1 malformation: review of evidences and proposal of a new hypothesis. *Neurosurg Rev.* 2010;33(3): 271–284; discussion 284–285.
3. Strahle J, Smith BW, Martinez M, et al. The association between Chiari malformation Type I, spinal syrinx, and scoliosis. *J Neurosurg Pediatr.* 2015;15(6):607–611.

12.22 Chiari II Malformation

Case History

A 2-month-old infant was noted to have head lag, feeding difficulties, and trouble tracking objects with her eyes.

Diagnosis: Chiari II Malformation

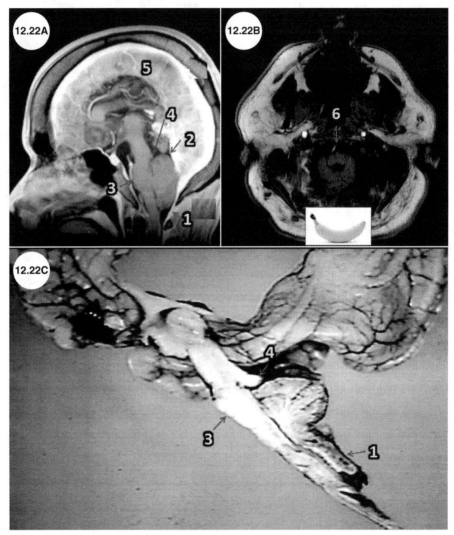

Images 12.22A and 12.22B: Postcontrast sagittal and axial T1-weighted images and gross pathology demonstrate the core features of a Chiari malformation type II. (1) Herniation of the medulla and cerebellar vermis and tonsils into the cervical canal. (2) Upward herniation of the cerebellum through the tentorium. (3) Elongation of the pons and fourth ventricle. (4) Tectal "beaking" due to fusion of the colliculi. (5) Supratentorial abnormalities such as partial agenesis of the corpus callosum (the splenium most commonly) and heterotopias are also common. (6) The cerebellar hemispheres envelop the brainstem forming the "banana" sign. **Image 12.22C:** Gross pathology demonstrates several of the features of a Chiari malformation type II (image credit www.wikidoc.org).

Introduction

- Chiari malformation type II (CMII) can have any of the features of CMI (downward displacement of the cerebellar tonsils 5 mm or more below the plane of foramen magnum, syringomyelia), along with noncommunicating hydrocephalus and lumbosacral spinal bifida.

- As a result of the downward displacement of the brainstem, a kink between the medulla and cervical spinal cord, and herniation of the cerebellar vermis, CSF circulation is blocked at the level of the foramen magnum. This results in obstructive hydrocephalus.

- Along with the obstructive hydrocephalus, there also appears to be a migration defect of cerebral cortical neurons. Possible failure of pontine flexion during embryogenesis has also been proposed to result in elongation of the fourth ventricle. There has also been evidence of brainstem hemorrhage, ischemia, or neuronal agenesis.

Clinical Presentation

- In the first few weeks of life, infants develop symptoms from lower cranial nerve palsies and impaired brainstem function (vocal cord paralysis, stridor, retrocollis, apnea, feeding difficulties, difficulty with secretions), and head lag, later followed by spastic paresis of the upper extremities and opisthotonus.

- Symptoms include difficulty swallowing (71%), stridor (59%), arm weakness (53%), apnea (29%), and aspiration (12%).

- CMII is commonly associated with myelomeningocele, which is exposure of spinal neural tissue in the lumbosacral region in 80% of the cases.

Radiographic Appearance and Diagnosis

- The core features of CMII are best appreciated on sagittal MRI. These are:

  1. Herniation of the medulla and cerebellar vermis and tonsils into the cervical canal
  2. Upward herniation of the cerebellum through the tentorium
  3. Elongation of the pons and fourth ventricle

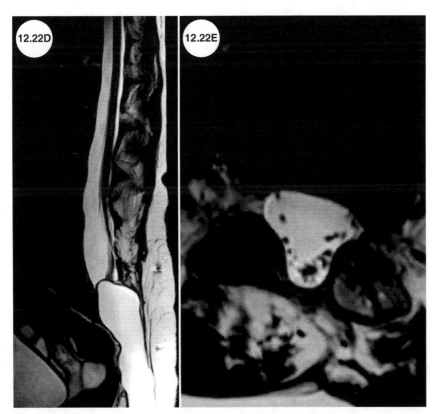

Images 12.22D and 12.22E: Sagittal and axial T2-weighted images of the lumbar spine demonstrate a myelomeningocele.

4. Tectal "beaking" due to fusion of the colliculi
5. Supratentorial abnormalities such as partial agenesis of the corpus callosum (the splenium most commonly) and heterotopias are also common
6. The cerebellar tonsils are low-lying and hemispheres envelop the brainstem forming the "banana" sign

▨ As a result of this displacement, the pons and cranial nerves are elongated and compressed, and the foramina of Luschka and Magendie and the basal cisterns can be occluded with resultant hydrocephalus. Additional findings include hypoplasia of the posterior fossa, absence of the septum pellucidum, poorly myelinated cerebellar folia, hypoplasia of the falx cerebri, degeneration of the lower cranial nerve nuclei, and cortical malformations including PMG, heterotopias, and cortical dysgenesis. A myelomeningocele, lying as low at L5, is common as well.

Treatment

▨ Surgical intervention for CMII is indicated for patients with critical neurological signs such as apnea, stridor, dysphagia, and disordered breathing. Surgical decompression and dividing a tight, fibrotic band at the C1 level can result in improvement. Typically, correction of the myelomeningocele and ventriculoperitoneal shunt placement for hydrocephalus occurs first. Despite surgical intervention, outcomes are generally poor, as the baseline brainstem and posterior fossa abnormalities are severe.

References

1. el Gammal T, Mark EK, Brooks BS. MR imaging of Chiari II malformation. *AJR Am J Roentgenol.* January 1988;150(1):163–170.
2. Wolpert SM, Anderson M, Scott RM, Kwan ES, Runge VM. Chiari II malformation: MR imaging evaluation. *AJR Am J Roentgenol.* November 1987;149(5):1033–1042.
3. Chiapparini L, Saletti V, Solero CL, Bruzzone MG, Valentini LG. Neuroradiological diagnosis of Chiari malformations. *Neurol Sci.* December 2011;32(Suppl. 3):S283–S286.

12.23 | Dandy–Walker Syndrome

Case History

A 4-day-old infant had an MRI as part of an evaluation for abnormalities found on a prenatal ultrasound. The baby had dysmorphic facial features and a cleft palate.

Diagnosis: Dandy–Walker Syndrome

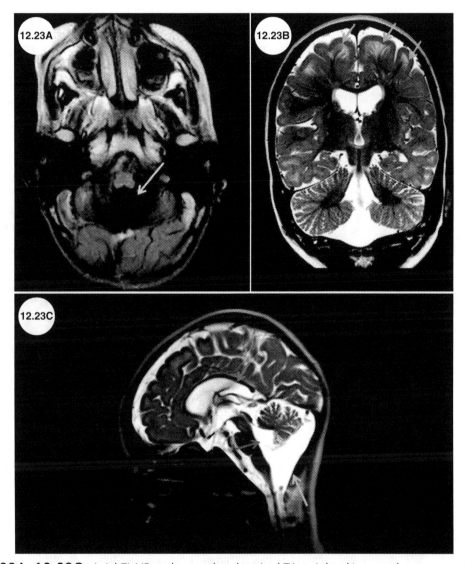

Images 12.23A–12.23C: Axial FLAIR and coronal and sagittal T1-weighted images demonstrate the characteristic features of Dandy–Walker syndrome. Enlargement of the fourth ventricle (red arrow), partial or complete agenesis of the cerebellar vermis (yellow arrow), and an enlarged cisterna magna (blue arrow). The corpus callosum is seen (pink arrow), and there are multiple cortical heterotopias (green arrows).

Introduction

■ Dandy–Walker Syndrome (DWS) is a disorder of cerebellar development characterized by the following triad:

1. Complete or partial agenesis of the cerebellar vermis
2. Cystic dilatation of the fourth ventricle
3. Enlarged posterior fossa

■ The incidence of DWS is 1 per 25,000 to 30,000 births, with a slight female predominance.

■ The exact embryologic malformation leading to DWS is not known, but is thought to result from a neural tube closure defect at the cerebellar level at approximately 4 weeks gestation. As a result, the roof of the fourth ventricle fails to form properly.

■ DWS is on a spectrum of developmental anomalies associated with trisomy 9 and mutations on the X chromosome. It is associated with many other clinical conditions, including Klippel–Feil syndrome, Cornelia de Lange syndrome, Rubinstein–Taybi syndrome, and hypertelorism.

Clinical Presentation

■ Macrocephaly, with bulging of the skull most prominent in the occiput, is the most common presenting sign. It is associated with hydrocephalus in 75% of infants at 3 months of age and 80% of infants at 1 year.

■ Compression of the structures of the posterior fossa results in recurrent attacks of pallor, ataxia, abnormal respirations, headache, vomiting, seizures, apnea, truncal ataxia, and cranial neuropathies. In older infants with hydrocephalus, symptoms of ICP such as headache and nausea and vomiting are seen. Mental retardation and spastic diplegia are common.

■ Physical examination may reveal macrocephaly, hypotonia, downwardly displaced eyes (sunsetting), spasticity, hemiparesis, enlarged posterior fossa, facial nerve palsies, ataxia, nystagmus, and lower extremity hyperreflexia. Dysmorphic facial features include cleft palate and low-set ears. Polydactyly (extra fingers or toes) and syndactyly (fusion of fingers or toes) are common. Cardiovascular malformations and polycystic kidneys may occur.

■ Up to 20% of patients do not present until late childhood or adulthood. Symptoms in these patients include headaches, gait ataxia, muscle spasms, facial paralysis, and cognitive and psychiatric disturbances.

Radiographic Appearance and Diagnosis

■ MRI is the ideal study because it can better identify other cerebral abnormalities, which may also be present.

■ It will show:

1. Enlargement of the fourth ventricle.
2. Partial or complete agenesis of the cerebellar vermis. The cerebellar hemispheres are preserved and are connected to a thin membrane at the roof of the fourth ventricle.
3. Enlarged cisterna magna. Over time, growth of the cyst pushes the torcula (the confluence of sinuses) superiorly, above the level of the lambdoid suture.

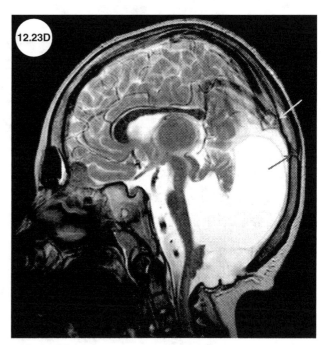

Image 12.23D: Sagittal T2-weighted image demonstrates the characteristic findings of DWS with the torcula (yellow arrow) above the lambdoid suture (red arrow) (image credit Hellerhoff; https://en.wikipedia.org/wiki/Dandy-Walker_malformation#/media/File:Dandy-Walker-Variante_-_MRT_T2_sagittal.jpg).

■ The vast majority of patients will also have hydrocephalus due to aqueductal stenosis by 3 months. DWS is associated with other malformations in two-thirds of children, the most common of which is agenesis of the corpus callosum. Other cortical malformations include

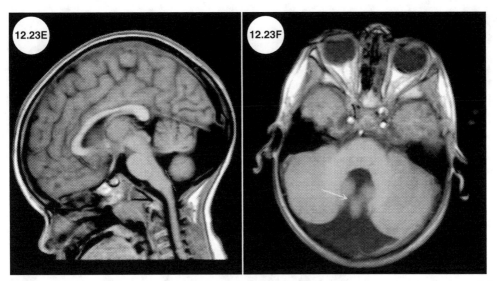

Images 12.23E and 12.23F: Axial and sagittal T1-weighted images demonstrate enlargement of the fourth ventricle (red arrow) and partial agenesis of the cerebellar vermis (yellow arrow). The cisterna magna is only mildly enlarged.

heterotopias, abnormal gyral formation, dysraphisms, holoprosencephaly, schizencephaly, and syringomyelia, congenital tumors, occipital encephalocele, and PMG.

■ In many cases, the diagnosis can be made by prenatal ultrasound.

■ There is a Dandy–Walker variant that is similar to DWS, but with minimal or no enlargement of the posterior fossa. This variant is much more common than classic DWS, and accounts for one-third of posterior fossa malformations. The clinical presentation is much milder.

Treatment

■ Decompression of the fourth ventricular cyst will alleviate symptoms, but hydrocephalus almost always recurs and a ventriculoperitoneal shunt is required in two-thirds of affected children. For patients in whom there is no communication between the Dandy–Walker cyst and the lateral ventricles, a posterior fossa shunt may be required as well.

■ Even after successful shunting, some children will experience transitory, but sometimes fatal episodes of lethargy, apnea, personality change, and vomiting. The mechanism of this is unknown, but is not related to shunt malfunction.

■ Approximately 70% of live fetuses die, usually due to non-neurological abnormalities.

■ Genetic counseling is important for parents considering future pregnancies.

References

1. Phillips JJ, Mahony BS, Siebert JR, Lalani T, Fligner CL, Kapur RP. Dandy-Walker malformation complex: correlation between ultrasonographic diagnosis and postmortem neuropathology. *Obstet Gynecol*. March 2006;107(3):685–693.
2. Forzano F, Mansour S, Ierullo A, Homfray T, Thilaganathan B. Posterior fossa malformation in fetuses: a report of 56 further cases and a review of the literature. *Prenat Diagn*. June 2007;27(6):495–501.

12.24 Tethered Cord Syndrome

Case History

A child presented with pain, weakness, and incontinence, which had progressed over several years.

Diagnosis: Tethered Cord Syndrome

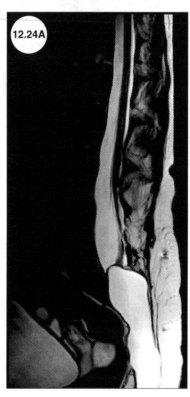

Image 12.24A: Sagittal T2-weighted image of the lumbar spine demonstrates a low-lying spinal cord in association with a sacral meningocele.

Introduction

■ Tethered spinal cord syndrome occurs when a fibrous attachment on the spinal cord causes abnormal stretching of the cord. It is usually secondary to neural tube malformation and occurs at the conus medullaris. It is closely linked to spina bifida. It also may occur after spinal cord trauma.

Clinical Presentation

■ It usually presents in children with progressive low back pain, numbness and weakness of the legs, and bowel/bladder incontinence. Cutaneous manifestations include hairy patches, dimples, or subcutaneous lipomas on the lower back. Syringomyelias may form in some patients. Spina bifida, scoliosis, and clubbed foot are common. Milder cases may not present until adulthood when it presents with pain, paraplegia, and bowel/bladder abnormalities.

Radiographic Appearance and Diagnosis

■ MRI is the preferred imaging modality. It can demonstrate the location of the tethering and whether there is a lower than normal position of the conus medullaris. MRI will also detect the presence of any tumor or lipoma. Ultrasounds may be used in young infants.

Treatment

- In children, early surgery can prevent further neurological deterioration. Almost all patients have decreased pain, and many have improvement in neurological function. Surgical detethering of the spinal cord is also the treatment of choice in most adults as well.

Reference

1. Lew SM, Kothbauer KF. Tethered cord syndrome: an updated review. *Pediatr Neurosurg.* 2007;43(3):236–248.

12.25 Vein of Galen Malformation

Case History

A 4-week-old baby presented with feeding difficulties and failure to thrive. On examination, the head circumference was in the 96th percentile and the baby was tachycardic.

Diagnosis: Vein of Galen Malformation

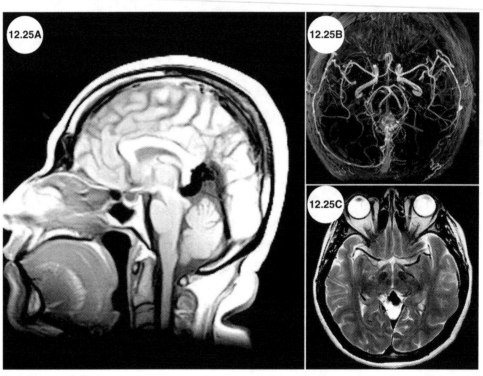

Images 12.25A–12.25C: Sagittal T1-weighted image, magnetic resonance angiography, and axial T2-weighted image demonstrate a vein of Galen malformation (red arrow).

Introduction

■ The vein of Galen is located under the cerebral hemispheres and drains the anterior and central brain areas of the brain into the sinuses of the posterior cerebral fossa. The median prosencephalic vein of Markowski (MProsV) is the primary venous drainage of the brain from 6 to 11 weeks gestation until the subependymal venous drainage system takes over. At that time, the MProsV should regresses into the vein of Galen.

■ In vein of Galen malformations (VGMs), the MProsV forms anomalous connections with the choroidal arteries around 8 weeks gestation, resulting in high flow pressure and hemodynamic

stress, which prevents the MProsV from regressing. It instead forms an aneurysm that drains into the vein of Galen. There is arteriovenous shunting of blood from the choroidal arteries draining into a dilated, persistent median prosencephalic MProsV.

■ VGMs are the most commonly seen cranial arteriovenous malformations in neonates, with an incidence of 1 per 25,000 births.

Clinical Presentation

■ The clinical presentation varies by age. Ninety percent of patients present in the neonatal period, most commonly with refractory high output heart failure. It is the result of high volume venous return to the right side of the heart. The right heart chamber dilates and eventually left-sided heart failure occurs secondary to preload volume overload. It manifests as cardiomegaly, difficulty feeding, failure to thrive, and tachycardia. Larger arteriovenous shunting and dysfunction present earlier and can result in cardiogenic shock. Other features include increasing head circumference, a loud intracranial bruit, and dilated orbital veins.

- Infants and young children present with hydrocephalus, cognitive delay, and seizures due to compression of adjacent brain structures with resultant hydrocephalus and parenchymal ischemia. Older children and adults present with headaches and subarachnoid hemorrhage.

Radiographic Appearance and Diagnosis

- Up to 30% of VGMs are diagnosed with prenatal ultrasound, as early as the second trimester, though most often during the third trimester. Ultrasound will show an anechoic, posterior, midline cystic lesion with significant flow on Doppler examination.

- Prenatal MRI can better the size and anatomy of the malformation and feeder veins. On T2WIs, the dilated MProsV will appear as a flow void. The brain parenchyma may show focal white matter lesions or diffuse brain destruction.

- Angiography is the gold standard for evaluating the malformation. It will demonstrate reflux into the choroidal arteries and congested cortical veins. The arterial phase will show persistent flow into the malformation. The venous phase will show progressive thrombosis of the sigmoid sinus and reflux into the subependymal veins. There may also be backflow into the cavernous sinus.

Treatment

- Conservative medical management of symptoms is the initial treatment. In neonatal cases of severe cardiac failure or hydrocephalus, partial embolization can be performed as early as 2 weeks of age as a temporizing measure.

- Once the cavernous sinus has matured, after 5 to 6 months of age, there are interventional options. These include transarterial embolization, venous embolization, and surgical ligation of the arterial feeders from the PCA and MCA with plication of the aneurysm. On average, patients require 2.5 treatments to correct the malformation. Ventriculoperitoneal shunting can also be done after embolization for hydrocephalus.

- In older children and adults, management of the hydrocephalus and hemorrhage is the cornerstone. For the hydrocephalus, one can place a ventriculoperitoneal shunt and third ventriculostomy.

- Without treatment, mortality rates from cardiac failure or cerebral dysfunction are extremely high. Neonates and patients with brain parenchymal changes, such as encephalomalacia, atrophy, and calcifications, have worse outcomes. Overall mortality rate, including those with embolization, is 15%. Fifty percent to seventy-five percent of those treated with embolization will have minimal to no developmental delays or permanent disabilities.

References

1. Yan J, Wen J, Gopaul R, Zhang CY, Xiao SW. Outcome and complications of endovascular embolization for vein of Galen malformations: a systematic review and meta-analysis. *J Neurosurg.* July 2015:1–19.
2. Chow ML, Cooke DL, Fullerton HJ, et al. Radiological and clinical features of vein of Galen malformations. *J Neurointerv Surg.* June 2015;7(6):443–448.

CHAPTER 13

NEUROCUTANEOUS SYNDROMES

13.1   Neurofibromatosis Type 1

Case History

A 5-year-old boy presented with headaches and "trouble seeing." Dermatological examination revealed multiple café-au-lait spots and axillary speckling. His visual acuity was 20/70 OD and 20/200 OS.

Diagnosis: Neurofibromatosis Type 1

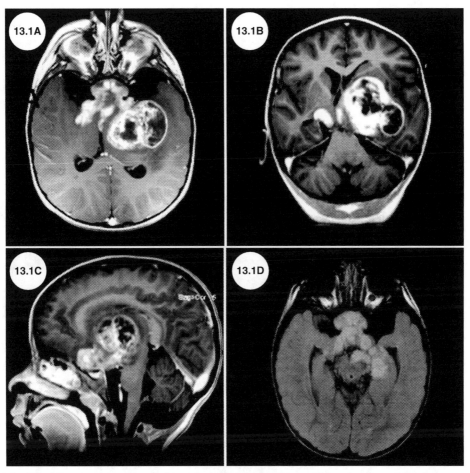

Images 13.1A–13.1D: Postcontrast axial, coronal, and sagittal T1-weighted and axial fluid-attenuated inversion recovery (FLAIR) images demonstrate a large, heterogeneously enhancing lesion arising from the optic nerves, chiasm, and tract, more so on the left, with mass effect on the temporal lobe and ventricular system.

Introduction

■ NF1 (von Recklinghausen disease) is an auto-somal-dominant condition caused by decreased production of the protein neurofibromin, which has a putative tumor suppressor function.

■ The *NF1* gene has been localized to the long arm of chromosome 17; a more severe phenotype has been observed in a subset of patients with a complete gene deletion. Only one *NF1* gene need be deleted or mutated to produce the condition.

■ Mutations in another gene (*SPRED1*) have been identified in a subset of patients described to have an NF-like syndrome, also known as Legius syndrome. These patients do not develop neuro-fibromas or Lisch nodules, unlike NF1.

Clinical Presentation

■ NF1 presents with a variable combination of cutaneous findings, benign neurofibromas, visual disturbances due to optic pathway gliomas, and abnormalities of the skeletal system. Patients develop symptoms by the age of 5.

■ Additional features include learning disabilities in about half of the patients, scoliosis, behavioral disturbances, hypertension, pheochromocytomas, hypoglycemia, iris fibromas glaucoma, seizures in 10% of patients, gliomas in the brain and brainstem, and glomus tumors. Congenital pseudoarthrosis and bowing of tibial bones can be evident at birth.

Radiographic Appearance and Diagnosis

■ The diagnosis requires the presence of at least two of seven criteria to confirm the presence of neurofibromatosis, type 1. The seven clinical criteria used to diagnose NF1 are as follows:

1. *Six or more café-au-lait spots or hyperpigmented macules greater than or equal to 5 mm in diameter in prepubertal children and 15 mm postpubertal*

2. *Axillary or inguinal freckles (>2)*

3. *Two or more typical neurofibromas or one plexiform neurofibroma*

4. *Optic nerve glioma*

5. *Two or more iris hamartomas (Lisch nodules), often identified only through slit-lamp examination*

6. *Sphenoid dysplasia or typical long-bone abnormalities such as pseudarthrosis*

7. *First-degree relative (eg, mother, father, sister, brother) with NF1*

■ Optic pathway gliomas often originate from the optic nerve, but may grow along the length of the visual pathways including the optic chiasm and tract. They homogeneously enhance with the administration of contrast, and there is often significant mass effect on adjacent structures. They are hyperintense on T2-weighted images.

■ The dermatological and ocular manifestations of NF1 are shown (see **Images 13.1E–13.1G**).

■ Plexiform neurofibromas appear as large masses on peripheral nerves.

■ Thinning of the long bones is visible on plain radiographs.

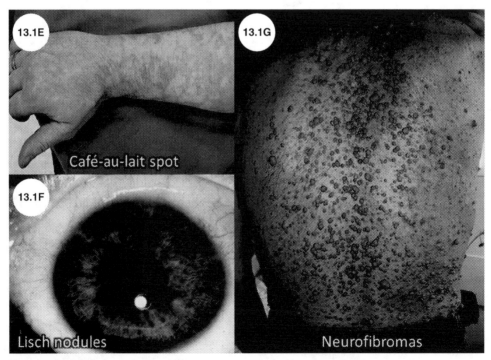

Image 13.1E: A café-au-lait spot (image credit Klaus D. Peter). **Image 13.1F:** Multiple Lisch nodules in a patient with NF1 (image: National Eye Institute). **Image 13.1G:** Multiple subcutaneous neurofibromas (image credit Klaus D. Peter).

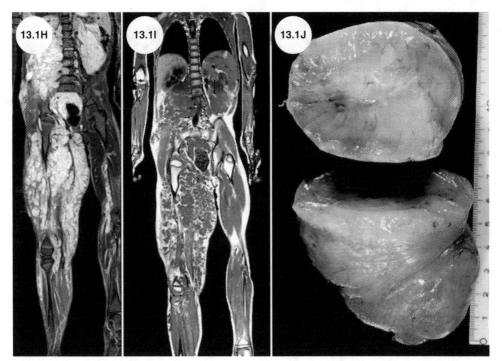

Images 13.1H and 13.1I: Coronal postcontrast T1-weighted and STIR images demonstrate an enormous plexiform neurofibroma extending from the retroperitoneum through the pelvis and right leg.
Image 13.1J: Gross pathology of a neurofibroma (image credit Jensflorian).

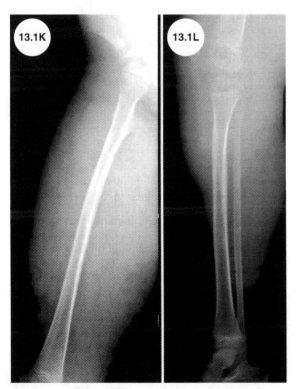

Images 13.1K and 13.1L: Lateral radiographs of the leg of a patient with NF1 demonstrate thinning of the long bones.

■ Another common finding is numerous foci of abnormal hyperintensity on T2-weighted images that are concentrated in the basal ganglia, cerebellum, and brainstem. These are referred to as "unidentified objects" or "UBOs." These lesions may represent areas of proliferation of glial cells. They may spontaneously resolve, but may be a marker for cognitive impairment.

■ The pathological findings of a neurofibroma are shown in **Image 13.1O**.

Treatment

■ Symptomatic skin neurofibromas can be treated with simple excision, carbon dioxide laser ablation, and electrocautery. Partial surgical excision of plexiform neurofibromas may be attempted, but total excision is often not possible. Resection of optic pathway gliomas may be attempted if only one nerve is affected, though there will be permanent visual loss in that eye.

■ Orthopedic surgery may be needed to correct limb overgrowth.

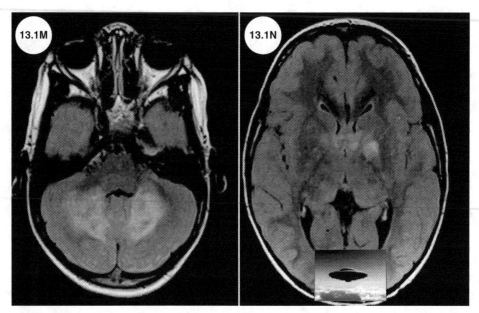

Images 13.1M and 13.1N: Axial FLAIR images demonstrate hyperintensities in the basal ganglia and cerebellum in a patient with NF1.

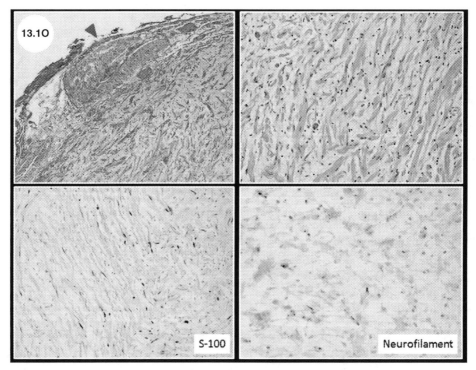

Image 13.1O: Top left: Low power view showing a well-circumscribed tumor in association with the peripheral nerve (red arrowhead). Top right: collagen bundles in a "shredded carrot" pattern in a myxoid (bluish) background. Bottom left: Patchy immunoreactivity for S-100. Bottom right: Neurofilament positive axons within the tumor. (Image courtesy of Dr. Seema Shroff, Fellow, Neuropathology, NYULMC.)

References

1. Hirbe AC, Gutmann DH. Neurofibromatosis type 1: a multidisciplinary approach to care. *Lancet Neurol.* August 2014;13(8):834–843.

2. Rosenbaum T, Wimmer K. Neurofibromatosis type 1 (NF1) and associated tumors. *Klin Padiatr.* November 2014;226(6–7): 309–315.

3. Ferner RE, Gutmann DH. Neurofibromatosis type 1 (NF1): diagnosis and management. *Handb Clin Neurol.* 2013;115:939–955.

13.2   Neurofibromatosis Type 2

Case History

A 23-year-old female developed hearing loss and tinnitus. On examination, she was found to have bilateral sensorineural hearing loss as well as mild weakness and hyperreflexia in her legs.

Diagnosis: Neurofibromatosis Type 2

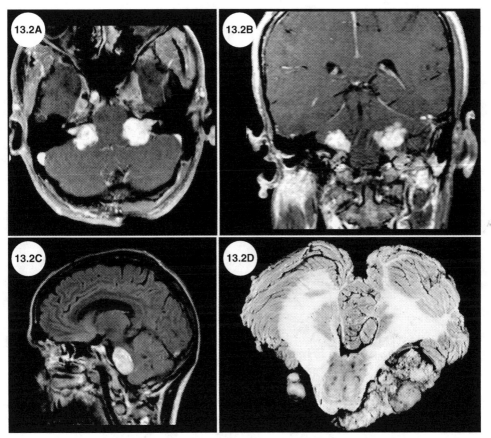

Images 13.2A–13.2C: Postcontrast axial and coronal T1-weighted and axial FLAIR images demonstrate bilateral vestibular schwannomas in a patient with neurofibromatosis type 2. **Image 13.2D:** Gross pathology of bilateral vestibular schwannomas (image credit The Armed Forces Institute of Pathology).

Introduction

■ Neurofibromatosis type 2 (NF2) is characterized by the growth of multiple, nonmalignant brain tumors. It is caused by a defect on chromosome 22 that gives rise to a product called *merlin* or *schwannomin*. It is a member of the ezrin, radixin, moesin (ERM) family of cytoskeleton–membrane linker proteins. The NF2 mutation is about 98% penetrant.

■ It affects about 1 in 60,000 people. Half of the cases are sporadic, and half are inherited in an autosomal-dominant fashion.

Clinical Presentation

■ Bilateral vestibular schwannomas are the hallmark of the disease, seen in over 90% of patients. The most common clinical presentation is slowly progressive, bilateral hearing loss in older children and young adults. Almost all patients are affected by the age of 30 years.

■ Schwannomas of other cranial nerves are seen most commonly in the trigeminal nerve. Multiple meningiomas are also characteristic and may present with seizures, headaches, or focal neurological symptoms from compression of the underlying brain or spinal cord.

■ Nearly half of the patients have spinal lesions, which present with a slowly progressive myelopathy.

■ More than 90% of patients have an opacity of the lens known as a juvenile subcapsular cataract.

■ In contrast to NF1, skin lesions are not common.

■ The formal diagnostic criteria for NF2 require one of the following clinical presentations:

  ▫ Bilateral vestibular schwannomas
  ▫ Unilateral vestibular schwannoma **and** any two of the following: meningioma, schwannoma, glioma, neurofibroma, posterior subcapsular lenticular opacity

  ▫ A first-degree relative with NF2 **and** either a unilateral vestibular schwannoma **or** any two of the following: meningioma, schwannoma, glioma, neurofibroma, posterior subcapsular lenticular opacity

  ▫ Multiple meningiomas **and** either a unilateral vestibular schwannoma **or** any two of the following: schwannoma, glioma, neurofibroma, cataract

Radiographic Appearance and Diagnosis

■ Imaging will often reveal bilateral vestibular schwannomas. These are extraaxial, enhancing masses that originate in the internal auditory canal and project into the cerebellopontine angle often with significant mass effect on the brainstem and cerebellum. Schwannomas can be seen on other cranial nerves as well, most commonly the trigeminal nerve.

■ Diagnostic technologies such as MRI and CT can reveal tumors as small as a few millimeters in diameter, thus allowing early treatment.

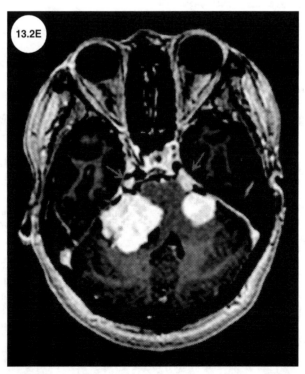

Image 13.2E: Postcontrast axial T1-weighted image demonstrates bilateral schwannomas originating from the trigeminal nerve (red arrows) in addition to bilateral vestibular schwannomas in a patient with NF2.

■ Meningiomas are extraaxial, homogeneously enhancing masses that frequently have a dural tail and externally compress the brain and spinal cord.

■ Lesions of the spinal canal include extramedullary lesions (meningiomas and schwannomas) and intramedullary lesions (astrocytomas or ependymomas).

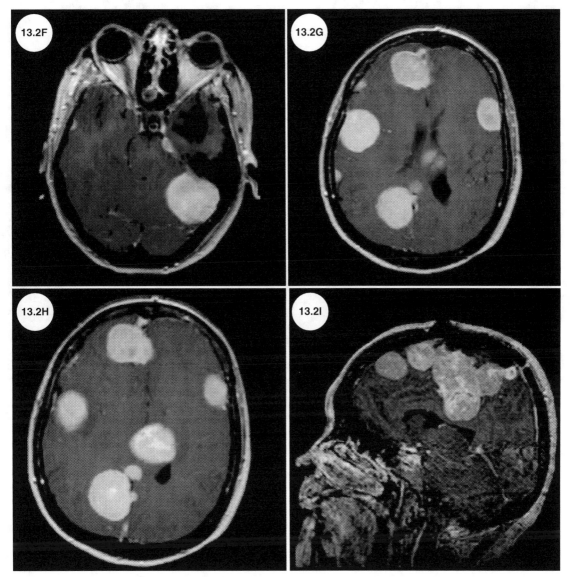

Images 13.2F–13.2I: Postcontrast axial and sagittal T1-weighted images demonstrate multiple meningiomas in a patient with NF2.

Treatment

■ At present, treatments are aimed at controlling the symptoms.

■ Surgical resection of symptomatic tumors is the mainstay of treatment. However, many tumors are not resectable due to their location and only partial removal of tumors is possible. Surgical removal of the tumors may result in hearing loss.

■ Radiation therapy (radiosurgery).

■ Watchful waiting—if tumors are not progressing rapidly or if the patient has other serious medical issues.

■ Genetic counseling is important as well.

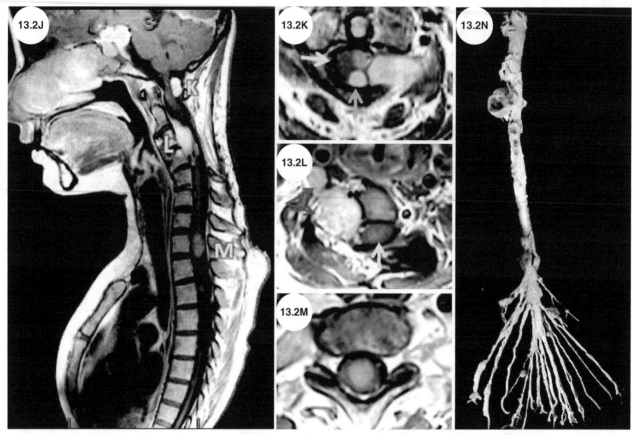

Images 13.2J–13.2N: Postcontrast sagittal and axial T1-weighted images of the cervical spine demonstrate an extradural meningioma (green arrow in Image 13.2K), the dumbbell shape of peripheral nerve schwannoma (red arrows in Image 13.2L), and an intramedullary tumor consistent with an intramedullary ependymoma (Image 13.2J). The spinal cord is indicated by the yellow arrows. Gross pathology of spinal cord in neurofibromatosis with multiple schwannomas (13.2N).

References

1. Evans DG. Neurofibromatosis type 2 (NF2): a clinical and molecular review. *Orphanet J Rare Dis.* June 2009;4:16.

2. Lloyd SK, Evans DG. Neurofibromatosis type 2 (NF2): diagnosis and management. *Handb Clin Neurol.* 2013;115: 957–967.

13.3 Sturge–Weber Syndrome

Case History

An 8-year-old boy presented with mental retardation and seizures since infancy. He had a large "port-wine stain" on his upper face on the right side.

Diagnosis: Sturge–Weber Syndrome

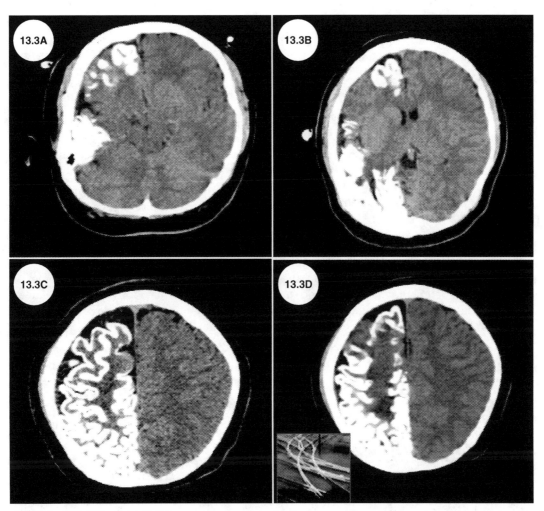

Images 13.3A–13.3D: Axial CT images demonstrate the "tram-track" calcifications of Sturge–Weber syndrome.

Introduction

■ Sturge–Weber syndrome is characterized by angiomas of the meninges, eye, face, and brain. It is unique among the neurocutaneous disorders in that it is sporadic, without a hereditary component.

Clinical Presentation

■ Patients present with seizures that usually start in infancy. There is often a port-wine stain birthmark, caused by an overgrowth of capillaries, usually in the ophthalmic nerve distribution. Malformation of blood vessels in the pia mater

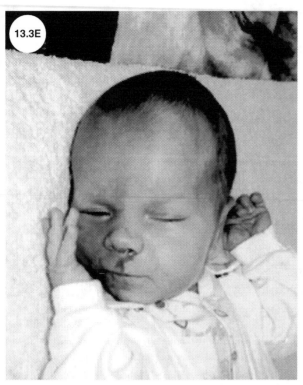

Image 13.3E: A port-wine stain in the distribution of the trigeminal nerve.

causes failure of venous drainage. This, in turn, leads to neuronal loss and calcification in the cerebral cortex ipsilateral to the birthmark. In most patients, the findings are unilateral. Stroke-like episodes, hemiparesis, visual field defects, headaches, and cognitive dysfunction are commonly encountered.

■ Ocular manifestations: glaucoma, buphthalmos, tomato-catsup fundus, iris heterochromia, tortuous retinal vessels, myopia, strabismus, amblyopia, visual field defects, conjunctival and choroid hemangiomas.

Radiographic Appearance and Diagnosis

■ Skull radiography shows classic double-lined gyriform pattern of calcifications paralleling cerebral convolutions referred to as "tram-track" or "railroad-track" calcifications.

■ Head CT and brain MRI typically reveal parietooccipital calcifications in a gyriform distribution. Most commonly the posterior portion of the brain is affected, and the frontal lobes are spared. However, in severe cases, all four lobes of the brain are involved. There may be cortical atrophy, abnormal draining veins, and an enlarged choroid plexus with prominent contrast enhancement.

■ CT or MRI may show hemiatrophy of the cerebral hemisphere; changes similar to those of the Dyke–Davidoff–Masson syndrome, including cerebral hemiatrophy with ipsilateral calvarial diploic space enlargement, may be seen in Sturge–Weber syndrome.

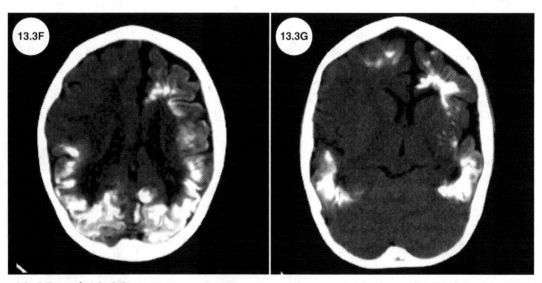

Images 13.3F and 13.3G: Axial CT images demonstrate the remarkable degree of "tram-track" calcification possible in Sturge–Weber syndrome.

■ With the addition of contrast, leptomeningeal enhancement and choroid plexus hypertrophy are commonly seen.

■ On catheter angiograms, superficial cortical veins are absent and the deep venous drainage is enlarged and abnormal.

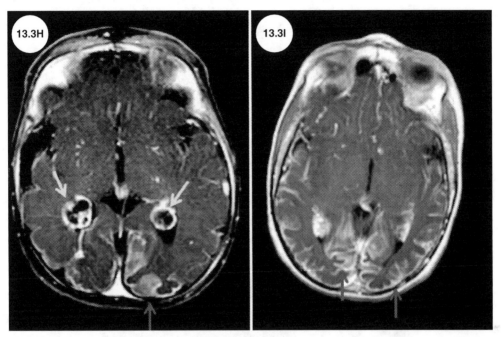

Images 13.3H and 13.3I: Postcontrast axial T1-weighted images demonstrate bilateral occipital lobe leptomeningeal enhancement (red arrows) compatible with angiomatosis. There is also enhancement and hypertrophy of the choroid plexus bilaterally (yellow arrows).

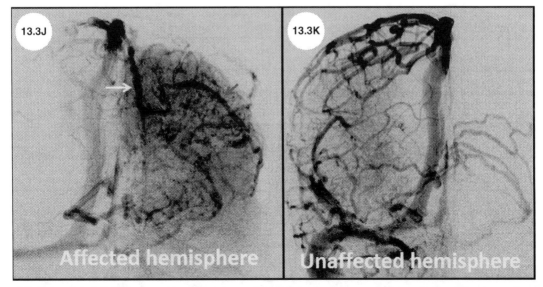

Images 13.3J and 13.3K: Anterior–posterior angiogram in the venous phase revealing that the surface medial and lateral convexity veins are absent, with exception of a single midfrontal convexity vein (red arrow) draining into the superior sagittal sinus (yellow arrow), a hallmark of Sturge–Weber syndrome. The contralateral side is normal for comparison.

Treatment

■ Seizures: Antiseizure medications, focal cortical resection, corpus callosotomy or vagal nerve stimulator (VNS). Hemispherectomy (anatomic hemispherectomy vs functional hemispherectomy vs hemidecortication) is recommended when seizures are intractable or when there is evidence of progressive cortical damage. VNS can be performed in patients who are not good candidates for other surgeries.

■ Cutaneous: dye laser anticoagulation.

■ Eyes: glaucoma surgery, radiotherapy for choroidal hemangiomas.

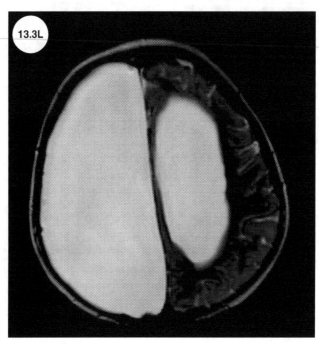

Image 13.3L: Axial T2-weighted image from a patient who underwent a right hemispherectomy to control seizures.

References

1. Sudarsanam A, Ardern-Holmes SL. Sturge-Weber syndrome: from the past to the present. *Eur J Paediatr Neurol.* May 2014;18(3):257–266.

2. Comi AM. Sturge-Weber syndrome and epilepsy: an argument for aggressive seizure management in these patients. *Expert Rev Neurother.* August 2007;7(8):951–956.

13.4 von Hippel–Lindau Syndrome

Case History

A 13-year-old presented with dizziness and ataxia.

Diagnosis: von Hippel–Lindau Syndrome

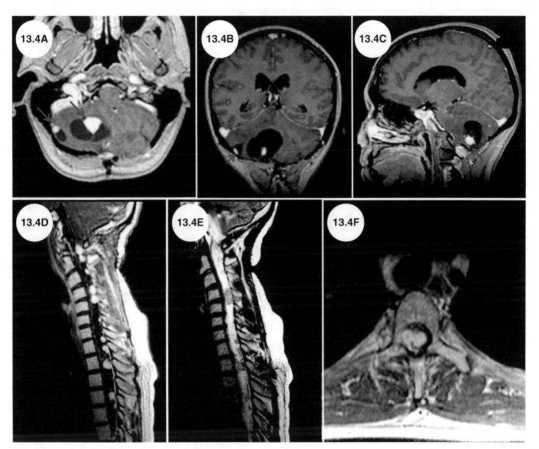

Images 13.4A–13.4C: Postcontrast axial, coronal, and sagittal T1-weighted images demonstrate two right cerebellar hemangiomas in a patient with von Hippel–Lindau syndrome. An enhancing nodule is seen at the margin of the lesions (red arrows). **Images 13.4D–13.4F:** Postcontrast sagittal T1-weighted and T2-weighted and postcontrast axial T1-weighted images demonstrate innumerable spinal hemangiomas.

Introduction

■ von Hippel–Lindau (VHL) syndrome is caused by an autosomal-dominant mutation in the *VHL* gene, which acts as a tumor suppressor. It is characterized by multiple hemangiomas of the eye and central nervous system (CNS).

Hemangioblastomas are noninfiltrative masses formed by the overgrowth of capillaries. They are the most common primary infratentorial neoplasm in adults. About 20% of all hemangioblastomas occur as part of VHL syndrome.

■ It occurs in about 1 in 35,000 to 1 in 50,000 persons.

Clinical Presentation

■ Patients present with symptoms of increased intracranial pressure (ICP) and cerebellar dysfunction. These include headache, ataxia, nausea, vomiting, and vertigo. If there is hemorrhage into the tumor, patients may experience sudden and severe neurological symptoms. Spinal hemangioblastomas present with a progressive myelopathy and are highly specific for VHL.

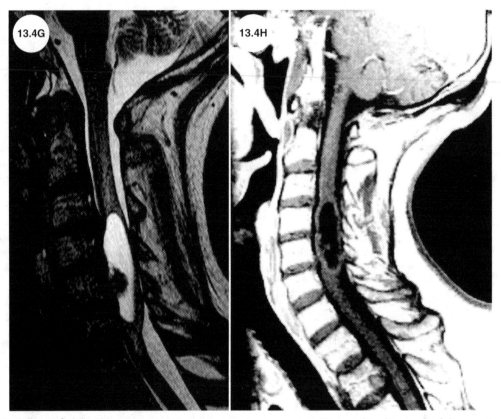

Images 13.4G and 13.4H: Sagittal T2-weighted and postcontrast T1-weighted images of the cervical spine demonstrate a hemangioblastoma, which is again cystic with a solid nodule (red arrow).

■ Retinal hemangiomas are a core feature of the disease and can cause visual loss.

■ On histology, hemangiomas are highly vascular tumors.

■ Other features include cysts of the pancreas, kidneys, liver, and reproductive organs. Clear-cell renal cell carcinomas, pancreatic neuroendocrine tumors, and pheochromocytomas also occur at an increased frequency. These tumors are a frequent cause of death for patients with VHL.

■ Approximately 10% of patients develop endolymphatic sac tumors, which can lead to sudden and severe hearing loss.

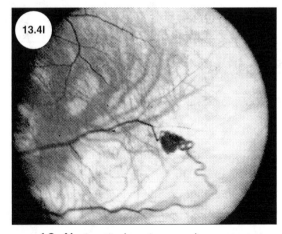

Image 13.4I: A retinal angiogram demonstrates an ocular hemangioma (image credit Dr. Stephen C. Pollack).

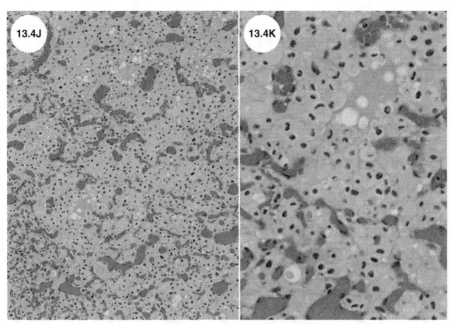

Images 13.4J and 13.4K: Low and high power magnification reveals the vascularity of a hemangioblastoma (image credit Dr. Seema Shroff, Fellow, Neuropathology, NYULMC).

Radiographic Appearance

- Hemangioblastomas are cystic masses with an enhancing nodule at the margin of the lesion 50% of the time. The contents of the cyst are isodense to cerebrospinal fluid (CSF) on all sequences. In the other 50% of cases, they are solidly enhancing masses.

- Seventy-five percent occur in the cerebellum, most often in the vermis, while the remainder occur in the spinal cord or medulla. Supratentorial hemangioblastomas are very rare.

Treatment

- It is important to screen patients with VHL for retinal angiomas, hemangioblastomas, renal carcinomas, and pheochromocytomas. Hemangioblastomas are benign, and surgery is curative if the entire tumor can be removed. The tumor will recur if resection is not complete. Treatment of retinal angiomas and renal carcinomas can reduce disability and increase life expectancy.

References

1. Friedrich CA. Von Hippel-Lindau syndrome. A pleomorphic condition. *Cancer.* December 1999;86: 2478–2482.
2. Maher ER, Neumann HP, Richard S. von Hippel-Lindau disease: a clinical and scientific review. *Eur J Hum Genet.* June 2011;19(6):617–623.
3. Chou A Toon C, Pickett J, Gill AJ. von Hippel-Lindau syndrome. *Front Horm Res.* 2013;41:30–49.

13.5 | Tuberous Sclerosis

Case History

An 8-year-old child with MR developed intractable seizures and mental retardation. The examination showed subungual fibromas of toenails, adenoma sebaceum, and a Shagreen patch. The patient had autistic features and language delays, but no focal motor or sensory deficits.

Diagnosis: Tuberous Sclerosis Complex

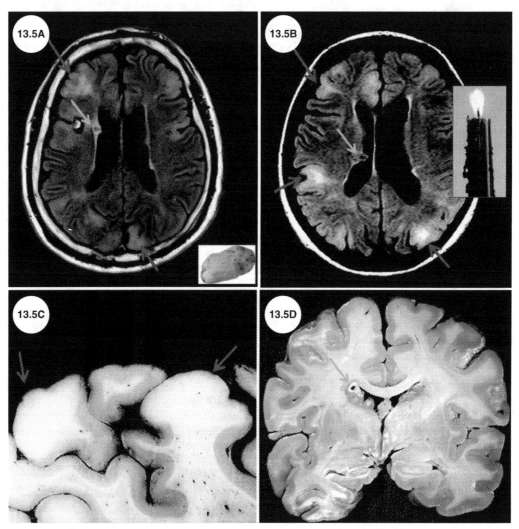

Images 13.5A and 13.5B: Axial FLAIR images demonstrate multiple cortical tubers (red arrows) and subependymal nodules (blue arrows) creating the "candle-guttering" sign. **Images 13.5C and 13.5D:** Gross pathology of cortical tubers (red arrow) and subependymal nodules (blue arrow). The cortex is thickened.

Introduction

■ Tuberous sclerosis complex (TSC) is a neurocutaneous disorder characterized by hamartomas in the brain, skin, heart, lung, liver, and kidney.

■ TSC is an autosomal-dominant disorder affecting children and adults; it results from mutations in one of two genes, *TSC1* (encoding hamartin) or *TSC2* (encoding tuberin).

Major Features of TSC

■ Facial angiofibromas or forehead plaque.

■ Nontraumatic ungual or periungual fibroma.

■ Hypomelanotic macules (>3).

■ Shagreen patch (connective tissue nevus).

■ Multiple retinal nodular hamartoma.

■ Cortical tuber: When cerebellar cortical dysplasia and cerebral white matter migration tracts occur together, they should be counted as one rather than two features of tuberous sclerosis (TS).

■ Subependymal nodules (SEN).

■ Subependymal giant cell astrocytoma (SEGA).

■ Cardiac rhabdomyoma, single or multiple.

■ Lymphangioleiomyomatosis: When both lymphangioleiomyomatosis (LAM) and renal angiomyolipomas (AMLs) are present, other features of TS should be present before a definite diagnosis is assigned. As many as 60% of women with sporadic LAM (and not TSC) may have renal or other AMLs.

■ Renal AML: When both LAM and renal AMLs are present, other features of TS should be present before a definite diagnosis is assigned (see previous remarks).

Minor Features of TSC

■ Multiple randomly distributed pits in dental enamel.

■ Hamartomatous rectal polyps: Histological confirmation is suggested.

■ Bone cysts: Radiographic confirmation is sufficient.

■ Cerebral white matter radial migration lines: Radiographic confirmation is sufficient. One panel member felt strongly that three or more radial migration lines should constitute a major sign.

■ Gingival fibromas.

■ Nonrenal hamartoma: Histological confirmation is suggested.

■ Retinal achromic patch.

■ "Confetti" skin lesions.

■ Multiple renal cysts.

Diagnostic Criteria for TSC

■ Definite TSC—Two major features or one major feature plus two or more minor features.

■ Possible TSC—Either one major feature or two or more minor features.

Clinical Presentation

■ TSC is characterized by a variable combination of mental retardation, autism, seizures, and a wide variety of dermatological abnormalities.

■ The kidneys, heart, eyes, lungs, and eyes may be affected by hamartomas.

  ▪ **Renal:** autosomal-dominant polycystic kidney disease, isolated renal cyst(s), AMLs, which are more common in women and may develop later in adulthood, and renal carcinoma.

  ▪ **Cardiac:** rhabdomyomas, which cause cardiac output failure.

  ▪ **Pulmonary:** multifocal micronodular pneumocyte hyperplasia (MMPH), pulmonary cysts, and LAM; LAM is inexorably progressive and more common in women.

  ▪ **Ocular:** retinal astrocytomas, hypopigmented areas of retina, iris, and even eyelashes.

  ▪ **Hepatic:** Cysts, typically asymptomatic and nonprogressive.

Radiographic Appearance

■ Radiographically, TS is characterized by:

  ▪ **Cortical tubers,** which are thought to be due to either poor myelination or dysplasia of the white matter. On CT images, the tubers are often calcified. On T2-weighted images, they appear as hyperdensities of the cortex and subcortical white matter. Tubers are characterized by dysplastic glial and neuronal elements and disorganized cortical lamination.

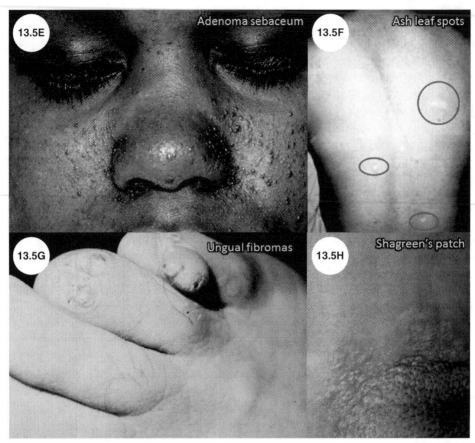

Image 13.5E: Adenoma sebaceum (image credit Herbert L. Fred, MD, and Hendrik A. van Dijk). **Image 13.5F:** Ash leaf spots (image credit Herbert L. Fred, MD, and Hendrik A. van Dijk). **Image 13.5G:** Ungual fibromas (image credit Dr. David G. Cogan). **Image 13.5H:** A shagreen's patch.

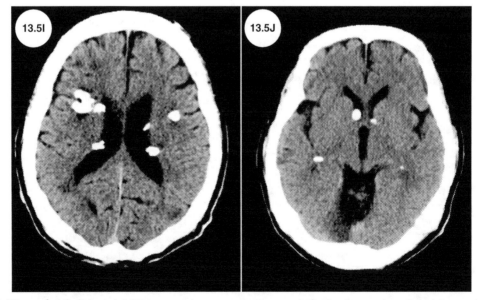

Images 13.5I and 13.5J: Axial CT images demonstrate many calcified subependymal nodules and lesions within the brain parenchyma.

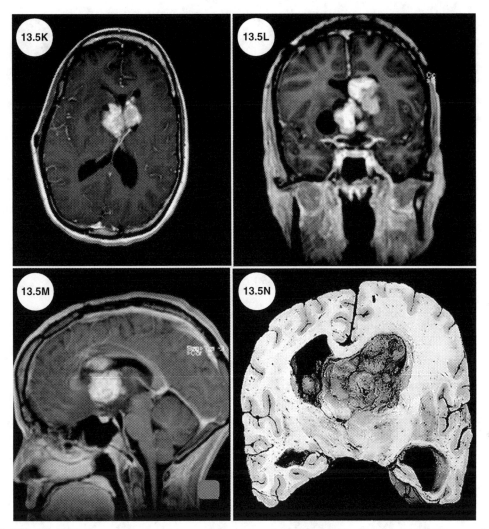

Images 13.5K–13.5M: Postcontrast axial, coronal, and sagittal T1-weighted images demonstrate a large SEGA in the left frontal horn and third ventricle with cystic portions extending into the right basal ganglia. **Image 13.5N:** Gross pathology of a SEGA (image credit The Armed Forces Institute of Pathology).

■ **Subependymal nodules (SENs).** These are projections into the walls of the lateral ventricles said to have a "candle-guttering" appearance. They are shown in **Images 13.5A and 13.5B**.

■ **Subependymal giant cell astrocytomas (SEGAs).** The generally benign SENs can degenerate into SEGAs in 5% to 10% of cases. SEGAs are benign tumors that arise from the subependyma and project into the lateral ventricle often abutting the septum pellucidum. They have variable signals on both CT and MRI depending on the degree of calcification. They are often clinically silent, but if large enough may lead to obstructive hydrocephalus and increased ICP.

■ **Cerebral aneurysms:** These have been reported intracranially as well as in the aorta and axillary arteries.

■ Extraneurological manifestations of TS include AMLs, which are benign tumors of the kidney composed of blood vessels, smooth muscle cells, and fat cells.

■ LAM is a proliferation of disorderly smooth muscle growth throughout the lungs and pulmonary vasculature.

Treatment

■ Seizures: antiseizure medications; note that vigabatrin (Sabril) is considered a first-line therapy for infantile spasms; ketogenic diet.

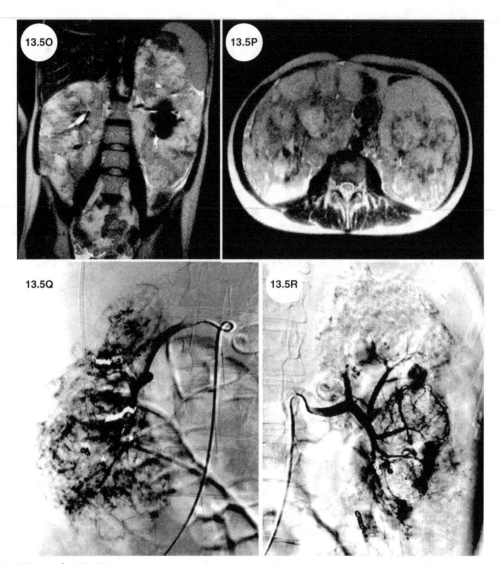

Images 13.5O and 13.5P: Coronal and axial T1-weighted images of the abdomen and pelvis showing massive renal enlargement due to innumerable angiomyolipomas. **Images 13.5Q and 13.5R:** Right and left renal angiograms demonstrate abnormal vessels associated with angiomyolipomas.

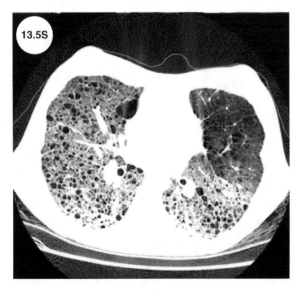

Image 13.5S: Axial chest CT image demonstrates severe cystic lung disease consistent with lymphangiomyomatosis.

- m-TOR inhibitors: rapamycin or sirolimus or everolimus (Afinitor) is used to treat various hamartomas or SEGAs.

- Surgery: surgical resection of tumors affecting various organs if symptomatic; focal cortical resection, corpus callosotomy, VNS, removal of SEGAs, shunt surgery for obstructive hydrocephalus.

- Facial angiofibromas: laser therapy, topical rapamycin.

References

1. Grajkowska W, Kotulska K, Jurkiewicz E, Matyja E. Brain lesions in tuberous sclerosis complex. Review. *Folia Neuropathol.* 2010;48(3):139–149.

2. Borkowska J, Schwartz RA, Kotulska K, Jozwiak S. Tuberous sclerosis complex: tumors and tumorigenesis. *Int J Dermatol.* January 2011;50(1):13–20.

3. Fallah A, Rodgers SD, Weil AG, et al. Resective epilepsy surgery for tuberous sclerosis in children: determining predictors of seizure outcomes in a multicenter retrospective cohort Study. *Neurosurgery.* October 2015;77(4):517–524.

CHAPTER 14

TRAUMA

14.1 | Epidural Hematoma

Case History

Patient 1: A 35-year-old woman was hit in the head during a fight. Though the patient was initially unconscious, she soon seemed to be fine and was able to talk and act normally. She returned home and about 3 hours later was taken to a local hospital after complaining of a headache. She was transferred from there by ambulance in critical condition and was admitted about 7 hours after the fall. She died the next day.

Patient 2: A 55-year-old man arrived unconscious after a car accident.

Patient 3: A 23-year-old man arrived unconscious after he was hit in the head with a blunt object.

Diagnosis: Epidural Hematoma

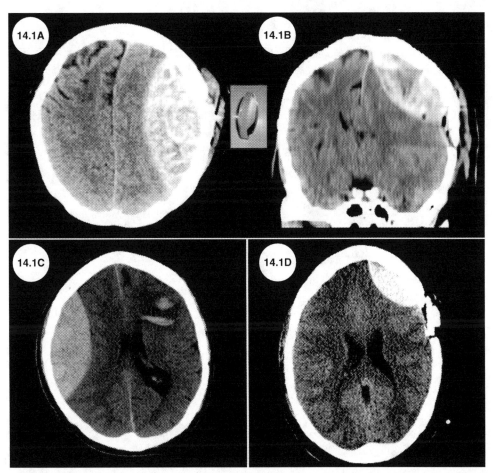

Images 14.1A and 14.1B: Axial and coronal CT images demonstrate a large, "lens-shaped" left epidural hematoma with midline shift and subfalcine herniation visible on the coronal image. **Image 14.1C:** Axial CT image demonstrates a large, right epidural hematoma with midline shift and hemorrhagic contusions in the left frontal lobe. **Image 14.1D:** Axial CT image demonstrates a left epidural hematoma with a skull fracture.

Introduction

■ Epidural hematomas occur when there is damage to the middle meningeal artery, a branch of the external carotid artery found in the epidural space.

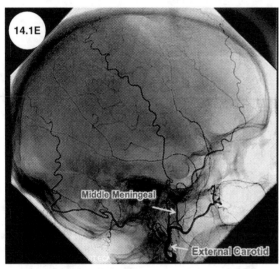

Image 14.1E: Catheter angiogram demonstrating the location of the middle meningeal artery.

Clinical Presentation

■ Patients present after head trauma or neurosurgical procedures. The degree of trauma required to produce an epidural hematoma causes a concussion severe enough to render the patient unconscious. After the patient awakens from this initial blow, there is a lucid period of several hours, after which there may be rapid neurological deterioration due to expansion of the hematoma.

■ The rapidity of the decline occurs as the expanding hematoma is from an arterial source, in contrast to subdural hematomas (SDHs), which originate from the lower pressure venous system. Additionally, the dura is firmly adherent to the skull at suture lines. As the hematoma expands, it cannot cross these suture lines, causing compression of the underlying brain.

Radiographic Appearance and Diagnosis

■ CTs are the imaging modality of choice for patients with head trauma. Epidural hematomas have a lens-shaped appearance. Depending on the size and location of the hematoma, there may be mass effect and brain herniation.

Treatment

■ The treatment for expanding epidural hematomas is immediate neurosurgical evacuation. Without treatment, large bleeds may be fatal in several hours.

References

1. Araujo JL, Aguiar Udo P, Todeschini AB, Saade N, Veiga JC. Epidemiological analysis of 210 cases of surgically treated traumatic extradural hematoma. *Rev Col Bras Cir*. July–August 2012;39(4):268–271.
2. Zink BJ. Traumatic brain injury outcome: concepts for emergency care. *Ann Emerg Med*. March 2001;37(3):318–332.
3. Graham DI, Gennareli TA. Pathology of brain damage after head injury. In: Cooper P, Golfinos G, eds. *Head Injury*. 4th ed. New York, NY: Morgan Hill; 2000:133–154.

14.2 Subdural Hematoma

Case History

An 80-year-old man presented to the hospital after falling down at home. He was discharged, but returned 21 days later with confusion and headaches.

Diagnosis: Subdural Hematoma

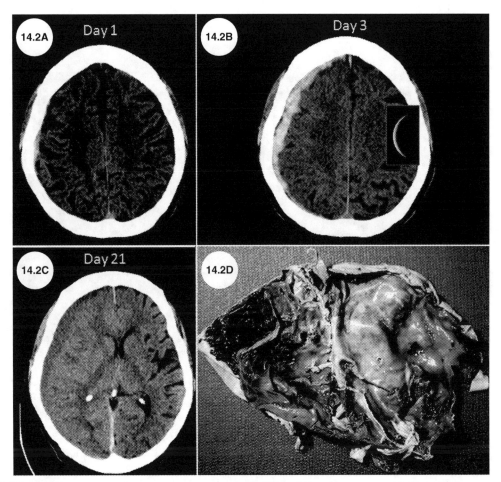

Image 14.2A: Axial CT image demonstrates a very small right subdural hematoma (red arrow). **Image 14.2B:** Axial CT image, taken 3 days later, demonstrates marked expansion of the hematoma. It is crescent-shaped. **Image 14.2C:** Axial CT image, taken 21 days later, demonstrates the evolution of the hematoma. As there is no longer acute blood, the appearance is isodense to brain parenchyma. **Image 14.2D:** Gross pathology of a subdural hematoma.

Introduction

■ SDHs are due to tearing of the bridging veins, which course through the dura and drain the underlying brain into the dural sinuses. Movement of the brain within the skull can tear the bridging veins and cause bleeding into the potential space between the dura and arachnoid layer.

Clinical Presentation

■ SDH presents with a headache, cognitive dysfunction, or progressive focal neurological deficits. Since the bleeding is under venous pressure, the hematoma can present quite slowly and grow to a large size before patients develop symptoms.

■ Elderly patients and alcoholics are especially vulnerable to SDHs as brain atrophy leads to stretching of the bridging veins. In this population, they are sometimes found incidentally, and large SDHs can accumulate with minor trauma or even without a known history of trauma.

Radiographic Appearance and Diagnosis

■ CT is the imaging modality of choice to investigate SDHs. Acute SDHs present with a crescent-shaped hyperdensity representing acute blood products. There may be significant mass effect and compression of the underlying brain depending on its size. Over the next few weeks to months, the blood is replaced by cerebrospinal fluid (CSF), and the fluid collection has a density similar to CSF. Patients may suffer recurrent bleeding, with both chronic and acute blood products.

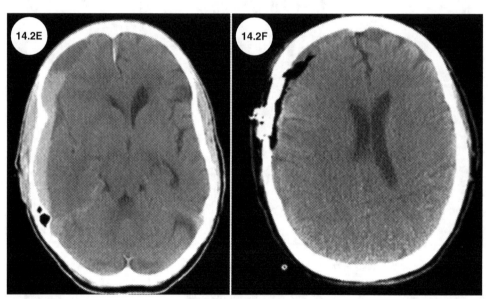

Image 14.2E: Axial CT scan demonstrates large right subdural hematoma with both acute blood and chronic fluid collection. There is a large amount of mass effect with midline shift. **Image 14.2F:** Axial CT scan, taken after neurosurgical evacuation reveals a decrease in the mass effect and pneumocephalus.

Treatment

■ Small SDHs may be monitored clinically and radiographically. Surgical evacuation is required to treat larger, symptomatic SDHs.

References

1. Iliescu IA. Current diagnosis and treatment of chronic subdural haematomas. *J Med Life*. July–September 2015;8(3):278–284.

2. Iliescu IA, Constantinescu AI. Clinical evolutional aspects of chronic subdural haematomas—literature review. *J Med Life*. 2015;8:26–33.

3. Adhiyaman V, Asghar M, Ganeshram KN, Bhowmick BK. Chronic subdural haematoma in the elderly. *Postgrad Med J*. February 2002;78(916):71–75.

14.3 | Hemorrhagic Contusions

Case History

A 43-year-old man arrived unconscious after a motor vehicle accident.

Diagnosis: Hemorrhagic Contusions

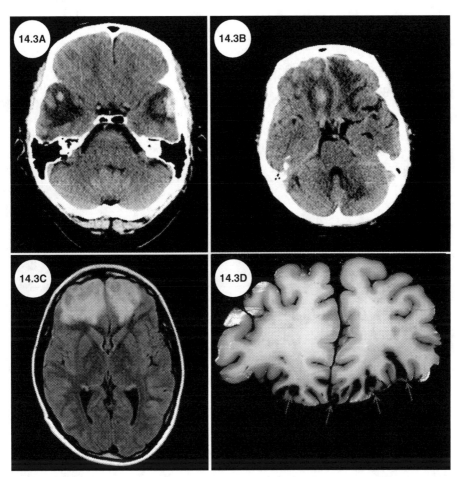

Images 14.3A and 14.3B: Axial CT images demonstrate hemorrhagic contusions in the temporal and frontal lobes bilaterally. **Image 14.3C:** Axial fluid-attenuated inversion recovery (FLAIR) image demonstrates hemorrhagic contusions in the frontal lobes. **Image 14.3D:** Hemorrhagic contusions are visible frontal lobes on gross pathology (red arrows).

Introduction

■ Trauma is one of the leading causes of intraparenchymal hemorrhage and cerebral contusion. The orbitofrontal cortex and anterior temporal lobes are especially vulnerable in acceleration–deceleration injuries, when the brain crashes into and is lacerated by bone at the base of the skull. The surface of the brain is most commonly affected.

■ Contusions that occur directly below the site of impact are referred to as coup injuries, while those that are on the opposite side of the skull are called contrecoup injuries. The impact accelerates first the skull (at this point the brain immediately subjacent to the point of impact may be damaged—so-called coup injury) and then its content away from it. As the skull stops, the brain then impacts on the internal surface of the skull, resulting in damage, called the contrecoup injury. Often, the contrecoup injury is larger than the coup injury.

Clinical Presentation

■ Patients with severe hemorrhagic contusions are always rendered unconscious by the trauma. Those with damage to the orbitofrontal cortex are frequently disinhibited and demonstrate poor executive function as a result of their injuries. Patients with damage to the temporal lobes have difficulty with memory consolidation and develop seizures as a result. Aphasia is commonly seen with left-sided lesions.

Radiographic Appearance and Diagnosis

■ CT scans are used initially in head trauma patients to visualize the blood. Their sensitivity approaches 100% in detected hemorrhagic contusions, though blood may appear isodense in patients with severe anemia. MRI is not often performed in such patients, but is more sensitive for contusions.

Treatment

■ Treatment is supportive. There is evidence that prophylactic anticonvulsants decrease the rate of seizures in the short term, but not in the long term.

Reference

1. Torbic H, Forni AA, Anger KE, Degrado JR, Greenwood BC. Use of antiepileptics for seizure prophylaxis after traumatic brain injury. *Am J Health Syst Pharm*. May 2013;70(9): 759–766.

14.4 | Diffuse Axonal Injury

Case History

A 35-year-old woman developed significant cognitive impairment after a motor vehicle accident.

Diagnosis: Diffuse Axonal Injury

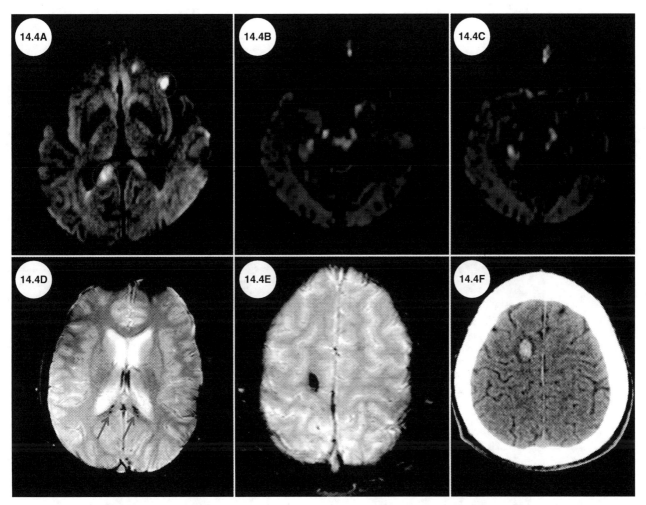

Images 14.4A–14.4C: Axial-diffusion-weighted images demonstrate areas of restricted diffusion, with several lesions in the corpus callosum and the grey–white junction, and midbrain characteristic of diffuse axonal injury.
Images 14.4D and 14.4E: Axial gradient echo images demonstrate foci of susceptibility secondary to prior microhemorrhages. The red arrows point to microhemorrhage in the corpus callosum, a typical location for such hemorrhages. **Image 14.4F:** Axial CT image demonstrates intraparenchymal hemorrhage in the right frontal lobe.

Introduction

- Diffuse axonal injury (DAI) occurs due to shear forces in patients with head injuries that involve angular rotation and acceleration–deceleration injuries, most commonly motor vehicle accidents.

- In such injuries, the cerebral hemispheres rotate around the upper brainstem. The tentorium cerebelli prevents movement of the cerebellum, and swinging motion of the cerebrum is prevented by the falx cerebri. As a result, axons are stretched, though not torn.

Clinical Presentation

■ Patients with injuries severe enough to produce DAI uniformly suffer immediate loss of consciousness. Many remain comatose or in a persistent vegetative state. The extent of the injury might not be appreciated until patients fail to improve as expected. Those who regain consciousness are left with severe cognitive deficits.

■ There is no treatment beyond supportive care.

Radiographic Appearance and Diagnosis

■ The lesions are typically oblong and located at the grey–white junction. They may also be seen in the corpus callosum and, in severe cases, the brainstem.

■ The initial imaging modality in trauma patients is a noncontrast CT. However, only large hemorrhages will be seen, and most DAIs are too small to be seen on CT. MRI is much more sensitive, and often multiple small microhemorrhages can be seen best on gradient echo imaging. Diffusion-weighted imaging is also very sensitive for revealing the DAI.

■ A grading system exists for DAI as follows:

   ■ **Grade I:** Involves the grey–white matter junction, primarily of the frontal and temporal lobes.

   ■ **Grade II:** Involves the corpus callosum, most commonly the splenium and posterior body.

   ■ **Grade III:** Involves the brainstem or cerebellum.

Treatment

■ Treatment is supportive.

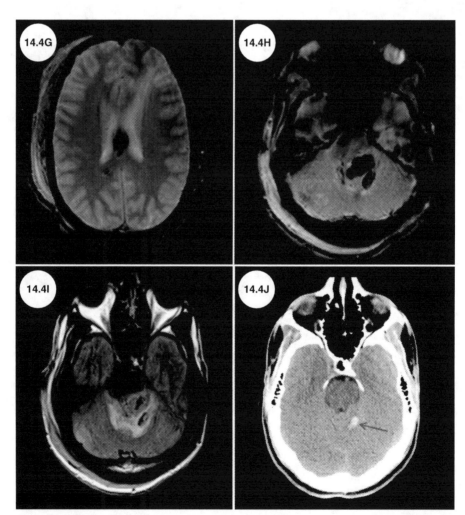

Images 14.4G and 14.4H: Axial gradient echo images demonstrate foci of susceptibility in the corpus callous, brainstem, and cerebellum in a patient with severe head trauma. Soft tissue swelling is evident over the right calvarium. **Images 14.4I and 14.4J:** Axial FLAIR and CT image demonstrate acute blood products (red arrow) in the cerebellum and edema throughout the cerebellum and pons.

14.5 | Gunshot Wound

Case History

A 45-year-old woman developed personality changes after being shot in the head.

A 25-year-old woman developed paraplegia after being shot in the back.

Diagnosis: Gunshot Wound

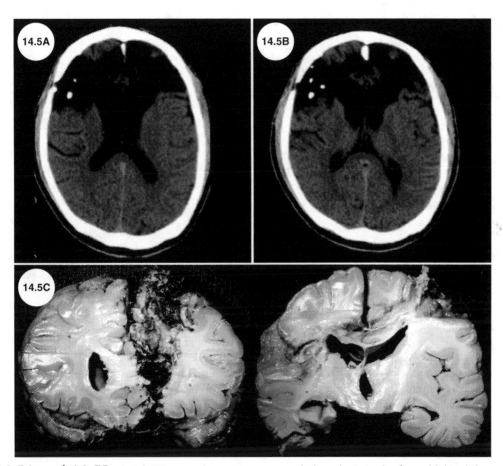

Images 14.5A and 14.5B: Axial CT scans demonstrate encephalomalacia in the frontal lobes bilaterally with residual bone fragments in the right frontal lobe in a patient who suffered a gunshot wound. **Image 14.5C:** Gross pathology of gunshot wounds in two different patients (image credit Roberta J. Seidman, MD).

Introduction

■ Trauma remains the leading cause of neurological disability in young people, and unfortunately, gunshot wounds are common in the United States. There are approximately 130,000 people shot annually in the United States, and over 30,000 deaths.

■ Approximately 62% of gun deaths are suicides. With homicides, African American men between the ages of 15 and 40 are by far most likely to be victims.

Clinical Presentation

■ The injury suffered by the patient depends on the type of weapon used, the bullet used, and the location of the injury. The brain and spinal cord are particularly vulnerable to gunshot wounds. Bullets fired from rifles have the greatest velocity,

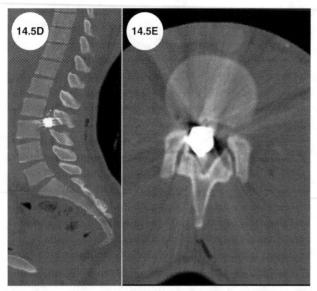

Images 14.5D and 14.5E: Sagittal and axial CT scans of the lumbar spine demonstrate a bullet in the upper lumbar spine, at the level of the conus medullaris.

and encased bullets that rotate around their short axes or deform upon impact cause more local tissue damage. Not surprisingly, many gunshot wounds to the head are instantly fatal.

Radiographic Appearance and Diagnosis

▓ CT is the modality of choice when imaging gunshot victims, though most bullets are safe to use with MRIs.

▓ Imaging is useful in gunshot injuries to determine the course of the bullet and assess for hemorrhage and air. The final location of the bullet may be quite distant from its entry point as internal structures alter its course. It the bullet is not found, the exit wound must be located.

Treatment

▓ In studies by Moraes et al and Vècsei V. et al, patients with lower admission scores on the Glasgow Coma Scale (GCS), a unilateral dilated pupil or medium fixed pupil, a transventricular or bihemispheric bullet trajectory, intraventricular hemorrhage, and bilobar or multilobar wounds were strong factors in predicting morbidity and mortality. In such patients, surgical treatment was only suggested in the presence of a hematoma with mass effect and the outcome is poor. In contrast, patients with a GCS score above 8, normal pupils, and injury to a single brain lobe may benefit from aggressive treatment.

References

1. Martins RS, Siqueira MG, Santos MT, Zanon-Collange N, Moraes OJ. Prognostic factors and treatment of penetrating gunshot wounds to the head. *Surg Neurol.* August 2003;60(2): 98–104.

2. Hofbauer M, Kdolsky R, Figl M, et al. Predictive factors influencing the outcome after gunshot injuries to the head-a retrospective cohort study. *J Trauma.* October 2010;69(4):770–775.

3. Kim TW, Lee JK, Moon KS, et al. Penetrating gunshot injuries to the brain. *J Trauma.* June 2007;62(6):1446–1451.

CHAPTER 15
MISCELLANEOUS

15.1 | Behcet's Disease

Case History

A 42-year-old man from Jordan presented with severe dysarthria, imbalance, and diplopia.

Diagnosis: Behcet's Disease

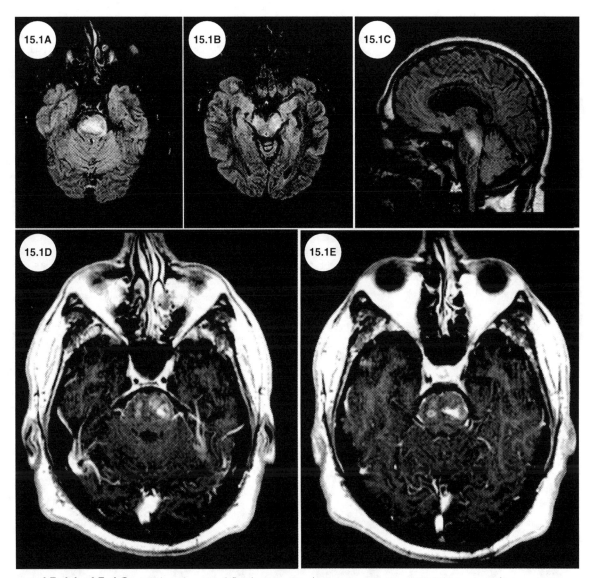

Images 15.1A–15.1C: Axial and sagittal fluid-attenuated inversion recovery (FLAIR) images demonstrate hyperintensity of the pontine tegmentum, midbrain, and pons. **Images 15.1D and 15.1E:** Postcontrast axial T1-weighted images demonstrate patchy enhancement of the lesions in the pons.

Introduction

- Behcet's disease is a systemic, necrotizing vasculitis, most commonly seen in the Middle East and Central Asia.

Clinical Presentation

- Patients develop oral and genital ulcers and can have ocular manifestations (uveitis or retinal vasculitis). Multiple organ systems, including the gastrointestinal, pulmonary, musculoskeletal, cardiovascular, and neurological systems can be involved.

- The formal diagnostic criteria for Behcet's disease are oral ulcers at least thrice (in any 12-month period), along with two out of the following four symptoms:

    1. Anal or genital ulcers (including orchitis or epididymitis in males).
    2. Dermatological lesion such as erythema nodosum, acne, or folliculitis.
    3. Ocular inflammation including uveitis, iritis, or retinal vasculitis.
    4. Positive pathergy reaction, defined as a papule larger than 2 mm, 24 to 48 hours after a needle prick.

- The central nervous system (CNS) is involved in 30% to 40% of patients, and only rarely are CNS manifestations the presenting symptom. The symptoms are not specific and include headache, lethargy, cranial neuropathies, ataxia, weakness, and sensory disturbances. Meningitis and sinus venous thrombosis are other possible presentations.

Radiographic Appearance and Diagnosis

- The most commonly involved areas are the basal ganglia, brainstem, and subcortical white matter. Lesions are hyperintense on T2-weighted images with mass effect and edema. There is a variable pattern of enhancement with the administration of contrast. As in this case, the pontomedullary junction is a common location for brainstem lesions. In patients without systemic manifestations of Behcet's disease, these lesions may be indistinguishable from neoplasms. Lesions may also be seen in the basal ganglia, thalami, optic nerves, and, rarely, the spinal cord.

- Sinus venous thrombosis will appear as clots in the venous system.

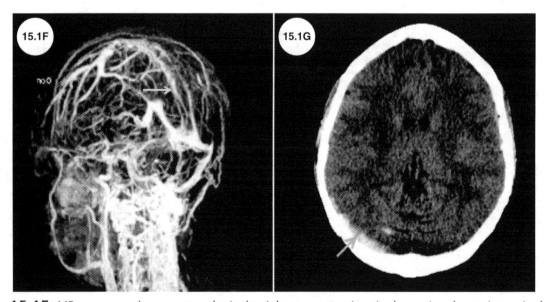

Image 15.1F: MR venogram demonstrates clot in the right transverse sinus (red arrow) and superior sagittal sinus (yellow arrow). **Image 15.1G:** Axial CT image demonstrates hyperdensity in the right transverse sinus corresponding to the clot (blue arrow).

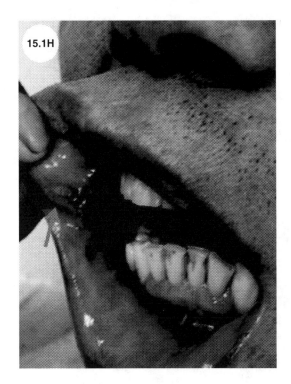

Image 15.1H: An oral ulcer in a patient with Behcet's disease (pink arrow) (image credit Drs. Ahmet Altiner and Rajni Mandal).

- It is associated with HLA-B51, and this is frequently tested.
- General examination may reveal oral or genital ulcers.

Treatment

- It is treated with immunosuppression or with tumor necrosis factor (TNF)-alpha inhibitors, such as etanercept or infliximab.

References

1. Peño IC, De las Heras Revilla V, Carbonell BP, et al. Neurobehçet: clinical and demographic characteristics. *Eur J Neurol.* September 2012;19(9):1224–1227.
2. Houman MH, Bellakhal S, Ben Salem T, et al. Characteristics of neurological manifestations of Behçet's: a retrospective monocentric study in Tunisia. *Clin Neurol Neurosurg.* October 2013;115(10):2015–2018.
3. Aguiar de Sousa D, Mestre T, Ferro JM. Cerebral venous thrombosis in Behçet's disease: a systematic review. *J Neurol.* May 2011;258(5):719–727.

15.2 Neurosarcoidosis

Case History

A 45-year-old man developed seizures and cognitive impairment.

Diagnosis: Neurosarcoidosis

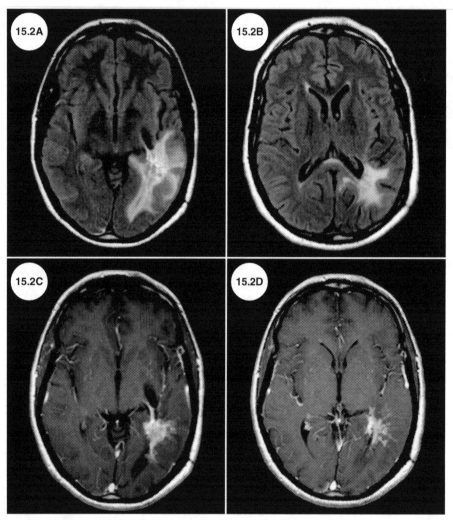

Images 15.2A–15.2D: Axial FLAIR and postcontrast T1-weighted images demonstrate an enhancing, spiculated lesion in the left temporal and parietal lobes with surrounding edema.

Introduction

■ Sarcoidosis is an idiopathic disease characterized by noncaseating granulomas, primarily in the lung. Approximately 10% of patients have involvement of the CNS, though isolated CNS involvement is unusual. It affects women more commonly than men, usually between the ages of 30 and 40.

Clinical Presentation

■ Neurosarcoidosis can present with a wide spectrum of clinical manifestations, which can prove a diagnostic challenge in patients without systemic manifestations. The most common form of CNS involvement is a basilar meningitis that presents with hydrocephalus and cranial neuropathies. The optic and facial nerves are the most commonly affected, and involvement of the facial nerve may be bilateral. Any of the cranial nerves may be affected, however, leading to diplopia, dysphagia, hearing loss, vertigo, and tongue weakness. Leptomeningeal involvement occurs in nearly 50% of patients and may lead to hydrocephalus.

◼ Involvement of the pituitary gland may lead to diabetes insipidus and other endocrinopathies, while hypothalamic involvement can lead to changes in appetite and temperature dysregulation.

◼ Parenchymal involvement can cause seizures, cognitive impairment, psychiatric disturbances, and focal neurological deficits.

◼ Involvement of the spinal cord and spinal nerve roots may cause a severe, painful myelopathy.

◼ The peripheral and autonomic nervous systems can be involved as well.

Radiographic Appearance and Diagnosis

◼ The imaging findings are highly variable, reflecting the diverse clinical picture in neurosarcoidosis. The imaging findings are nonspecific and may mimic neoplastic or demyelinating disease. CNS disease takes several forms: parenchymal involvement, leptomeningeal involvement, and involvement of the pituitary gland/stalk, hypothalamus, and cranial nerves. The spinal cord may also be involved.

Parenchymal Involvement

There are different patterns of parenchymal involvement in neurosarcoidosis.

◼ **Enhancing mass:** As seen in **Images 15.2A–15.2D**, neurosarcoidosis may present as an enhancing mass that is hyperintense on T2-weighted images with nodular or solid enhancement.

◼ **White matter disease:** White matter disease with perivascular enhancement may be difficult to distinguish from multiple sclerosis. Examples from two different patients are shown in **Images 15.2E–15.2J**.

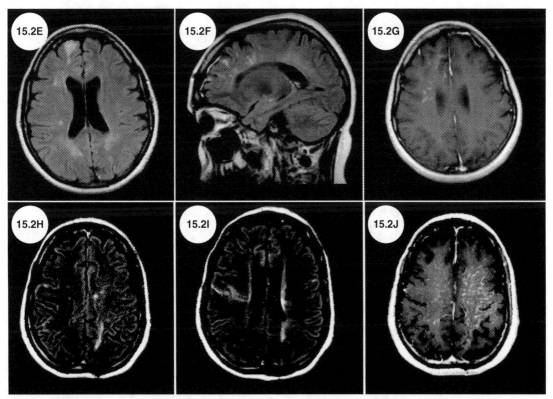

Images 15.2E–15.2G: Axial and sagittal FLAIR and postcontrast axial T1-weighted images demonstrate multiple white matter lesions with a cortical lesion in the right frontal lobe. Many of the lesions enhance. **Images 15.2H–15.2J:** Axial FLAIR and postcontrast T1-weighted images from another patient demonstrate extensive white matter and cortical hyperintensities with linear streaks of enhancement predominantly in the left frontal lobe.

Leptomeningeal Involvement

Leptomeningeal enhancement is common, particularly around the basal cisterns. The enhancement may be smooth or nodular. It can cause a vasculitis with resultant infarction, and over time there may be significant hydrocephalus.

Pituitary Gland and Stalk, Hypothalamus, Cranial Nerves

Pituitary/hypothalamic and cranial nerve involvement is seen in 40% of the cases. The facial and optic nerves are most commonly involved, though any cranial nerve can be affected. Involvement of the 'cranial nerves, pituitary gland, and hypothalamus often occurs with extensive involvement of the basilar meninges, but may occur in isolation. Examples from two different patients are shown in **Images 15.2O–15.2T.**

Spinal Cord

The myelopathy of sarcoidosis leads to a swollen spinal cord, with intramedullary enhancement and often of the meninges surrounding the cord. It preferentially affects the cervical spine. This form of neurosarcoidosis has the worst prognosis.

■ Cerebrospinal fluid (CSF) analysis commonly reveals a moderate lymphocytic pleocytosis and elevated protein. A low CSF glucose (hypoglycorrhachia) is highly suggestive of this diagnosis. Oligoclonal bands will be present in about 30% of cases. Serum angiotensin converting enzyme (ACE) is elevated in half of the patients.

■ In cases without systemic manifestations, the diagnosis may be difficult, and a chest CT or PET scan should be performed in suspected cases to screen for occult disease in the lungs or lymph nodes. A biopsy is often required to confirm the diagnosis.

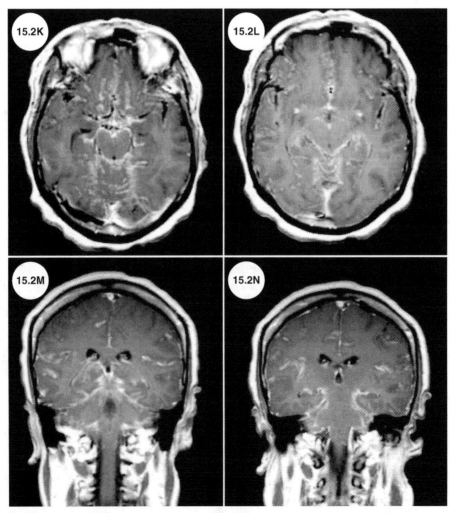

Images 15.2K–15.2N: Postcontrast axial and coronal T1-weighted images demonstrate extensive leptomeningeal enhancement, primarily in the basal cisterns.

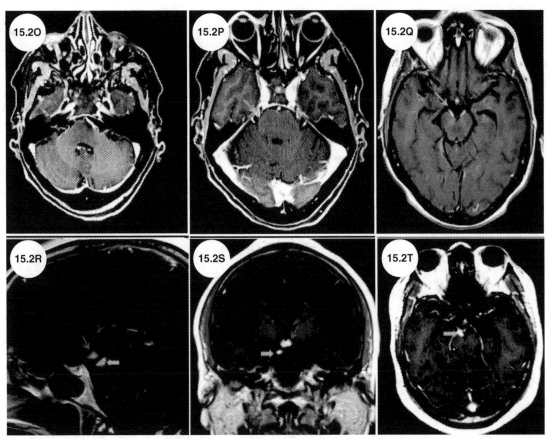

Images 15.2O–15.2Q: Postcontrast axial T1-weighted images demonstrate enhancement of the facial (red arrow), trigeminal (orange arrow), and oculomotor (blue arrow) nerves bilaterally in a patient with sarcoidosis.
Images 15.2R–15.2T: Postcontrast sagittal, coronal, and axial T1-weighted images demonstrate enhancement of the hypothalamus (red arrows) and oculomotor nerve (blue arrows).

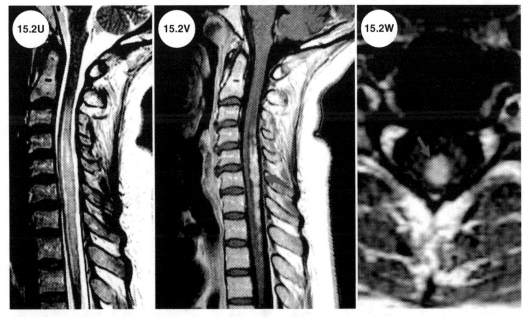

Images 15.2U–15.2W: Sagittal T2-weighted and postcontrast sagittal and axial T1-weighted images demonstrate a longitudinally extensive myelitis with cord swelling and enhancement (red arrows) of the dorsal columns in a patient with neurosarcoidosis.

Treatment

- It is treated with a combination of steroids and immunosuppression. Infliximab has been used in treatment-refractory cases.

References

1. Tavee JO, Stern BJ. Neurosarcoidosis. *Continuum (Minneap Minn)*. June 2014;20(3 Neurology of Systemic Disease):545–559.

2. Schwendimann RN, Harris MK, Elliott DG, et al. Neurosarcoidosis: clinical features, diagnosis, and management. *Am J Ther.* May–June 2013;20(3):292–299.

3. Vargas DL, Stern BJ. Neurosarcoidosis: diagnosis and management. *Semin Respir Crit Care Med.* August 2010;31(4): 419–427.

4. Stjepanović MI, Vucinić VM, Jovanović D, Mijajlović M, Trifunović VS, Stjepanović MM. Treatment of neurosarcoidosis: innovations and challenges. *Med Pregl.* May–June 2014; 67:161–166.

15.3 Langerhans Cell Histiocytosis

Case History

A 17-year-old girl presented with bone pain, hearing loss, and excessive urination.

Diagnosis: Langerhans Cell Histiocytosis

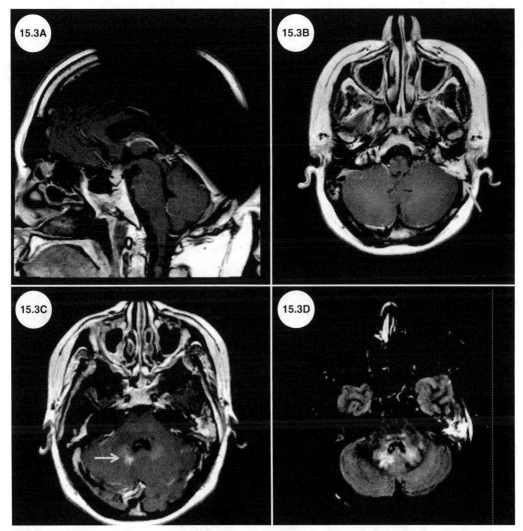

Images 15.3A–15.3C: Postcontrast sagittal and axial T1-weighted images demonstrate enhancement of the infundibulum and hypothalamus (red arrow), an enhancing mass in the temporal bone (blue arrow), and enhancement of the dentate nuclei (yellow arrow). **Image 15.3D:** Axial FLAIR image demonstrates symmetrical hyperintensity in the dentate nuclei and medial lemniscus in the pons.

Introduction

■ Langerhans cell histiocytosis is a multiorgan disease that usually occurs in young children. Excess immature Langerhans cells form granulomas.

■ It is a rare disease affecting only about 1 to 2 in 100,000 people.

Clinical Presentation

■ It most commonly affects the bones, leading to pain, swelling, and fractures. Patients with involvement of the CNS present with a degenerative course of highly variable severity and speed. CNS disease usually manifests as diabetes insipidus due to involvement of the hypothalamic–pituitary axis. Cranial-facial involvement due to bone destruction of the skull and orbits is also common.

Radiographic Appearance

■ The most common findings are bony lesions of the skull or craniofacial bones. Dural-based masses, cystic lesions of the pineal gland, infundibular thickening, choroid-plexus lesions, prominent, dilated *Virchow–Robin spaces*, T2 hyperintensity of the pons and dentate nucleus of the cerebellum, and brain atrophy are all well described.

■ Histology is needed to confirm the diagnosis.

Treatment

■ Systemic disease requires treatment with steroids and chemotherapy. Even with treatment, mortality may approach 10%.

References

1. Gabbay LB, Leite Cda C, Andriola RS, Pinho Pda C, Lucato LT. Histiocytosis: a review focusing on neuroimaging findings. *Arq Neuropsiquiatr*. July 2014 Jul;72(7):548–558.
2. Prayer D, Grois N, Prosch H, Gadner H, Barkovich AJ. MR imaging presentation of intracranial disease associated with Langerhans cell histiocytosis. *AJNR Am J Neuroradiol*. May 2004;25(5):880–891.
3. Gabbay LB, Leite Cda C, Andriola RS, Pinho Pda C, Lucato LT. Histiocytosis: a review focusing on neuroimaging findings. *Arq Neuropsiquiatr*. July 2014;72(7):548–558.
4. Prayer D, Grois N, Prosch H, Gadner H, Barkovich AJ. MR imaging presentation of intracranial disease associated with Langerhans cell histiocytosis. *AJNR Am J Neuroradiol*. May 2004;25(5):880–891.

15.4 Tolosa–Hunt Syndrome

Case History

A 35-year-old man developed severe facial pain and double vision.

Diagnosis: Tolosa–Hunt Syndrome

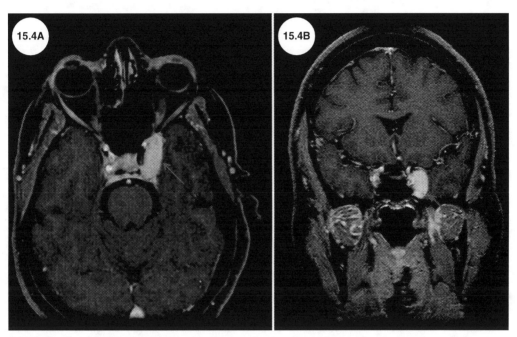

Images 15.4A and 15.4B: Postcontrast, fat-suppressed axial and coronal T1-weighted images demonstrate an enhancing lesion (red arrows) in the left cavernous sinus.

Introduction

■ Tolosa–Hunt syndrome is an idiopathic granulomatous disease of the cavernous sinus and orbital apex.

Clinical Presentation

■ It presents as a painful, unilateral ophthalmoplegia. Involvement of the optic nerve occurs in 25% of patients, and sensory loss in the distribution of the first two divisions of the trigeminal nerve is common. The symptoms typically present over the course of days to weeks.

■ The International Headache Society criteria for Tolosa–Hunt syndrome are:

1. One or more episodes of unilateral orbital pain persisting for weeks if untreated.

2. Paresis of one or more of the third, fourth, and/or sixth cranial nerves and/or demonstration of granuloma by MRI or biopsy.

3. Paresis coincides with the onset of pain or follows it within 2 weeks.

4. Pain and paresis resolve within 72 hours when treated adequately with corticosteroids.

5. Other causes have been excluded by appropriate investigations.

Radiographic Appearance and Diagnosis

■ MRI typically shows an enhancing, inflammatory lesion in the cavernous sinus and orbital apex. The lesion is hyperintense on T2-weighted images. Imaging findings are nonspecific, and it is a diagnosis of exclusion. In some patients, a biopsy may be needed to exclude neoplastic processes (lymphomas or meningiomas), which have a similar presentation.

Treatment

■ It is highly responsive, both clinically and radiographically, to corticosteroids. If there is no improvement, the diagnosis should be reconsidered. Immunosuppressive agents may be needed in treatment-refractory cases. It is recurrent after months to years in nearly half of the patients.

References

1. Jain R, Sawhney S, Koul RL, Chand P. Tolosa-Hunt syndrome: MRI appearances. *J Med Imaging Radiat Oncol.* October 2008;52(5):447–451.
2. Kline LB, Hoyt WF. The Tolosa-Hunt syndrome. *J Neurol Neurosurg Psychiatry.* November 2001;71(5):577–582.
3. Sánchez Vallejo R, Lopez-Rueda A, Olarte AM, San Roman L. MRI findings in Tolosa-Hunt syndrome (THS). *BMJ Case Rep.* November 2014;2014.

15.5 Orbital Pseudotumor

Case History

A 23-year-old woman presented with double vision, proptosis, and pain of her right eye.

Diagnosis: Orbital Pseudotumor

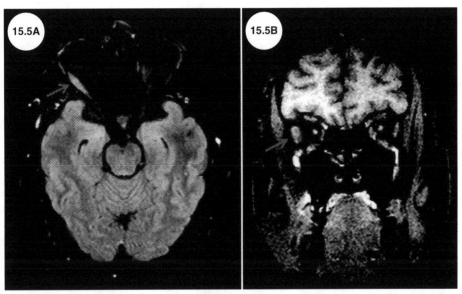

Images 15.5A and 15.5B: Axial FLAIR and coronal T1-weighted images demonstrate hyperintensity and enlargement of the right lateral rectus muscle (red arrows).

Introduction

- Idiopathic orbital inflammatory disease or **orbital pseudotumor** is an idiopathic inflammatory condition of the orbit. It most commonly involves the extraocular muscles, but may also affect the sclera, uvea, lacrimal glands, and retrobulbar soft tissue.

Clinical Presentation

- Patients develop painful proptosis, redness, and diplopia. Symptoms develop rapidly and are unilateral in the vast majority of patients. It often occurs in conjunction with other autoimmune, inflammatory, or rheumatologic conditions.

- A classification scheme has been proposed depending on which part of the orbit is most involved:

  1. Myositic
  2. Lacrimal
  3. Anterior—involvement of the globe, retrobulbar orbit
  4. Diffuse—multifocal intraconal involvement with or without an extraconal component
  5. Apical—involving the orbital apex and with intracranial involvement

Radiographic Appearance and Diagnosis

- Radiographic features depend on which part of the orbit is affected. For a myositis presentation, as depicted previously, imaging will reveal enlargement of one or more of the extraocular muscles. The muscles are slightly hyperintense on T2-weighted images and hypointense on T1-weighted images. There is often avid enhancement with the administration of contrast. In contrast to myositis associated with thyroid disease, the muscle tendons are affected.

■ It is a diagnosis of exclusion, once other causes have been ruled out.

Treatment

■ There is dramatic response to steroids, and the diagnosis should be reconsidered in patients who do not respond.

References

1. Montagnese F, Wenninger S, Schoser B. "Orbiting around" the orbital myositis: clinical features, differential diagnosis and therapy. *J Neurol.* 2016;263(4):631–640.
2. Costa RM, Dumitrascu OM, Gordon LK. Orbital myositis: diagnosis and management. *Curr Allergy Asthma Rep.* July 2009;9(4):316–323.

15.6 | Orbital Cavernous Venous Malformation

Case History

A 40-year-old woman presented with double vision and proptosis.

Diagnosis: Orbital Cavernous Venous Malformation

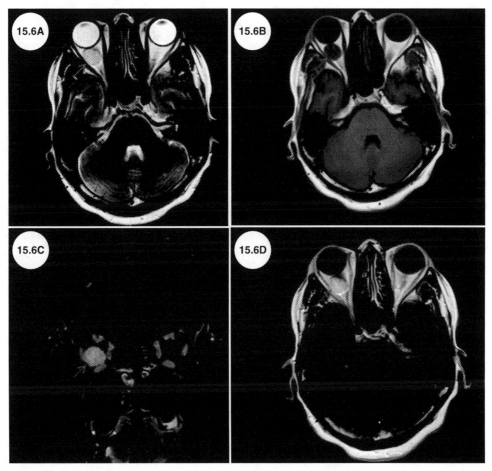

Images 15.6A–15.6D: Axial T2-weighted, noncontrast T1-weighted, and postcontrast coronal and axial T1-weighted images demonstrate an avidly enhancing ovoid intraconal mass in the right inferolateral orbit, which is separate from the optic nerve and displaces it superomedially.

Introduction

■ Cavernous venous malformations of the orbit (also known as cavernous hemangiomas) are the slow-growing, benign, vascular lesions of the orbit. They are the most common vascular lesions of the orbit in adults, though overall, they are an uncommon finding.

Clinical Presentation

- They most commonly present in middle-aged females with proptosis and double vision. Visual loss due to optic nerve dysfunction occurs in about one-third of patients. They may be found as incidental findings on imaging done for other reasons.

Radiographic Appearance and Diagnosis

- MRI is the imaging modality of choice. These lesions are most commonly found in the lateral aspect of the intraconal space. They are well-circumscribed, round or oval, masses that are iso-intense on T1-weighted images and hyperintense on T2-weighted images. Contrast enhancement is common.

Treatment

- Surgical removal of the lesion is curative. Incidental lesions may be monitored with clinical and radiographic monitoring.

References

1. Rootman DB, Heran MK, Rootman J, White VA, Luemsamran P, Yucel YH. Cavernous venous malformations of the orbit (so-called cavernous haemangioma): a comprehensive evaluation of their clinical, imaging and histologic nature. *Br J Ophthalmol.* July 2014;98(7):880–888.
2. Khan SN, Sepahdari AR. Orbital masses: CT and MRI of common vascular lesions, benign tumors, and malignancies. *Saudi J Ophthalmol.* October 2012;26(4):373–383.

15.7 Dilated Perivascular Spaces

Case History

A 90-year-old man presented with mild cognitive impairment.

Diagnosis: Dilated Perivascular Spaces—"Etat Crible"

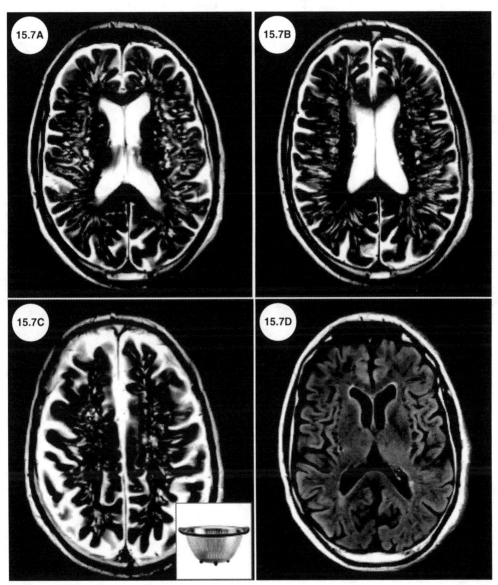

Images 15.7A–15.7D: Axial T2-weighted and FLAIR images demonstrate the "colander-like" appearance of multiple dilated perivascular spaces and mild white matter disease.

Introduction

■ Perivascular spaces, also called Virchow–Robin spaces, are fluid-filled continuations of the subarachnoid space along the blood vessel walls that penetrate the base of the brain into the cerebral cortex and basal ganglia. Perivascular spaces play an important role in the maintenance of the blood–brain barrier and regulation of fluid drainage in the CNS.

Clinical Presentation

■ Enlarged perivascular spaces are common, particularly in elderly patients with hypertension. They may be enlarged to a diameter of 5 millimeters normally and are usually of no clinical consequence, though they can occasionally lead to hydrocephalus.

■ They can be seen as a feature of the mucopolysaccharidoses (Hunter and Hurler disease).

Radiographic Appearance

■ On MR imaging, dilated perivascular spaces are ovoid, cystic cavities that are most commonly bilateral and symmetric. They follow the appearance of CSF on all sequences and there is no mass effect, edema, calcification, or enhancement. They are categorized into three types:

1. **Type 1:** found in the basal ganglia along the course of the lenticulostriate arteries
2. **Type 2:** found in the cortex along the course of the medullary arteries
3. **Type 3:** found in the midbrain

■ They may be difficult to distinguish from lacunar infarctions; however, lacunar infarctions are more commonly located in the upper putamen, while dilated perivascular spaces are located in the inferior part.

■ In certain cases, innumerable dilated perivascular spaces take on a "colander-like" appearance condition, termed "etat crible."

Treatment

■ There is no direct treatment beyond controlling hypertension and other vascular risk factors.

References

1. Akiguchi I, Shirakashi Y, Budka H, et al. Disproportionate subarachnoid space hydrocephalus—outcome and perivascular space. *Ann Clin Transl Neurol.* August 2014;1(8): 562–569.
2. Román GC. On the history of lacunes, etat criblé, and the white matter lesions of vascular dementia. *Cerebrovasc Dis.* 2002;13(Suppl. 2):1–6.

15.8   Fibrous Dysplasia of the Skull

Case History

A 20-year-old woman presented with slowly progressive decreased visual acuity.

Diagnosis: Fibrous Dysplasia of the Skull

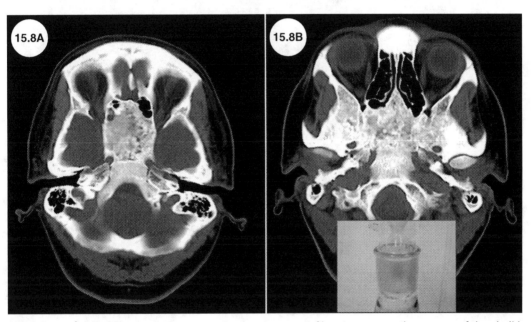

Images 15.8A and 15.8B: Axial CT images demonstrate an infiltrative, expansile process of the skull base with "ground glass" matrix mineralization consistent with fibrous dysplasia.

Introduction

■ Craniofacial fibrous dysplasia is a congenital, idiopathic bone disorder, characterized by failure of the osteoblasts to undergo normal development and maturation. It can occur anywhere throughout the calvarium, though the anterior craniofacial bones are most commonly affected. The ethmoids are most commonly involved followed by the sphenoid frontal, maxilla, and temporal bones.

Clinical Presentation

■ It presents with headache and facial pain in teenagers and young adults. Craniofacial deformity and nasal stuffiness are common symptoms as well.

■ When there is involvement of the maxillary, sphenoid, ethmoid, and frontal bones, there is exophthalmos and decreased visual acuity due to involvement of the optic nerves. Involvement of other cranial nerves is common as well. Patients have a much higher likelihood of developing malignant bone tumors.

■ McCune–Albright syndrome is defined by the triad of fibrous dysplasia, café-au-lait skin macules with a "jagged coast of Maine" appearance, and endocrinopathies often leading to precocious puberty.

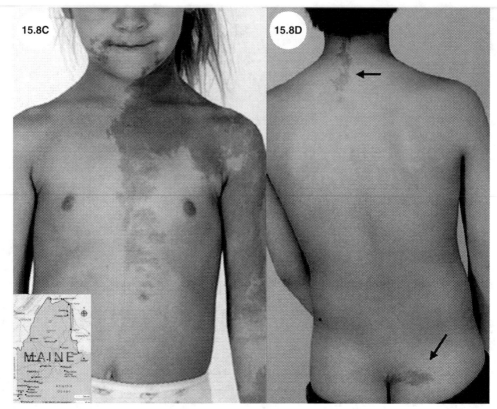

Images 15.8C and 15.8D: Café-au-lait skin macules with a "jagged coast of Maine" appearance in McCune–Albright syndrome.

Source: Dumitrescu CE, Collins MT. McCune-Albright syndrome. *Orphanet J Rare Dis.* 2008;3:12.

Radiographic Appearance and Diagnosis

■ On CT scans, the affected bones are expanded with a "ground glass" appearance. Though the bones are expanded, the cortex is intact.

Treatment

■ Surgery is reserved for symptomatic patients; however, complete resection is not possible.

References

1. Bowers CA, Taussky P, Couldwell WT. Surgical treatment of craniofacial fibrous dysplasia in adults. *Neurosurg Rev.* January 2014;37(1):47–53.
2. Salenave S, Boyce AM, Collins MT, Chanson P. Acromegaly and McCune-Albright syndrome. *J Clin Endocrinol Metab.* June 2014;99(6):1955–1969.
3. Frisch CD, Carlson ML, Kahue CN, et al. Fibrous dysplasia of the temporal bone: a review of 66 cases. *Laryngoscope.* June 2015;125(6):1438–1443.
4. Dumitrescu CE, Collins MT. McCune-Albright syndrome. *Orphanet J Rare Dis.* 2008;3:12.

15.9 | Hyperostosis Frontalis

Case History

A 46-year-old woman presented with a seizure. She was obese and had been diagnosed with depression and diabetes several years earlier.

Diagnosis: Hyperostosis Frontalis Interna/ Morgagni–Stewart–Morel Syndrome

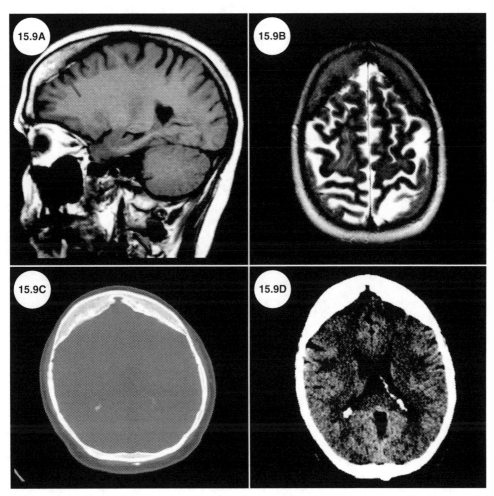

Images 15.9A–15.9D: Sagittal T1-weighted and axial T2-weighted images and axial CT images in bone and brain windows demonstrate bony overgrowth (red arrows) in the frontal lobes consistent with hyperostosis frontalis interna.

Introduction

- Hyperostosis frontalis interna is a benign overgrowth of the inner side of the frontal bone of the skull. It is a not uncommon finding, seen mostly in women after menopause.

Clinical Presentation

- It is usually asymptomatic and an incidental finding. However, it can be seen as part of Morgagni–Stewart–Morel syndrome. This rare syndrome also includes a variety of endocrinopathies (diabetes mellitus, diabetes insipidus, and hyperparathyroidism hirsutism, menstrual disorders, galactorrhea) as well as headaches, transient hemiparesis, obesity, vertigo, depression, and seizures.

Radiographic Appearance and Diagnosis

■ Imaging will show increased bone growth over the frontal lobes bilaterally.

Treatment

■ No treatment is necessary for incidentally discovered hyperostosis frontalis interna. The endocrine dysfunction of patients with Morgagni–Stewart–Morel syndrome requires treatment.

References

1. Raikos A, Paraskevas GK, Yusuf F, et al. Etiopathogenesis of hyperostosis frontalis interna: a mystery still. *Ann Anat.* October 2011;193(5):453–458.
2. She R, Szakacs J. Hyperostosis frontalis interna: case report and review of literature. *Ann Clin Lab Sci.* Spring 2004;34(2):206–208.

15.10 | Idiopathic Intracranial Hypertension

Case History

An obese 30-year-old female presented with severe headaches and visual loss. On exam, she had an enlarged blind spot and papilledema.

Diagnosis: Idiopathic Intracranial Hypertension

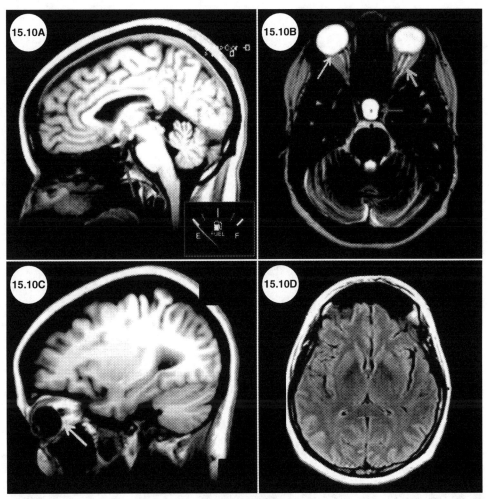

Images 15.10A–15.10C: Sagittal T1-weighted and axial T2-weighted images demonstrate an empty sella (red arrows), papilledema with flattening of the posterior globe (yellow arrows), distension of the optic nerve sheath in the subarachnoid spaces (blue arrow), and tortuous optic nerves consistent with the diagnosis of idiopathic intracranial hypertension. **Image 15.10D:** Axial FLAIR image demonstrates "slit-like ventricles" and effacement of the basal cisterns in another patient with idiopathic intracranial hypertension.

Introduction

- The total volume of CSF is about 150 ml, and about 600 to 700 ml are produced daily. It is formed in the arachnoid granulations and flows through the foramens of Luschka and Magendie into the subarachnoid space, where it is reabsorbed into the venous system by the arachnoid villi. The normal intracranial pressure (ICP) is 5 to 15 mmHg.

- Idiopathic intracranial hypertension (IIH) is due to either impaired absorption or increased production of CSF. It affects about 1 to 4 in 100,000 people.

- It classically presents in young, overweight females. Various endocrinopathies, polycystic ovarian syndrome, excess vitamin A, and withdrawal from steroids are risk factors. It can occur in children and adults, and the average age of diagnosis is 30.

Clinical Presentation

- Patients present with a throbbing headache over the entire head, which is often worse in the morning. Other symptoms include double vision, nausea, vomiting, and pulsatile tinnitus. Patients may have episodes of visual loss due to transiently increased ICP. These can be brought on by heavy lifting, laughing, sneezing, or coughing. Visual loss is the most feared complication and can occur as blind spot enlargement or visual field constriction.

- Patients with increased ICP due to mass lesions have a similar presentation. It is for this reason that IIH is also known as pseudotumor cerebri.

- Formal diagnostic criteria are known as the modified Dandy criteria:

  1. Symptoms of raised ICP (headache, nausea, vomiting, transient visual obscurations, or papilledema)
  2. No localizing signs with the exception of abducens nerve palsy
  3. The patient is awake and alert.
  4. No imaging evidence of thrombosis
  5. Cerebrospinal fluid opening pressure greater than 25 cmH$_2$O and otherwise normal CSF
  6. No other explanation for the raised intracranial pressure

Radiographic Appearance and Diagnosis

- The classic imaging finding in IIH is a decrease in the size of the ventricles, described as "slit-like" ventricles, though imaging can also be normal. Another finding is the "empty sella" sign, where there is flattening of the pituitary gland due to chronic increased ICP. Other findings include distension of the optic nerve sheath subarachnoid spaces, tortuous optic nerves, and flattening of the posterior part of the globes. An MR venogram may reveal narrowing of the lateral portions of the transverse sinuses.

- Fundoscopic examination is crucial in any patient with a complaint of headache. In patients with IIH, exam may reveal papilledema, which is defined as swelling of the optic disc due to increased ICP. Abducens nerve palsies are also common.

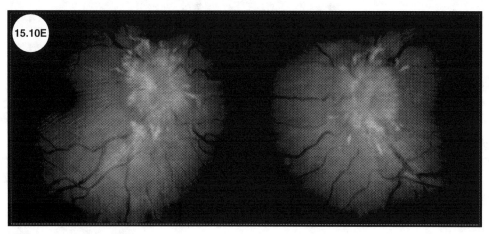

Image 15.10E: Severe papilledema.

Source: Garcia T, Bonnay G, Tourbah A, Arndt C. Optical coherence tomography in neuro-ophthalmology. In: Kawasaki M, ed. *Optical Coherence Tomography.*

■ An LP demonstrating increased ICP is needed to confirm the diagnosis.

Treatment

■ Medical treatment includes acetazolamide, a carbonic anhydrase inhibitor, to reduce CSF production. Furosemide, a loop diuretic, may be added as well. Surgical intervention is used in treatment-refractory cases. This includes optic nerve sheath fenestration to relieve pressure on the optic nerve and shunting of the ventricular system. Ultimately, weight loss, including possible bariatric surgery, may be needed. Stenting of the venous system has shown success in some case series, but is not yet a standard treatment.

References

1. Kosmorsky GS. Idiopathic intracranial hypertension: pseudotumor cerebri. *Headache.* February 2014;54(2):389–393.
2. Wall M. Idiopathic intracranial hypertension. *Neurol Clin.* August 2010;28(3):593–617.
3. Thurtell MJ, Wall M. Idiopathic intracranial hypertension (pseudotumor cerebri): recognition, treatment, and ongoing management. *Curr Treat Options Neurol.* February 2013;15(1): 1–12.

15.11 Intracranial Hypotension

Case History

A 45-year-old female developed a severe headache after a lumbar puncture.

Diagnosis: Intracranial Hypotension

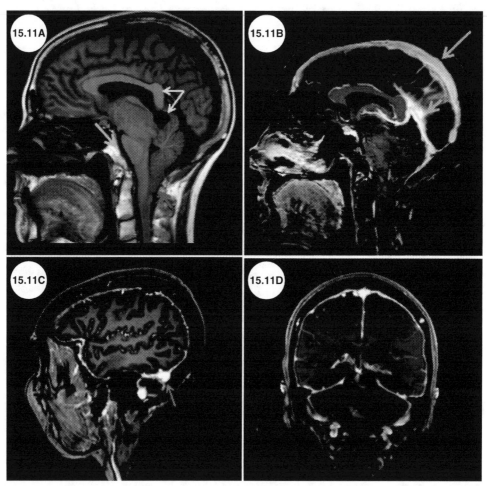

Image 15.11A: Sagittal T1-weighted image demonstrates "brain sagging" including descent of the cerebellar tonsils with crowding the foramen magnum (red arrow), flattening of the ventral pons against the clivus (blue arrow), inferior displacement of the third ventricle and drooping of the splenium of the corpus callosum (yellow arrows), and near complete effacement of the basal cisterns. **Images 5.11B and 15.11C:** Postcontrast sagittal T1-weighted images demonstrate prominent engorgement of the dural venous sinuses (green arrows). The transverse sinus is rounded, with a convex inferior margin (pink arrow), the venous distension sign. **Image 15.11D:** Postcontrast coronal T1-weighted image demonstrates diffuse meningeal enhancement.

Introduction

■ Intracranial hypotension can occur after a lumbar puncture, trauma, neurosurgical procedures, or spontaneously due to a CSF leak in the subarachnoid space.

Clinical Presentation

■ It is characterized by an excruciating headache that is worsened when standing and relieved by lying down. Other symptoms include horizontal diplopia, vertigo, hearing loss, nausea/vomiting, visual loss or photophobia, and neck/interscapular pain.

Radiographic Appearance and Diagnosis

■ In patients with prolonged intracranial hypotension there is "brain sagging" with downward herniation of the cerebellar tonsils into the foramen magnum, flattening of the pons against the clivus, drooping of the splenium of the corpus callosum, and effacement of the basal cisterns. With the administration of contrast, the venous system is engorged and the transverse sinus is rounded and convex. This finding is known as the "venous distension" sign, and it is highly sensitive and specific for intracranial hypotension. These findings are best seen on sagittal MRI images. Other findings include brain edema and swelling of the pituitary gland. In severe cases, there may be subdural fluid collections.

■ In cases without a history known to produce intracranial hypotension, an LP can document

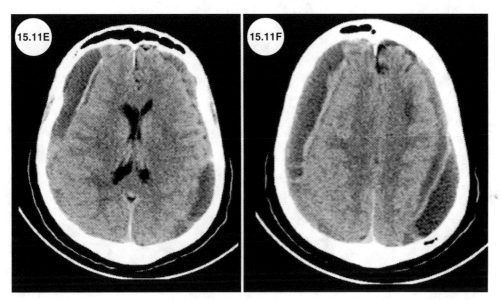

Images 15.11E and 15.11F: Axial CT images demonstrate chronic bilateral subdural collections with mass effect in a patient with prolonged intracranial hypotension.

the hypotension (less than 7 cm CSF). Spinal cisternography can be used to locate the site of the leakage.

Treatment

■ Many cases resolve spontaneously. Epidural blood patches are highly effective in relieving the headache in a majority of patients. In refractory cases with a defined leak, surgical repair may be required.

References

1. Urbach H. Intracranial hypotension: clinical presentation, imaging findings, and imaging-guided therapy. *Curr Opin Neurol.* August 2014;27(4):414–424.
2. Spears RC. Low-pressure/spinal fluid leak headache. *Curr Pain Headache Rep.* June 2014;18(6):425.
3. Mokri B. Spontaneous intracranial hypotension. *Curr Neurol Neurosci Rep.* March 2001;1(2):109–117.
4. Schievink WI, Maya MM, Moser FG, Tourje J. Spectrum of subdural fluid collections in spontaneous intracranial hypotension. *J Neurosurg.* October 2005;103(4):608–613.

15.12 | Copper-Beaten Skull

Case History

A 12-year-old child presented with severe headaches and visual loss. She had papill-edema on fundoscopic exam and a lumbar puncture revealed an increased opening pressure.

Diagnosis: Copper-Beaten Skull

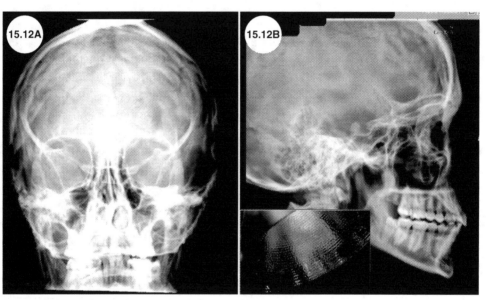

Images 15.12A and 15.12B: Skull radiographs reveal a "copper-beaten" skull.

Introduction

■ Any pathology that leads to an increased ICP can leave gyral impressions on the skull's inner table. The resulting pattern appears similar to hand-worked metal and is referred to as a "copper-beaten skull."

Clinical Presentation

■ The clinical presentation is related to the underlying cause. This can be obstructive hydrocephalus, craniosynostosis, or mass lesions.

■ It is usually seen in children, and, when localized to the posterior part of the skull, can occasionally be a normal finding.

Radiographic Appearance

■ Normally, the inner table of the skull is smooth. In some patients with severe, prolonged increased ICP, the skull develops a mottled appearance, known as a "copper-beaten skull," reflecting the underlying gyri.

Treatment

■ The treatment depends on the underlying cause.

References

1. Tuite GF, Evanson J, Chong WK, et al. The beaten copper cranium: a correlation between intracranial pressure, cranial radiographs, and computed tomographic scans in children with craniosynostosis. *Neurosurgery*. October 1996;39(4): 691–699.
2. Agrawal D, Steinbok P, Cochrane DD. Significance of beaten copper appearance on skull radiographs in children with isolated sagittal synostosis. *Childs Nerv Syst*. December 2007;23(12):1467–1470.

15.13 | Tension Pneumocephalus

Case History

A 65-year-old man developed a severe headache and decreased level of consciousness after a neurosurgical procedure.

Diagnosis: Tension pneumocephalus, Mount Fuji Sign

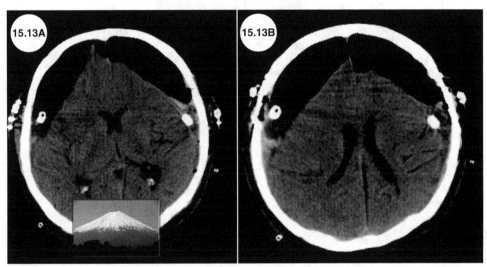

Images 15.13A and 15.13B: Axial CT images demonstrate pneumocephalus with severe compression of the frontal lobes bilaterally: the "Mount Fuji" sign.

Introduction

- Pneumocephalus refers to gas, most commonly air, within the skull. The most common cause is traumatic injury, which results in a skull fracture and a tear in the dura. It may occur after surgical procedures, particularly those involving the paranasal sinuses. If the intracranial pressure is lower than the extracranial pressure, air flows into the intracranial compartment. Often, there is a ball-valve mechanism, and air can only flow inwards into the skull.

Clinical Presentation

- Air acts like any other intracranial mass, producing symptoms of increased ICP (headache, nausea, vomiting) and focal neurological symptoms due to compression of the underlying brain.

Radiographic Appearance

- CT scans are very sensitive for detecting even small amounts of air as it appears completely black. Fat has an identical appearance on soft tissue windows, but can be differentiated on bone windows or by measuring the Hounsfield units. It can be extraaxial, intraaxial, or intraventricular. A particular pattern of pneumocephalus involves compression of the frontal lobes. This is termed the "Mount Fuji sign" due to its resemblance to this Japanese mountain.

Treatment

- Tension pneumocephalus is a neurosurgical emergency where release of the air and repair of any cranial defect are required. In contrast, small amounts of air are expected after neurosurgical procedures.

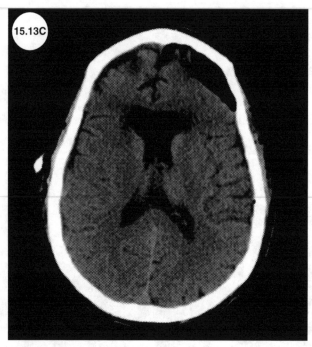

Image 15.13C: Axial CT image demonstrates hypodensity in the frontal horns of the lateral ventricles and in the subdural space over the left frontal lobe consistent with air.

References

1. Pulickal GG, Sitoh YY, Ng WH. Tension pneumocephalus. *Singapore Med J*. March 2014;55(3):e46–e48.
2. Naraghi M, Ghazizadeh M. Tension pneumocephalus: a life-threatening complication of septoplasty and septorhino-plasty. *B-ENT*. 2012;8(3):203–205.
3. Haran RP, Chandy MJ. Symptomatic pneumocephalus after transsphenoidal surgery. *Surg Neurol*. December 1997;48(6):575–578.

15.14 | Cervical Spondylotic Myelopathy

Case History

A 66-year-old man presented with several falls over the course of the past few months. He said that his legs felt weak and his walking speed and endurance had declined significantly over the past few years. On examination, he had symmetrical weakness of his legs and mild weakness of his hand. He had a "scissoring" gait. His reflexes were extremely brisk in his legs with upgoing toes bilaterally.

Diagnosis: Cervical Spondylotic Myelopathy

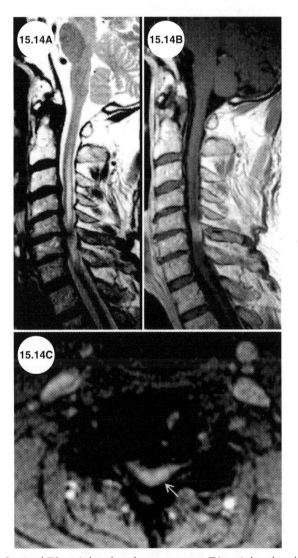

Images 15.14A–15.14C: Sagittal T2-weighted and postcontrast T1-weighted and axial T1-weighted images demonstrate severe cervical spondylosis with intrinsic spinal cord hyperintensity on T2-weighted images and enhancement (red arrow) on postcontrast imaging. On the axial image, the spinal cord (yellow arrow) is flattened with effacement of the surrounding cerebrospinal fluid.

Introduction

■ Cervical spondylotic myelopathy (CSM) is the most common spinal cord disorder in older adults. Spondylosis refers to the degenerative changes that occur in the spine, and myelopathy due to narrowing of the spinal canal is known as spondylotic myelopathy.

Clinical Presentation

■ Patients present with the gradual onset of leg weakness and stiffness with difficulty walking. They also have neck stiffness and the insidious onset of pain in the neck, subscapular region, and shoulders, often radiating to the arms and hands. Bladder urgency, frequency, and/or retention, and weakness of the upper extremities may be seen in severe, longstanding cases.

■ Neurological exam will reveal weakness and spasticity of the legs, and weakness and atrophy of the hands and arms in advanced cases. Patients will be hyperreflexic with pathological reflexes (ankle clonus, Babinski sign, Hoffman's sign). The gait will be spastic, and this is sometimes referred to as a "scissoring" gait as patients appear to walk with their legs crossing each other. There will be a variable and asymmetric pattern of sensory abnormalities. Sensory loss may follow dermatomal distribution, while other patients have a sensory level.

Radiographic Appearance and Diagnosis

■ MRI is the imaging modality of choice. It will reveal narrowing of the spinal canal with the absence of the normal CSF around the spinal cord. The cord itself is compressed and distorted. There is often intrinsic hyperintensity within the spinal cord on T2-weighted images. It is important to note that enhancement can be seen due to CSM. It is most common at the C5–C6 levels.

Treatment

■ Surgical decompression of the spinal cord is necessary once frank myelopathy occurs.

■ Medical therapies include: cervical immobilization (collar or neck brace), cervical traction, skull traction, and physical therapy.

15.15 | Spinal Disc Herniation

Case History

A 46-year-old woman developed pain in her left arm and weakness of elbow extension.

Diagnosis: Disc Herniation

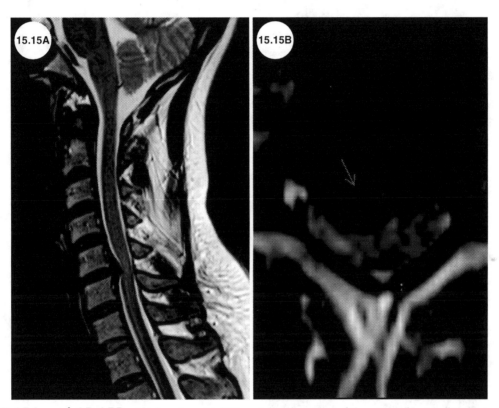

Images 15.15A and 15.15B: Axial and sagittal T2-weighted images of the cervical spine demonstrate a herniated disc at C5–C6, eccentric to the right, with mass effect of the thecal sac and spinal cord compression. Note that there is hyperintensity in the cord indicating edema or myelomalacia.

Introduction

■ A herniated disc occurs when there is displacement of material, typically the nucleus pulposus, with mass effect on the spinal cord or spinal nerve roots as they enter the intervertebral foramen. A tear in the outer, fibrous ring of an intervertebral disc allows the central portion to herniate out of the damaged annulus fibrosus. Contained herniations occur when the outer fibers of annulus fibrosus and posterior longitudinal ligament are intact. In contrast, with herniations that are not contained, there is a tear of outer fibers of annulus fibrosus and posterior longitudinal ligament (**Illustration 15.15.1**).

■ Additionally, cartilage, fragmented bone, and annular tissue may also herniate.

■ Displacements less than 25% of the disc circumference are called focal herniations, while those between 25% and 50% of the disc circumference are called "broad-based" (**Illustration 15.15.2**).

■ There are four locations for disc herniations (**Illustration 15.15.3**):

1. **Median:** Thickness of the posterior longitudinal ligament prevents most herniations in this area.

2. **Paramedian:** This is the most common area for disc herniations as the posterior longitudinal ligament is thin.

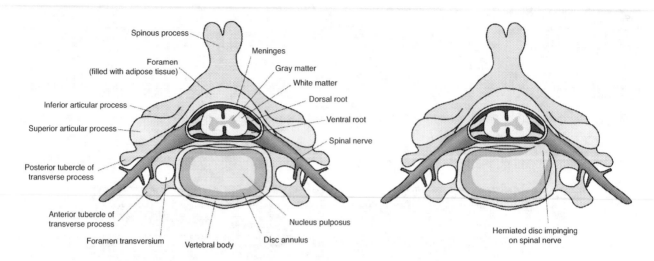

Illustration 15.15.1: Normal vertebral anatomy and a herniated disc (image credit debivort; https://commons.wikimedia.org/wiki/File:ACDF_coronal_english.png).

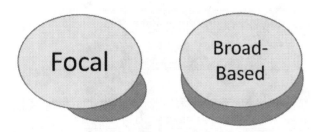

Illustration 15.15.2: Focal and broad-based disc herniations.

- Compression or irritation of a nerve root as it exits the spine is known as a radiculopathy. This occurs most often in the cervical and lumbar portions of the spine due to the mobility of the neck and lower back. Cervical disc herniation most commonly occurs between C5 and C6 or C6 and C7 vertebral bodies. In the lumbar spine, herniations most commonly occur between L4 and L5 or L5 and S1 vertebral bodies.

- In contrast to herniations, disc bulges involve over 25% of the circumference of an intervertebral disc. They occur gradually and are a near universal radiographic feature in older individuals.

Clinical Presentation

- The symptoms of a herniation vary depending on which nerve root is affected, but most commonly include, pain (local or radicular), weakness, and numbness and tingling along the course of the nerve. The neurological examination similarly varies depending on which nerve is affected, but includes: sensory loss in the distribution of a nerve root; and weakness and atrophy of muscles innervated by the compressed nerve in more severe cases. Diminished or absent reflex can be seen as well. Specific symptoms of cervical radiculopathies are as follows:

  - **C5:** pain and weakness in the shoulders and upper arms
  - **C6:** pain along the lateral aspect of the forearm and thumb, weakness of the biceps, wrists, thumb, and index finger

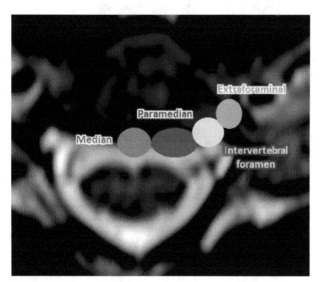

Illustration 15.15.3: Localization of herniated discs on the axial plane.

3. **Intervertebral foramen:** These account for less than 10% of disc herniations, but are highly symptomatic.

4. **Extraforaminal:** Disc herniations in this area are not common.

- **C7:** pain from the neck to the middle of the hand and triceps weakness
- **C8:** pain from the neck to lateral aspect of the forearm and hand, weakness in hand grip

- In the lumbar region, the sciatic nerve is the most commonly affected nerve, causing unilateral pain shooting down the back on one leg.

- In adults, the spinal cord ends in the upper part of the vertebral column. The cauda equina (or "horse's tail") contains about 10 nerve fiber pairs, (five lumbar, five sacral, and a single coccygeal nerve). Compression of these nerves, often by a herniated disk at L4–L5 or L5–S1, causes a constellation of findings known as the cauda equina syndrome. These are:

  - Localized low back pain with or without unilateral or bilateral sciatica (radicular pain). In some patients pain may be completely absent.

  - Numbness in the genitals, buttocks, and anus due to compression of the sacral nerve roots. This pattern is often termed saddle anesthesia.

  - Lower extremity weakness, which is often asymmetrical.

  - Absent or diminished knee or ankle jerks, and diminished bulbocavernosus reflexes.

  - Loss of anal sphincter tone and anal wink.

  - Bowel and bladder dysfunction (typically, urinary manifestations begin with retention and are later followed by an overflow incontinence); constipation.

Radiographic Appearance and Diagnosis

- MRI is the imaging modality of choice. It will reveal the disc herniation and demonstrate any compression of the spinal cord, nerve roots, or cauda equina.

Treatment

- Cervical radiculopathies are initially treated with NSAIDs, muscle relaxants, and physical therapy. For severe pain, steroid injections may provide further relief. Surgical removal of the disc (discectomy) is an option for those with symptoms that are refractory to medical management.

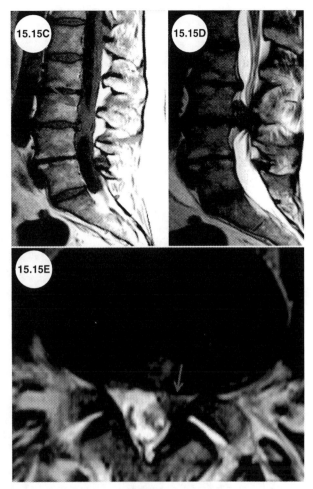

Images 15.15C–15.15E: Sagittal T1-weighted and sagittal and axial T2-weighted images of the lumbar spine demonstrate a large herniated disc (red arrows) with superior and inferior extension. There is mass effect on the thecal sac and lower cauda equina.

- In contrast, cauda equina syndrome (CES) is a neurosurgical emergency. Urgent surgical decompression of any herniated disc is indicated as soon as possible.

References

1. Schmid SL, Wechsler C, Farshad M, et al. Surgery for lumbar disc herniation: analysis of 500 consecutive patients treated in an interdisciplinary spine centre. *J Clin Neurosci.* January 2016;27:40–43.
2. Wong JJ, Côté P, Quesnele JJ, Stern PJ, Mior SA. The course and prognostic factors of symptomatic cervical disc herniation with radiculopathy: a systematic review of the literature. *Spine J.* August 2014;14(8):1781–1789.
3. Bhagawati D, Gwilym S. Neck pain with radiculopathy. *BMJ Clin Evid.* December 23, 2015;2015. pii: 1103.

15.16 | Ankylosing Spondylitis

Case History

A 23-year-old man presented with back stiffness and pain, particularly in the morning.

Diagnosis: Ankylosing Spondylitis

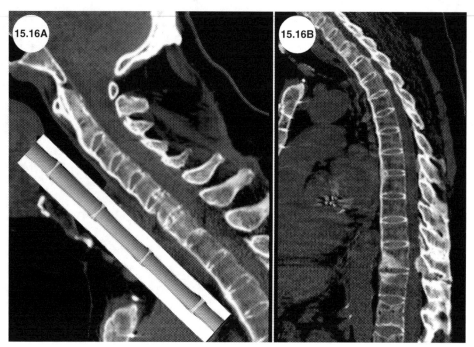

Images 15.16A and 15.16B: Sagittal CT images of the cervical and thoracic spine reveal straightening of the spine, the so-called "bamboo spine" appearance of ankylosing spondylitis.

Introduction

■ Ankylosing spondylitis (AS), a spondyloarthropathy, is a chronic, multisystem inflammatory disorder primarily involving the sacroiliac (SI) joints and the axial skeleton. There is a strong association in patients who are HLA-B27 positive, which is seen in about 90% of affected individuals. Patients are usually younger than 40 and have symptoms for over 3 months. It is more common in men than women.

Clinical Presentation

■ Patients present with the insidious onset of low back pain and stiffness. The symptoms are worse in the morning or with inactivity. There is improvement with exercise. In severe cases, a persistently flexed posture may lead to dyspnea. Patients are at increased risk of death from cardiovascular disease.

Radiographic Appearance and Diagnosis

■ In AS, there is ossification of the outer rim of the annulus fibrosus of the intervertebral discs. This leads to marginal syndesmophytes (bony growths that develop inside a ligament) and vertebral body fusion, which in turn creates the characteristic "bamboo spine."

■ Involvement of the SI joint, which is most often seen on conventional x-rays, is mandatory for the diagnosis of AS. Imaging of the SI joints, spine, and peripheral joints may reveal evidence of early sacroiliitis, erosions, and enthesitis.

Treatment

- No definite disease-modifying therapy exists, although TNF-alpha inhibitors appear to have potential. Symptomatic management includes pain control, exercise, and physical therapy.

Surgical intervention may be necessary to stabilize fracture and prevent neurological deficit.

References

1. Elalouf O, Elkayam O. Long-term safety and efficacy of infliximab for the treatment of ankylosing spondylitis. *Ther Clin Risk Manag.* November 2015;11:1719–1726.
2. Braun J, Sieper J. Ankylosing spondylitis. *Lancet.* April 2007;369(9570):1379–1390.

15.17 | Brain Herniation Syndromes

Case History

A 16-year-old boy presented with headaches and became unconscious.

Diagnosis: Tonsillar Herniation

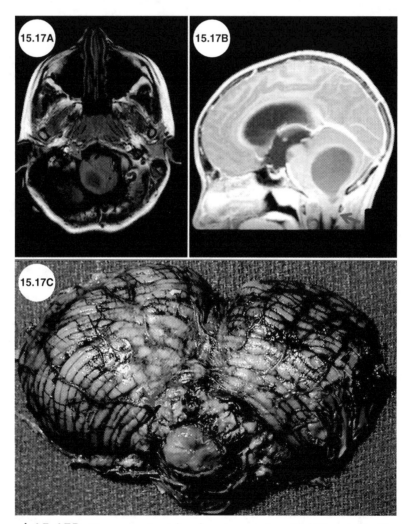

Images 15.17A and 15.17B: Noncontrast axial and postcontrast sagittal T1-weighted images demonstrate tonsillar herniation (red arrow) and flattening of the pons against the clivus in a patient with a large, cystic cerebellar mass. There is also upward herniation of the cerebellum. **Image 15.17C:** Gross image demonstrating tonsillar herniation (red arrow).

Introduction

■ Herniation of the brain from one compartment to another usually occurs as a result of increased ICP. There are several patterns of herniation of both the supratentorial and infratentorial compartments. They are uncal (transtentorial), central, subfalcine, extracranial, upward, and tonsillar (**Illustration 15.17.1**).

Radiographic Appearance and Clinical Presentation

Uncal (Transtentorial) Herniation

■ It occurs due to a supratentorial mass or due to swelling after a large infarct or anoxic brain injury. There is downward displacement of medial brain structures through the tentorial notch. The innermost part of the temporal lobe, the uncus, herniates through the tentorium cerebelli.

■ The downward displacement puts pressure on the underlying structures, including the brainstem and upper cranial nerves. Compression of the corticospinal tract as it runs through the cerebral peduncle causes contralateral weakness. In certain cases, compression of the contralateral cerebral peduncle can cause ipsilateral weakness. This is a false localizing sign and is known as "Kernohan's notch" phenomenon. The oculomotor nerve is frequently compressed as it emerges from the brainstem. As this is a compressive palsy, patients develop pupillary dilation prior to the ophthalmoplegia. Patients have usually suffered a devastating neurological event, and a "blown pupil" is often a sign of neurological decline. There can also be compression and infarction of the ipsilateral posterior cerebral artery (PCA).

■ Duret hemorrhages are small areas of bleeding in the midbrain and pons brainstem caused by downward displacement of the brainstem secondary to hippocampal gyrus herniation through the tentorial notch.

Central Herniation

■ A downward shift of the brainstem and the diencephalon due to a supratentorial mass. It results in Cheyne–Stokes respirations and pinpoint, nonreactive pupils.

Subfalcine (Cingulate) Herniation

■ Subfalcine (cingulate) herniation is a shift of the cingulate gyrus below the falx cerebri. This is the most common type of herniation pattern and is due to a mass in the frontal, parietal, or occipital lobes. Branches of the anterior cerebral artery may be compressed with subsequent infarction

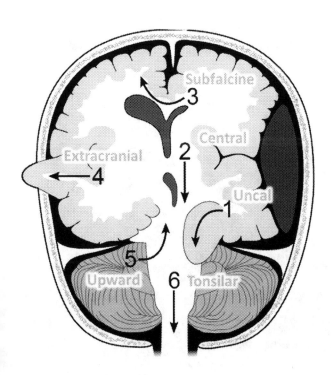

Illustration 15.17.1: Illustration of the herniation syndromes (image credit Rupert Millard).

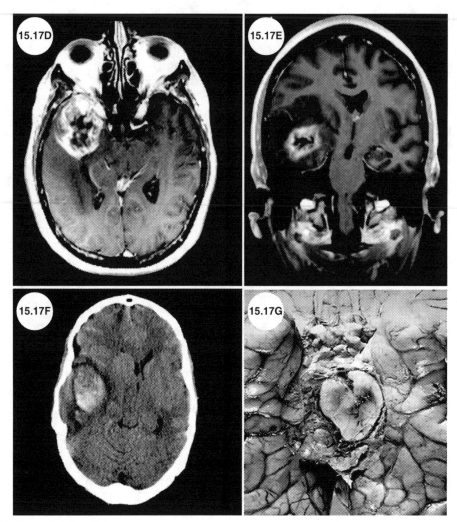

Images 15.17D and 15.17E: Postcontrast axial and coronal T1-weighted images demonstrate uncal herniation in a patient with a right temporal lobe glioma. **Image 15.17F:** CT image demonstrates uncal herniation in a patient with a right temporal lobe hemorrhage. **Image 15.17G:** Gross pathology demonstrating (red arrow) compression of the midbrain (image 15.17G credit Dimitri Agamanolis, MD).

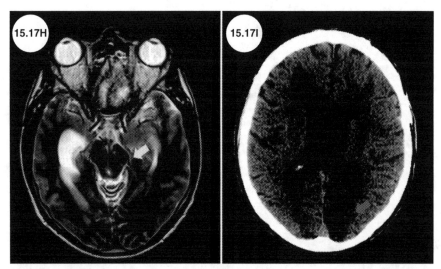

Images 15.17H and 15.17I: Axial T2-weighted image demonstrates uncal herniation compressing the left posterior cerebral artery (yellow arrow). A follow-up CT image 2 weeks later shows infarction in the left PCA territory (red arrow).

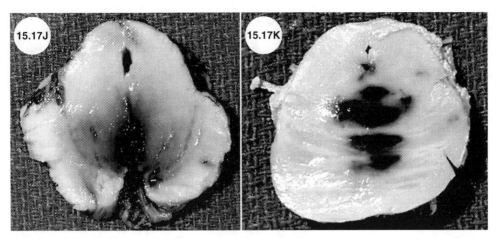

Images 15.17J and 15.17K: Gross specimens demonstrate Duret hemorrhages of the midbrain and pons.

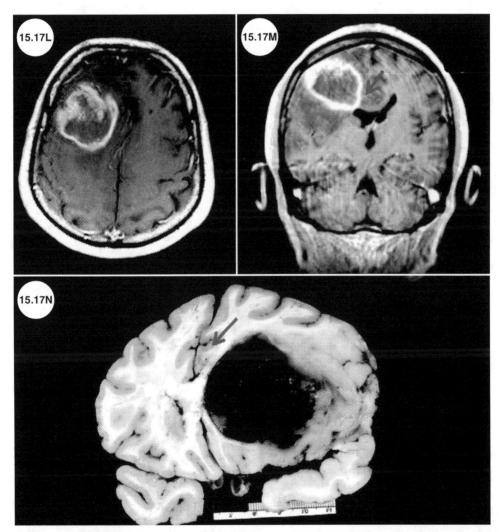

Images 15.17L and 15.17M: Postcontrast axial and coronal T1-weighted images demonstrate subfalcine (cingulate) herniation (red arrows) in a patient with a right frontal lobe glioma. **Image 15.17N:** Gross pathology demonstrates subfalcine (cingulate) herniation (red arrow) due to hemorrhagic tumor (image credit www.wikidoc.org via Professor Peter Anderson, DVM, PhD, and published with permission © PEIR, University of Alabama at Birmingham, Department of Pathology).

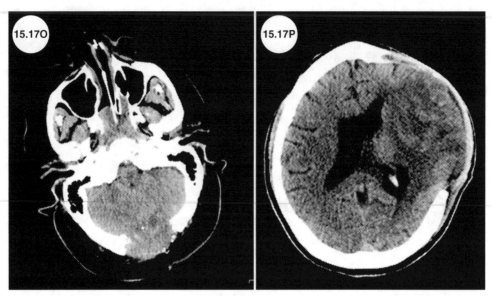

Image 15.17O: Axial CT scan demonstrates herniation of the cerebellum outside of a surgical defect.
Image 15.17P: Axial CT scan demonstrates brain herniation after a left hemicraniectomy in a patient with a large MCA infarct.

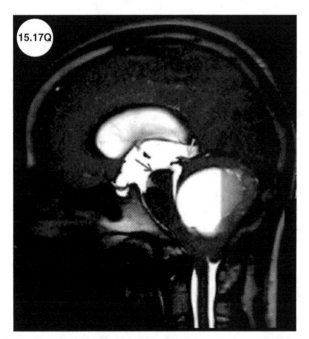

Image 15.17Q: Sagittal T2-weighted image demonstrates upward herniation of the midbrain (red arrow) and cerebellum (blue arrow) in a patient with a cerebellar mass.

and contralateral leg weakness. There may be contralateral hydrocephalus if there is obstruction at the foramen of Monro.

Extracranial (Transcalvarial) Herniation

■ In extracranial herniation, the brain herniates through a defect in the skull, usually as a result of trauma or a neurosurgical procedure. In certain cases, such as lobar hemorrhages, subarachnoid hemorrhage, or malignant middle cerebral artery (MCA) infarcts, allowing for external herniation may be lifesaving, as it prevents other, fatal herniation syndromes. Similarly, patients with large cerebellar infarcts may occlude the fourth ventricle and suffer fatal obstructive hydrocephalus. A decompressive craniectomy may be lifesaving in such patients.

Upward (Transtentorial) Herniation

■ Mass effect in the posterior fossa can cause the cerebellum and midbrain to move superiorly through the tentorial opening.

Tonsillar Herniation

■ In tonsillar herniation there is protrusion of the cerebellar tonsils through the foramen magnum due to pressure in the posterior fossa. An example is shown in **Images 15.17A–15.17C.** Patients develop a headache and neck stiffness. Compression of the brainstem centers for respiration and cardiac function may result in cardiac or respiratory arrest. Blood pressure instability is common.

Reference

1. Crudele A, Shah SO, Bar B. Decompressive Hemicraniectomy in Acute Neurological Diseases. *J Intensive Care Med.* August 2015.

15.18   Brain Death

Case History

An 85-year-old female was found unconscious at home and was nonresponsive on exam without brainstem reflexes.

Diagnosis: Brain Death

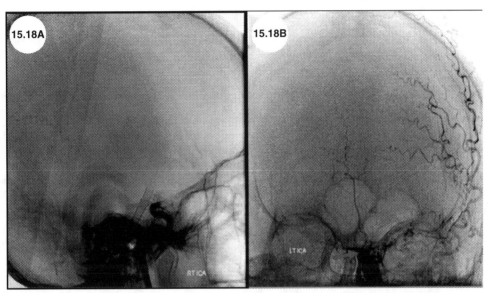

Images 15.18A and 15.18B: Catheter angiogram reveals no cerebral flow with injection of either internal carotid artery (red arrows) in a patient after a severe hypoxic event. Flow is seen in the external carotid artery and its branches. This is evidence of brain death.

Introduction

▦ Brain death is defined as the complete and irreversible loss of functions of the brain and brainstem. Brain dead patients are clinically dead, though other organs may continue to function only with mechanical support.

Clinical Presentation

The American Academy of Neurology Guidelines for brain death determination are summarized as follows:

▦ **Establish irreversible and proximate cause of coma by history, examination, and neuroimaging.** The presence of a CNS-depressant drug must be excluded. There should be no severe electrolyte, acid–base, or endocrine disturbances.

▦ **Core temperature must be normal.**

▦ **Achieve normal systolic blood pressure.**

▦ **Perform neurological examination confirming:**

1. **The patient is comatose:**
   ▦ Patients should not respond to noxious stimuli, though spinal reflexes may be retained

2. **Brainstem reflexes are absent:**
   ▦ Absence of pupillary response to a bright light in both eyes
   ▦ Absence of ocular movements using oculocephalic testing and oculovestibular reflex testing
   ▦ Absence of corneal reflex
   ▦ Absence of facial movement to a noxious stimulus
   ▦ Absence of the pharyngeal and tracheal reflexes

3. **Apnea:**

   - Absence of a respiratory drive is tested with a CO_2 challenge. If respiratory movements are absent and arterial PCO_2 is 60 mmHg or greater or there is a 20 mmHg increase above the baseline, the results support brain death.

   - Any physician may declare brain death, though certain specialties have more experience, and requirements may vary at different hospitals or in different states. In most cases, a single examination suffices, whereas some states and institutions require two different examinations by different doctors separated in time.

Radiographic Appearance

- Though brain death is a clinical diagnosis, several tests can be used as confirmatory measures. These include electroencephalography, technetium 99m scans, transcranial Doppler ultrasonography, and cerebral angiography, though electroencephalogram is not routinely recommended due to frequency of artifact. These tests are not required and do not replace neurological examination.

- With cerebral angiography, contrast is injected under high pressure in both anterior and posterior circulation. In brain dead patients, there will be no intracerebral flow, though there will be flow through the external carotid artery.

References

1. Scott JB, Gentile MA, Bennett SN, Couture M, MacIntyre NR. Apnea testing during brain death assessment: a review of clinical practice and published literature. *Respir Care*. March 2013;58(3):532–538.
2. Wijdicks EF, Varelas PN, Gronseth GS, Greer DM. American Academy of Neurology. Evidence-based guideline update: determining brain death in adults: report of the Quality Standards Subcommittee of the American Academy of Neurology. *Neurology*. June 2010;74(23):1911–1918.
3. Teitelbaum J, Shemi SD. Neurologic determination of death. *Neurol Clin*. November 2011;29(4):787–799.
4. Webb A, Samuels O. Brain death dilemmas and the use of ancillary testing. *Continuum (Minneap Minn)*. June 2012;18(3): 659–668.

Printed in the United States
By Bookmasters